D1571209

Copyright © 1998 American Psychiatric Press, Inc.

ALL RIGHTS RESERVED

Manufactured in the United States of America on acid-free paper

First Edition   01   00   99   98   4   3   2   1

American Psychiatric Press, Inc.
1400 K Street, N.W., Washington, DC   20005

Library of Congress Cataloging-in-Publication Data

Melatonin in psychiatric and neoplastic disorders / edited by Mohammad
    Shafii and Sharon Lee Shafii. — 1st ed.
        p.   cm. — (Progress in psychiatry)
    Includes bibliographical references and index.
    ISBN 0-88048-919-7 (alk. paper)
        1. Melatonin—Therapeutic use.   2. Mental illness—Chemotherapy.
    3. Tumors—Chemotherapy.   4. Melatonin—Physiological effect.
    I. Shafii, Mohammad.   II. Shafii, Sharon Lee.   III. Series.
        [DNLM: 1. Melatonin—therapeutic use.   2. Affective Disorders—
    drug therapy.   3. Sleep Disorders—drug therapy.   4. Neoplasms—
    drug therapy.   WK 350 M5177 1998]
    RC483.5.M44M45   1998
    616.89'18—dc21
    DNLM/DLC
    for Libarary of Congress   97-3183
                                                                                            CIP

British Library Cataloguing in Publication Data
A CIP record is available from the British Library.

To
Judith and Frank Beltman,
Samieh Shaffi-Dayan,
and
Carol Vander Wall Robinson

Very special family members
and longtime friends

Truth is the daughter of time.

—Formerly on the portal
of Strasburg Cathedral, 1699[1]

---

[1] From Eden HKF, Lloyd E: *The Book of Sun-Dials,* 4th Edition. London, UK, George Bell and Sons, 1900, p. 463.

Contents

Contributors xiii

Introduction to the Progress in
Psychiatry Series xvii
  David Spiegel, M.D.

Introduction xix
  Mohammad Shafii, M.D., and
  Sharon Lee Shafii, R.N., B.S.N.

Part I
Evolutionary Development and Neurobiology of the Pineal Gland

1   **Changes in Melatonin Throughout the Life
Cycle: Implications for Neurobiology and
Psychiatry** 3
  Russel J. Reiter, Ph.D., D.Med.

2   **The Structure and Evolutionary Development
of the Pineal Gland** 27
  Kunwar P. Bhatnagar, Ph.D.

Part II
Melatonin in Psychiatric Disorders in Adults

3   **Melatonin in Adult Depression** 43
  Lennart Wetterberg, M.D., Ph.D.

4   Melatonin in Circadian Phase Sleep and
Mood Disorders 81
Alfred J. Lewy, M.D., Ph.D., Robert L. Sack,
M.D., Neil L. Cutler, B.A., Vance K. Bauer,
M.A., and Rod J. Hughes, Ph.D.

5   Melatonin and Circadian Rhythms in
Bipolar Mood Disorder 105
Aimee Mayeda, M.D., and
John I. Nurnberger Jr., M.D., Ph.D.

6   Melatonin in Eating and Panic Disorders 125
Gregory M. Brown, M.D., Ph.D., M.R.C.C.,
Richard P. Swinson, M.D., F.R.C.P.C., and
Sidney H. Kennedy, M.D., F.R.C.P.C.

Part III
Melatonin in Children and Adolescents

7   Melatonin in Healthy and Depressed
Children and Adolescents 149
Mohammad Shafii, M.D., and
Sharon Lee Shafii, R.N., B.S.N.

8   Melatonin in Sleep Disorders in Children
With Neurodevelopmental Disabilities 169
James E. Jan, M.D., F.R.C.P.C.,
Hilary Espezel, R.N., B.S.N., and
Keith J. Goulden, M.D., F.R.C.P.C.

Part IV
Melatonin and Neoplastic Disorders

9   Melatonin at the Neoplastic Cellular Level 191
Steven M. Hill, Ph.D., Prahlad T. Ram, Ph.D., Tina
M. Molis, Ph.D., and Louaine L. Spriggs, Ph.D.

10   **The Melatonin Rhythm in Cancer Patients** **243**
David E. Blask, M.D., Ph.D.

11   **Meditation, Melatonin, and Cancer** **261**
Ann O. Massion, M.D., Jane Teas, Ph.D., and
James R. Hebert, Sc.D.

Index **295**

Contributors

Vance K. Bauer, M.A.
Research Associate, Sleep and Mood Disorders Laboratory, Oregon Health Sciences University, Portland, Oregon

Kunwar P. Bhatnagar, Ph.D.
Professor of Anatomy, Department of Anatomical Sciences and Neurobiology, Health Sciences Center, University of Louisville, Louisville, Kentucky

David E. Blask, M.D., Ph.D.
Senior Research Scientist, Mary Imogene Bassett Hospital, Research Institute, Cooperstown, New York

Gregory M. Brown, M.D., Ph.D., M.R.C.C.
Professor of Psychiatry, University of Toronto; Head, Neuroendocrinology Research Section, Clarke Institute of Psychiatry, Toronto, Canada

Neil L. Cutler, B.A.
Senior Research Assistant, Sleep and Mood Disorders Laboratory, Oregon Health Sciences University, Portland, Oregon

Hilary Espezel, R.N., B.S.N.
Program Coordinator, Visually Impaired Program, Sunny Hill Health Center, Vancouver, British Columbia, Canada

Keith J. Goulden, M.D., F.R.C.P.C.
Associate Professor of Pediatrics, University of Alberta; Medical Director, Division of Pediatric Education and Research, Glenrose Rehabilitation Hospital, Edmonton, Alberta, Canada

James R. Hebert, Sc.D.
Professor of Medicine and Epidemiology and Associate
Director of the Division of Preventive and Behavioral
Medicine, Department of Medicine, University of
Massachusetts Medical Center, Worcester, Massachusetts

Steven M. Hill, Ph.D.
Associate Professor of Anatomy and Medicine, Department of
Anatomy, Tulane University School of Medicine, New
Orleans, Louisiana

Rod J. Hughes, Ph.D.
Assistant Professor of Psychiatry, Sleep and Mood Disorders
Laboratory, Oregon Health Sciences University, Portland,
Oregon

James E. Jan, M.D., F.R.C.P.C.
Professor and Coordinator, Visually Impaired Program,
Children's Hospital, Vancouver, British Columbia, Canada

Sidney H. Kennedy, M.D., F.R.C.P.C.
Professor of Psychiatry, University of Toronto; Head, Mood
and Anxiety Division, Clarke Institute of Psychiatry, Toronto,
Canada

Alfred J. Lewy, M.D., Ph.D.
Professor of Psychiatry, Ophthalmology, and Pharmacology,
Sleep and Mood Disorders Laboratory, Oregon Health
Sciences University, Portland, Oregon

Ann O. Massion, M.D.
Assistant Professor, University of Massachusetts Medical
Center, Department of Psychiatry, Worcester, Massachusetts

Aimee Mayeda, M.D.
Assistant Professor of Psychiatry, Department of Psychiatry,
Indiana University School of Medicine; Medical Director,
Comprehensive Day Hospital Program, Mental Health Patient
Focused Care Team, Department of Veterans Affairs,
Roudebush Veterans Administration Medical Center,
Indianapolis, Indiana

Tina M. Molis, Ph.D.
Adjunct Assistant Professor, Department of Zoology, Weber State University, Ogden, Utah

John I. Nurnberger Jr., M.D., Ph.D.
Professor of Psychiatry and Director, Institute of Psychiatric Research, Indiana University Medical Center, Indianapolis, Indiana

Prahlad T. Ram, Ph.D.
Graduate student, Department of Anatomy, Tulane University School of Medicine, New Orleans, Louisiana

Russel J. Reiter, Ph.D., D.Med.
Professor of Neuroendocrinology, Department of Cellular and Structural Biology, The University of Texas, Health Science Center at San Antonio, San Antonio, Texas

Robert L. Sack, M.D.
Professor of Psychiatry, Sleep and Mood Disorders Laboratory, Oregon Health Sciences University, Portland, Oregon

Mohammad Shafii, M.D.
Professor of Psychiatry and Director, Child and Adolescent Psychiatry Residency Training Program, Department of Psychiatry and Behavioral Sciences, University of Louisville School of Medicine, Louisville, Kentucky

Sharon Lee Shafii, R.N., B.S.N.
Editor-in-Residence; Former Assistant Head Nurse, Adolescent Service, Neuropsychiatric Institute, University of Michigan Medical Center, Ann Arbor, Michigan

Louaine L. Spriggs, Ph.D.
Research Assistant Professor, Department of Anatomy and Tulane Cancer Center, Tulane University School of Medicine, New Orleans, Louisiana

Richard P. Swinson, M.D., F.R.C.P.C.
Professor, Department of Psychiatry, University of Toronto;
Head, Anxiety Disorders Clinic, Clarke Institute of Psychiatry,
Toronto, Canada

Jane Teas, Ph.D.
Research Assistant Professor, Department of Medicine,
Division of Preventive and Behavioral Medicine, University of
Massachusetts Medical Center, Worcester, Massachusetts

Lennart Wetterberg, M.D., Ph.D.
Professor and Head, Department of Psychiatry, Karolinska
Institute, St. Göran's Hospital, Stockholm, Sweden

Introduction to the Progress in Psychiatry Series

The Progress in Psychiatry Series is designed to capture in print the excitement that comes from assembling a diverse group of experts from various locations to examine in detail the newest information about a developing aspect of psychiatry. This series emerged as a collaboration between the American Psychiatric Association's (APA) Scientific Program Committee and the American Psychiatric Press, Inc. Great interest is generated by a number of the symposia presented each year at the APA annual meeting, and we realized that much of the information presented there, carefully assembled by people who are deeply immersed in a given area, would unfortunately not appear together in print. The symposia sessions at the annual meetings provide an unusual opportunity for experts who otherwise might not meet on the same platform to share their diverse viewpoints for a period of 3 hours. Some new themes are repeatedly reinforced and gain credence, whereas in other instances disagreements emerge, enabling the audience and now the reader to reach informed decisions about new directions in the field. The Progress in Psychiatry Series allows us to publish and capture some of the best of the symposia and thus provide an in-depth treatment of specific areas that might not otherwise be presented in broader review formats.

Psychiatry is, by nature, an interface discipline, combining the study of mind and brain, of individual and social environments, of the humane and the scientific. Therefore, progress in the field is rarely linear—it often comes from unexpected sources. Furthermore, new developments emerge from an array of viewpoints that do not necessarily provide immediate agreement but rather expert examination of the issues. We intend to present innovative ideas and data that will enable you, the reader, to participate in this process.

We believe the Progress in Psychiatry Series will provide you with an opportunity to review timely, new information in specific fields of interest as they are developing. We hope you find that the excitement of the presentations is captured in the written word and that this book proves to be informative and enjoyable reading.

David Spiegel, M.D.
Series Editor
Progress in Psychiatry Series

Introduction

Since the publication of our earlier book, *Biological Rhythms, Mood Disorders, Light Therapy, and the Pineal Gland,* in the Progress in Psychiatry Series in 1990, melatonin, a hormone of the pineal gland, has become a household word. Dissemination of knowledge in the media about melatonin is a welcome sign but also brings the potential for overexpectation and unsubstantiated claims of being a miracle drug. Now more than ever, scientists and clinicians need to become aware of the synthesis, metabolism, and function of melatonin in animals and humans in health and disease. Up-to-date knowledge of melatonin will help clinicians convey accurate information to their patients and the public.

During the last few years, our knowledge of the function and effect of melatonin has greatly expanded. Melatonin receptor sites have been located in the suprachiasmatic nuclei of the hypothalamus and at the intracellular level in many cells throughout the body. Recently, melatonin's function as a natural potent antioxidant at an intracellular level has been discovered. Also, it has been observed that cancer cells grow much more rapidly in the breast, gastrointestinal tract, and prostate of pinealectomized animals. Based on these findings, it is postulated that the pineal gland, and particularly its hormone, melatonin, has anticancer qualities. If future studies confirm the oncostatic qualities of melatonin, measurement of melatonin for use as a diagnostic tool and the prescription of melatonin as a treatment modality could become a possibility.

In psychiatric disorders, particularly in most studies of adult major depression, there is evidence of a decrease in serum melatonin. In contrast, some studies of major depression in children and adolescents and a few studies in adults show a significant increase in serum or urine melatonin. These divergent findings might reflect biologically different subtypes of major depression rather than the invalidity of the studies. Although phenomenologically, symptoms of major depression are similar, biologically they might be different. We need to transcend the "either-or" dualistic thinking and consider the possibility of biological divergence in apparently similar clinical phenomena.

Again, if future studies confirm the relationship between melatonin and psychiatric disorders, particularly in mood disorders and specifically in major depression, measurement of nocturnal serum melatonin and nocturnal urine melatonin and/or its metabolite 6-hydroxymelatonin sulfate (aMT6s) might help us to develop biologically objective tests to diagnose some forms or subtypes of major depression in adults or children and adolescents.

The use of melatonin for inducing sleep and for jet lag has increased significantly during the last few years. However, melatonin for use as a drug has not been rigorously tested or approved by the Federal Drug Administration. Also, quality control regarding purity is not ensured. In the United States, melatonin, in the form of capsules, pills, and sublingual tablets, can be purchased in drug stores as over-the-counter medication and in health food stores. However, in some European countries, the sale of melatonin is banned because it has not been tested as a pharmaceutical agent. Generally, it is believed that pharmaceutical companies are reluctant to test melatonin because, as a natural product, it would be difficult to patent. Some major drug companies have or are in the process of synthesizing melatonin analogues to be used as powerful chronobiotic or possible oncostatic agents. Over the next decade, we will probably be hearing much more about these agents.

Melatonin in Psychiatric and Neoplastic Disorders is written for adult, child, and adolescent psychiatrists, oncologists, endocrinologists, pediatricians, and other health professionals. This book is divided into four parts.

In Part I, "Evolutionary Development and Neurobiology of the Pineal Gland," the synthesis of melatonin and the change in melatonin levels throughout the life cycle from conception to advanced age are reviewed. Brief references are made to the anatomy, cellular structure, and evolution of the pineal gland in vertebrates, including mammals and humans.

In Part II, "Melatonin in Psychiatric Disorders in Adults," some of the pioneers in the field of pineology succinctly summarize their lifelong findings concerning melatonin in the areas of adult depression, sleep disorders, chronobiological mood disorders, bipolar disorders, eating disorders, panic disorders, shift-work maladaptation, and jet lag.

In Part III, "Melatonin in Children and Adolescents," we look at the pineal gland and melatonin in healthy infants, children, and adolescents. Recent studies on serum and/or urine melatonin and its metabolite, aMT6s, in children and adolescents with major depression are reviewed. The use of melatonin as an experimental sleep-inducing agent in developmentally disabled children, including those with autistic disorders who suffer from severe chronic sleep disorders, is discussed.

In Part IV, "Melatonin and Neoplastic Disorders," we review comprehensively but succinctly the in vitro and in vivo studies of the effects of melatonin as an antioxidant on cancer cells. Melatonin rhythm in animals and humans who suffer from various forms of cancer, including breast, prostate, and gastrointestinal, are discussed. The potential diagnostic and therapeutic value of melatonin in oncology is touched on.

The question arises whether or not one can increase his or her melatonin level through nonpharmacological means other than sleep. In the final chapter, preliminary studies are summarized showing that individuals regularly involved in the practice of mindful meditation had significantly more nocturnal serum melatonin and urinary aMT6s than nonmeditating control subjects. If future studies confirm this finding, various forms of meditation could be used to increase nocturnal serum melatonin as an adjunct in the treatment of patients who suffer from breast, prostate, or gastrointestinal tract cancers. Also, it might be possible to prescribe meditation for individuals who are at high risk for these types of cancer with the hope of prevention.

The idea for this book began with our studies on nocturnal

serum melatonin profile in major depression in children and adolescents (Shafii et al. 1996), which was made possible by a grant from the Alliant Community Trust Fund, Louisville, Kentucky. We appreciated this support, especially at a time when federal funds for research declined significantly. The editing and reediting of *Melatonin in Psychiatric and Neoplastic Disorders* became possible because of our sabbatical from the University of Louisville School of Medicine during the fall and winter of 1995 and 1996. We are grateful to Allan Tasman, M.D., professor and chair, department of psychiatry and behavioral sciences, University of Louisville, for his support and encouragement; to Robert F. Baxter, M.D., associate professor of psychiatry and director of the division of child and adolescent psychiatry, for his receptivity and help; to Sandra Elam, M.D., director of the Ackerly Child Psychiatric Inpatient Service, for clinical coverage during our absence; to Amy Willard, B.A., for her diligence in word processing and checking references; and to the faculty, staff, and residents of the division of child and adolescent psychiatry, University of Louisville School of Medicine, Louisville, Kentucky.

David Spiegel, M.D., professor of psychiatry, Stanford University, and editor of the Progress in Psychiatry Series, although himself on sabbatical in France, immediately and enthusiastically responded to our proposal for this book. We deeply appreciate his openness and receptivity to our ideas and his constructive editorial review and helpful suggestions.

From inception to conclusion, *Melatonin in Psychiatric and Neoplastic Disorders* has been a joint effort, with many hours of discussion, planning, research activities, collection of data, writing, rewriting, and editing. The future of research on melatonin and the pineal gland, with its possible implications for clinical psychiatry, oncology, endocrinology, and other areas of medicine, is very promising. We hope that this book will stimulate further research and clinical interest in this fertile area.

Mohammad Shafii, M.D., and Sharon Lee Shafii, R.N., B.S.N.

Reference

Shafii M, MacMillan DR, Key MP, et al: Nocturnal serum melatonin profile in major depression in children and adolescents. Arch Gen Psychiatry 53:1009–1013, 1996

Part I

Evolutionary Development and Neurobiology of the Pineal Gland

Chapter 1

Changes in Melatonin Throughout the Life Cycle: Implications for Neurobiology and Psychiatry

Russel J. Reiter, Ph.D., D.Med.

The pineal gland, after years of languishing with an image of physiological insignificance, is now entering "center stage" on the basis of its functional importance and diversity. The hormone of the pineal gland, melatonin (N-acetyl-5-methoxytryptamine), has been found to have a remarkable array of functions that unequivocally link it to neurological and behavioral disorders. Besides demonstrated effects on endocrine and circadian physiology, melatonin now appears related to the intracellular metabolism of all cells because of its ability to neutralize highly toxic free radicals (Reiter 1995b; Reiter et al. 1995). This scavenging action of melatonin is especially relevant to the brain because the indole readily crosses the blood-brain barrier and is taken up by neural tissues (Menendez-Pelaez and Reiter 1993; Menendez-Pelaez et al. 1993) and because the brain generates large numbers of toxic free radicals that are highly destructive to neurons (Beal 1994; Graham 1978). It is clear from a variety of studies that free-radical damage to cells is either a primary or secondary feature of several major neurobiological and behavioral disorders, including parkinsonism (Fahn and Cohen 1992) and Alzheimer's disease (Cotman 1994). Besides melatonin's receptor-independent antioxidative actions, the indole has obvious effects on neuroendocrine and circadian physiology (Reiter 1991b) and gene transcription (Carlberg and Wiesenberg 1995), which are presumably mediated by membrane (Reppert et al. 1994; Stankov and Reiter 1990) and nuclear receptors (Acuña-Castroviejo et al. 1994; Becker-Andre et al. 1994), respectively.

In this chapter, I summarize the recent advances related to the role of melatonin in neurobiology and describe the marked changes in the production and secretion of melatonin throughout the life cycle. Because the brain appears to be the primary target for melatonin, the results have clear implications for psychiatric disorders. (See Bhatnagar, Chapter 2, for a discussion of the neuroanatomy and evolutionary development of the pineal gland.)

Melatonin Production and Secretion

Although there are several organs that synthesize melatonin, the melatonin found in the blood is primarily derived from the pineal gland. Melatonin is a product of the metabolism of tryptophan, an amino acid taken up from the circulation by the pinealocytes. Tryptophan is quickly converted to 5-hydroxytryptophan in a reaction catalyzed by tryptophan hydroxylase (Reiter 1991b). The enzyme aromatic L-amino acid decarboxylase promotes the conversion of 5-hydroxytryptophan to 5-hydroxytryptamine (serotonin); the latter compound is in very high concentrations within the pineal gland (Giarman et al. 1960). The metabolic pathway by which serotonin is converted to melatonin initially involves the N-acetylation of serotonin to N-acetylserotonin and O-methylation of the latter compound by the enzyme hydroxyindole-O-methyltransferase (Figure 1–1). The acetylation of serotonin, which is catalyzed by the enzyme N-acetyltransferase, is generally considered rate limiting in melatonin production. Once produced, melatonin is quickly released into the systemic circulation. Thus, the levels of melatonin in the blood are an index of the synthetic activity of the pineal gland at virtually the same time (Reiter 1991b).

Melatonin production within the pineal gland occurs in a distinctly circadian manner, with the bulk of the synthesis occurring during the night. Because melatonin synthesis is essentially restricted to the daily dark period, it has been referred to as the chemical expression of darkness (Reiter 1991a). The nocturnal pro-

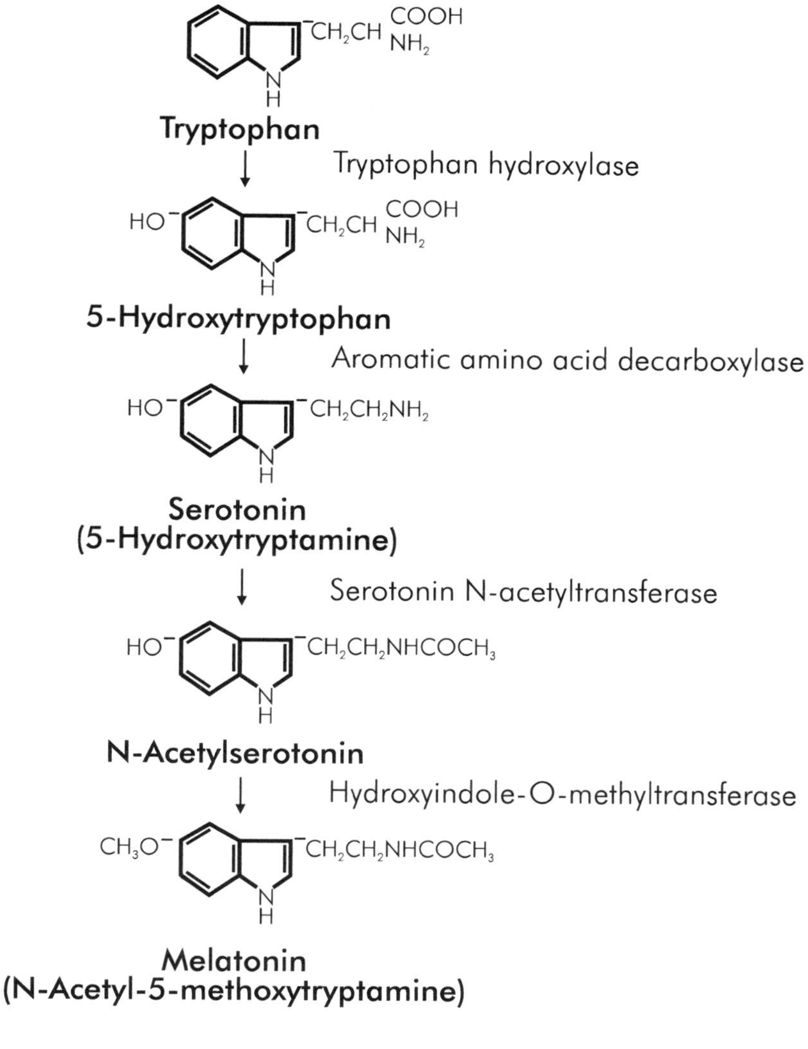

Figure 1–1. The metabolism of the amino acid tryptophan to melatonin in the pineal gland. The serotonin concentration in the pineal gland is about 100-fold greater than that in the brain. The rate-limiting enzyme in melatonin production seems to be serotonin *N*-acetyltransferase.

duction of melatonin is a consequence of a neural message that arrives in the pineal gland from the suprachiasmatic nucleus (SCN) of the hypothalamus. The activity of the SCN, an endogenous circadian-rhythm generator, is capable of activating the pineal gland at night with light, detected by the eyes, being inhibitory to the SCN. Because of this, the acute exposure of animals or man to light at night causes a precipitous decline in pineal melatonin production and a drop in circulating levels of the hormone (Lewy et al. 1980). Likewise, the extension of light into the normal period of darkness prevents the nighttime increase in pineal melatonin synthesis. The degree of suppression of nocturnal melatonin synthesis by acute light exposure is light-intensity dependent, with higher light levels being most inhibitory (McIntyre et al. 1989). Finally, adjusting the duration of the daily dark period also determines the duration of elevated melatonin because the length of time melatonin levels remain elevated at night is proportional to the length of the dark period (DeVries et al. 1993). Thus, light can be used as a "drug" to manipulate or totally suppress the circadian melatonin rhythm and therefore the quantity of melatonin produced.

The neural connections between the eyes and the pineal gland have been defined in a variety of mammals (DeVries et al. 1993), and it is assumed the same pathway exists in humans (Bruce et al. 1991; Kneisley et al. 1978; Vaughan 1984). This pathway involves photoreceptor cells in the retina, projections via the retinohypothalamic tract to the SCN, connections to the intermediolateral cell column of the upper thoracic cord, preganglionic sympathetic fibers to the superior cervical ganglia, and postganglionic projections to the pineal gland. Within the pineal gland, the sympathetic neurons end in the vicinity of the pinealocytes. Some of the neurotransmitters in the pathway include the excitatory amino acid glutamate at the retinohypothalamic tract–SCN interface and norepinephrine (NE) at the level of the postganglionic sympathetic neuron–pinealocyte interface. NE released from the postganglionic neurons within the pineal gland act via well-described metabolic pathways to promote the nocturnal rise in melatonin synthesis (Reiter 1991a, 1991b).

Once produced, melatonin quickly escapes from the pinealo-cytes, presumably by simple diffusion, to enter the blood. This generates a nighttime rise in blood melatonin levels (Figure 1–2) similar to that seen in the pineal gland itself. Presumably because of its high lipid solubility, melatonin also gains access to every other bodily fluid, where it exhibits a circadian rhythm, albeit at a reduced amplitude, such as that in the blood. Likewise, it is be-lieved that melatonin is taken up by every cell, where it may be partially compartmentalized (Menendez-Pelaez and Reiter 1993; Menendez-Pelaez et al. 1993). In particular, preliminary findings suggest that, intracellularly, highest concentrations of melatonin

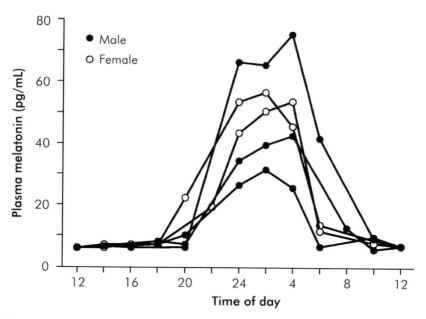

Figure 1–2. The circadian blood melatonin rhythm as measured in three adult males and three adult females, all of roughly the same age. There are no gender differences in the melatonin cycle, but there are great variations in the amplitude of the nocturnal melatonin peak among individuals of the same age, as illustrated here. Throughout a lifetime, those individuals with an attenuated melatonin rhythm are exposed to much less melatonin than individuals with a robust melatonin cycle.

exist in the nucleus. None of the morphophysiological barriers existing in the body (e.g., the blood-brain barrier) is an impediment to the passage of melatonin. Its ability to enter every cell is important for melatonin's function as an antioxidant. Presumably, intracellular levels of melatonin vary in a circadian manner, as they do in the pineal gland and in bodily fluids.

Besides light at night, pharmacological agents can be used to manipulate melatonin production. At least in nonhuman animals, the administration of MK-801, an N-methyl-D-aspartate (NMDA) receptor blocker at the level of the SCN, prevents light from inhibiting pineal melatonin production (Colwell et al. 1991; Poeggeler et al. 1995). Agents that block the interaction of NE with its receptors on the pinealocyte membrane (e.g., propranolol) depress melatonin synthesis (Arendt et al. 1985; Brismar et al. 1988). Conversely, β-adrenergic receptor agonists(e.g., isoproterenol) and drugs that delay NE reuptake into postganglionic sympathetic neurons in the pineal gland (e.g., desipramine) promote melatonin production (Demisch 1993; Polazidou et al. 1989). Other drugs that alter circulating melatonin levels in humans include benzodiazepines (Monteleone et al. 1989) and methoxypsoralen (Mauviard et al. 1991); the former depresses melatonin levels, whereas the latter increases them. It is likely that a variety of neurally active drugs also may impact the ability of the pineal gland to synthesize and secrete melatonin in a circadian manner, although this ability has rarely been an endpoint in studies where such drugs were used (Demisch 1993).

Melatonin Levels From Newborn to Advanced Age

While in utero, the fetus receives a circadian melatonin message from the maternal pineal via its placenta transfer (Kenneway et al. 1987). Following parturition, the newborn is deprived of the significant rhythm for several months, during which the infant pineal produces little if any melatonin. The circadian melatonin cycle in the newborn gradually develops, beginning at 3–4 months of age so that in a 1-year-old infant the melatonin cycle is well developed (Gupta 1988; see also Shafii and Shafii, Chapter 7, in this volume). Children who die of sudden infant death syndrome (SIDS) reportedly have a poorly developed pineal gland (Sparks and Hunsaker 1988) and low levels of melatonin (Sturner et al. 1994). Typically, children who die of SIDS do so at the age their melatonin rhythms should be developing; however, whether the reported observations in pineal development and the melatonin cycle relate to the condition of SIDS is unknown, although this speculation has been made (Maurizi 1988).

During childhood (i.e., ages 1–10 years), the melatonin rhythm is generally believed to be robust, with the largest day versus night differences in melatonin being present at this time. In general, children have been sparingly studied in terms of their circadian melatonin cycle, but one condition in which a rhythm is reportedly absent is in children with infantile lipofuscinosis (Gupta 1993). Lipofuscin, a product of lipid peroxidation, abundantly accumulates in children with this condition, suggesting that the low levels of melatonin may relate to the disease. Melatonin is known to be a potent scavenger of the hydroxyl (Tan et al. 1993) and peroxyl (Pieri et al. 1994) radicals, which initiate and propagate, respectively, lipid peroxidation (Kehrer 1993). Thus, low melatonin levels would be expected to be related to lipofuscin accumulation, but whether the low levels are in fact related to the extensive lipid damage these children sustain remains unknown.

Over the 3- to 5-year period when individuals are undergoing sexual maturation, there is substantial reduction in nocturnal melatonin levels (Waldhauser et al. 1993). This reduction may be permissive to normal sexual maturation. Certainly the maintenance of an exaggerated circadian melatonin rhythm beyond the normal age of puberty has been associated with delayed sexual maturation, a condition that was overcome when melatonin levels were reduced to the normal adult values (Puig-Domingo et al. 1992). The reduction in blood melatonin concentrations with the attenuation of nocturnal peak is generally believed to be a consequence of reduced production of the indole within the gland, although some believe it is due to the marked increase in body mass and blood volume during the period, which merely leads to a dilution of the available melatonin.

After adulthood is achieved, most individuals maintain a circadian melatonin cycle. However, the amplitude of the nocturnal melatonin peak varies widely (Figure 1–2), although there is no gender difference in mean blood melatonin levels. The melatonin rhythm is genetically determined (Wetterberg et al. 1983), with the amplitude of the nighttime peak being highly reproducible from night to night. Thus, if a person is seen to have an attenuated melatonin cycle, it is believed that this low-amplitude rhythm will be maintained throughout life. This means that the pineal gland of some individuals produces much less melatonin during a lifetime than does the gland of another person.

There seems to be no life event that is associated with the loss of the circadian melatonin cycle during aging; rather, after puberty, it is accepted that the melatonin rhythm gradually wanes, with the eventual consequence that in advanced age a day versus night difference in melatonin levels may be barely discernible (Reiter 1992, 1995c). The drop in melatonin during aging is likely due to a reduction in its production in the pineal gland because the enzymes that catalyze its formation, as well as the levels of this constituent in the gland, are reduced in old animals (Reiter et al. 1980a, 1980b, 1981).

The human pineal gland does not fare any better than that of animals in advanced age. Because the biosynthetic activity of the human pineal deteriorates during adulthood, blood levels of melatonin suffer a similar fate (Iguchi et al. 1982; Touitou et al. 1981). Figure 1–3 illustrates the gradual reduction of peak blood melatonin levels after puberty. The age-related drop in melatonin in the blood is reflected in a similar depression in the levels of its chief urinary metabolite, 6-hydroxymelatonin sulfate (Sack et al. 1986). Besides a reduction in nighttime peak levels of melatonin, the duration it remains elevated also is reduced (Nair et al. 1986). These reductions may be important because both the duration of elevated melatonin and the maximal level achieved may be essential elements of the message the cycle conveys.

Few experimental attempts have been made to maintain a youthful melatonin rhythm into advanced age. In Fisher 334 rats, which are often used for experimental studies on aging, calorie restriction (by 25%–40%), which prolongs life, also substantially maintains the melatonin rhythm well past the age it is normally lost (Stokkan et al. 1991). Whether the preserved rhythm has any functional significance for the old animals remains unknown.

Melatonin Levels in Relation to Jet Lag and Sleep Disorders

The condition of jet lag typically develops when individuals quickly cross several time zones, creating a situation where the body's circadian rhythms are temporarily not properly synchronized to the light-dark cycle (Bellamy 1986). During the period

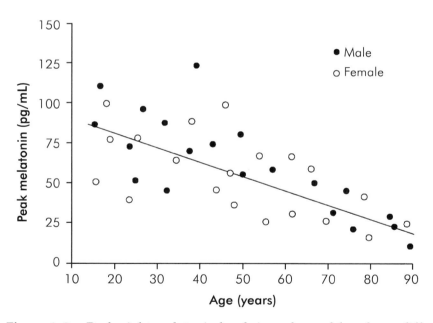

Figure 1–3. Peak night melatonin levels in males and females at different ages. There is gradual deterioration of the melatonin cycle after puberty, such that in elderly individuals the nighttime rise is barely discernible. Considering melatonin's potent antioxidant activity, the drop in melatonin may be related to aging and the onset of age-related diseases.

when the rhythms are being readjusted to the new time zone, among several signs of the lethargic condition humans experience is difficulty in sleeping. Considering melatonin's sleep-enhancing quality (Dawson and Encel 1993), it is believed that a disturbance of the melatonin rhythm is partially responsible for the phenomenon of jet lag (Arendt et al. 1987; Fevre-Montange et al. 1981). As a result, taking melatonin to combat the condition has become commonplace (Petrie et al. 1989, 1993). Like jet lag, shift work, which compromises endogenous circadian rhythms, also disturbs the melatonin cycle (Madakoro et al. 1993). Thus, melatonin also may be useful in the treatment of these individuals. Supplemental melatonin may benefit these conditions because it has acute sleep-promoting effects, as well as a rhythm-entraining effect (Arendt et al. 1984), with the latter consequence following a phase-response curve opposite to that induced by light (Lewy et al. 1992).

Besides its usefulness in the conditions already described, melatonin may be useful in a large number of other sleep disorders, including delayed sleep phase syndrome (Dahlitz et al. 1991), altered sleep-wake cycles in blind individuals (Dawson and Encel 1993), sleep disorders associated with dyssynchronized circadian rhythms (Tzischensky et al. 1992), and age-related sleep ineffi-ciency (Haimov et al. 1994). Melatonin is easily administered by a variety of means and has a seemingly limitless margin of safety as a drug (Norlund and Lerner 1977). Indeed, virtually no toxicity has been described.

Melatonin in Relation to
Neurodegenerative Diseases

Recently, melatonin was found to be a powerful hydroxyl (Tan et al. 1993) and peroxyl (Pieri et al. 1994) radical scavenger (Table 1–1). Free radicals are toxic agents generated within cells that damage macromolecules such as lipids, proteins, and deoxyribo-nucleic acid (DNA) (Floyd 1990). The brain is highly susceptible to free-radical damage because processes collectively referred to as the antioxidative defense system, which the body uses to protect itself against such oxidant damage, are not particularly well developed in the brain (Halliwell 1992). Some of the noteworthy neural conditions that cause the brain either to generate large numbers of radicals or exhibit excessive damage when they are produced include the high utilization of oxygen (Reiter 1995b) by the brain and excitatory amino acid neurotransmission (Figure 1–4) (Choi 1991; Schulz et al. 1995). Additionally, the brain contains copious amounts of polyunsaturated fatty acids, which are easily oxidized by free radicals (Proyer and McCoy 1991).

Considering the efficient antioxidant activity of melatonin (Hardeland et al. 1993; Reiter 1995a; Reiter et al. 1995), the ease with which it enters the brain (Menendez-Pelaez and Reiter 1993; Menendez-Pelaez et al. 1993), and the fact that it already has proven effective in protecting neural tissue from free-radical attack (Giusti et al. 1995; Melchiorri et al. 1995; Sewerynek et al. 1995), it may be an important molecule in protecting against neurodegenerative conditions that involve free radicals as potential agents contributing to the disease (Giusti et al. 1995; Poeggeler et al. 1993; Reiter 1995b; Reiter et al. 1994a, 1994b). This proposal is especially germane, considering that virtually all degenerative

Table 1–1.   Some of the free radicals and reactive oxygen species that damage neuronal tissue

Chemical species	Symbol	Half-life[a] (sec) at 37°
Superoxide anion radical	O_2^-	1×10^{-6}
Singlet oxygen	$^1O_2$	1×10^{-6}
Hydroxyl radical	$\bullet OH$	1×10^{-9}
Lipid peroxide	ROOH	$> 10^2$
Alkoxyl radical	$RO\bullet$	1×10^{-6}
Peroxyl radical	$ROO\bullet$	1×10^{-2}

[a]The half-life generally indicates the toxicity of these compounds. Using this criterion, the hydroxyl radical ($\bullet OH$) is the most toxic, a point on which there is widespread agreement. The pineal hormone melatonin is an efficient scavenger of a number of free radicals.

neurological conditions are related to advancing age, a period when the protective effects of melatonin are being lost due to diminished production of the indole (Reiter 1992; Reiter 1995c).

There are a large number of neurological disorders in which free radicals have been implicated (Table 1–2). For example, oxygen-derived reactive species have been linked to epilepsy and other seizure disorders in experimental animals (Armstead et al. 1989; Bozan et al. 1986). Neuroactive chemicals, which also alter antioxidative enzyme activities in the brain, are commonly found to induce seizures (Singh and Pathak 1990), and hyperbaric oxygen exposure in animals often induces convulsions and the associ-

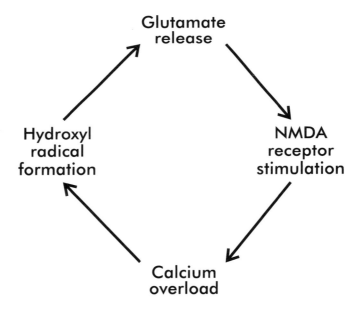

Figure 1–4.   Release of the excitatory amino acid neurotransmitter glutamate activates NMDA receptors in the postsynaptic neural membrane, opening calcium channels in the postsynaptic neuron. The $[Ca^{2+}]i$ leads to the generation of free radicals, promoting glutamate release and leading to the further production of free radicals that are highly toxic to the neurons in which they are produced.

ated lipid peroxidation in the brain (Torbati et al. 1992). This latter response to hyperbaric oxygen was recently found to be inhibited by treating rats with melatonin before their hyperbaric oxygen exposure (M. I. Pablos, R. J. Reiter, J. I. Chang, J. M. Guerrero, T. Agapito, unpublished data, December 1996). Also germane to this issue are observations, made more than two decades ago, that the acute loss of melatonin (due to surgical removal of the pineal gland) induces severe convulsions and sometimes death in parathyroidectomized rats (Reiter et al. 1973).

Cerebral ischemia due to hemorrhage into the brain or the transient interruption of the blood supply to the central nervous system (CNS) leads to severe postischemic neural damage. Free-radical generation during cerebral ischemia may be a major factor in neural death that often is associated with this condition (Kitagawa et al. 1990). Following ischemia, reperfusion of the tissue with blood leads to additional damage, presumably due to a rise in intracellular calcium levels, which results in an elevation in free-radical generation (Murphy et al. 1989). Antioxidants and calcium channel blockers are known to afford protection against ischemia/reperfusion injury, but melatonin is yet to be tested as a protective agent. Nitric oxide also seems to be involved in neuronal destruction associated with reperfusion injury in the brain, with inhibitors of nitric oxide synthase reducing the damage (Wu and Li 1993). Melatonin, at physiological concentrations, was

Table 1–2.   Some of the neural conditions in which free radicals may be involved in the disease process

Aluminum-induced neuropathy	Myasthenia gravis
Alzheimer's disease	Neurotoxic damage
Amyotrophic lateral sclerosis	Parkinson's disease
Batten's disease (lipofuscinosis)	Tardive dyskinesia
Down's syndrome	Traumatic brain injury
Hyperbaric hyperoxic injury	Vitamin E deficiency
Ischemia-reperfusion injury	Werdnig-Hoffmann disease
Muscular dystrophy	Xenobiotic nerve damage

recently found to inhibit nitric oxide synthase and therefore nitric oxide levels in brain homogenates (Pozo et al. 1994), suggesting this may be another means by which melatonin may protect against ischemia/reperfusion injury.

Free radicals often have been implicated as a causative factor in neuronal degeneration associated with Parkinson's disease (PD) (Fahn and Cohen 1992; Youdim et al. 1993). There are four biochemical features of the substantia nigra, the region of the brain that degenerates, which are linked to free-radical generation. These features include monoamine oxidase (MAO) activity, auto-oxidation, accumulation of iron, and the presence of neuro-melanin. MAO catalyzes the oxidative deamination of dopamine, giving rise to hydrogen peroxide, which can quickly be converted to the hydroxyl radical ($\bullet$OH) in the presence of a transition metal (Figure 1–5). Also, catecholamines are known to react with oxygen nonenzymatically in a process known as auto-oxidation. This process results in the formation of quinones and semiquinones, as well as hydrogen peroxide. The substantia nigra is rich in iron, which catalyzes the formation of $\bullet$OH, thereby leading to extensive damage to the associated dopaminergic neurons. Finally, the high levels of neuromelanin are believed to be a consequence of the auto-oxidation of dopamine, which, as already noted, results in toxic oxygen radical production. Antioxidants have been considered potentially beneficial in delaying PD onset, but melatonin has yet to be tested for this effect. There is an animal model of PD involving the injection of the neurotoxin 1-methyl-4-phenyl-

$$H_2O_2 + Fe^{2+} \longrightarrow Fe^{3+} + OH^- + \bullet OH$$

$$H_2O_2 + Cu^+ \longrightarrow Cu^{2+} + OH^- + \bullet OH$$

Figure 1–5.   The hydroxyl radical ($\bullet$OH) is readily generated when hydrogen peroxide (H_2O_2) is exposed to a transition metal such as Fe^{2+} or Cu^+; the process is known as the Fenton reaction.

1,2,3,6-tetrahydropyridine (MPTP) into the brain of mammals, leading to the generation of radicals, with the animals eventually developing Parkinson-like symptoms (Heikilla et al. 1989). Melatonin also has not been tested for its preventive action in this model.

Like PD, Alzheimer's disease (AD) may be related to oxidative damage by free radicals (Beal 1994; Cotman 1994). Protein oxidation products, which are a consequence of oxidative stress, are increased as is the level of lipid peroxidation in the brains of AD patients (Subbarao et al. 1990). These pathological changes may lead to the aggregation of amyloid and to damage to cytoskeletal proteins such as tau (Dyrks et al. 1992). Because of the complexity of this disease, it has been difficult to unravel the special role that free radicals play in AD, and there are no good models in which to test these interactions. There are no reports on the administration of melatonin to AD patients; however, there is one study on melatonin levels in the pineal gland of individuals who died of AD. According to Skene et al. (1990), these individuals have very low levels of melatonin in their pineal glands, a change that theoretically would aggravate the disease if free radicals are in fact involved. This study was not well controlled, and therefore the findings require confirmation.

The evidence of a link between oxidative stress and Huntington's disease (HD) is not compelling. However, excessive glutamate stimulation of postsynaptic receptors may be involved in the pathology of HD (Olney and Gubareff 1978). Because excitatory neurotransmitters stimulate oxygen-radical production intracellularly that could be neutralized by an antioxidant that readily crosses the blood-brain barrier, it is conceivable that antioxidants, including melatonin, could have utility in reducing the severity of HD.

Several forms of amyotrophic lateral sclerosis (ALS) have inadequate activity of the radical detoxifying enzyme superoxide dismutase (Bowling et al. 1993) in the afflicted motor neurons. This finding suggests that excessive radical production may be involved in this disorder. An oxidative component to multiple sclerosis (MS) is inferred by the observation that the iron chelator, desferrioxamine, has been reported to have therapeutic value in individuals with MS (Le Vine 1992). Due to its ability to neutralize iron, desferrioxamine reduces the formation of the highly toxic •OH. This demyelinating disease ultimately results in a block in axonal neurotransmission. Because melatonin readily enters the CNS and effectively scavenges •OH, it could have protective effects against MS.

Besides their potential relationship to the previously mentioned neurodegenerative conditions, oxygen radicals are suggested to be involved in schizophrenia and tardive dyskinesia. There are, of course, several theories of neuronal dysfunction to explain the symptoms of schizophrenia, with the involvement of free radicals being considered in only a minority of the theories (Cadet and Kohler 1994). The free-radical hypotheses stem from the proposed involvement of dopamine in schizophrenia. As pointed out earlier in this chapter, catecholamines are commonly associated with toxic oxygen by-products, such as semiquinone, hydrogen peroxide, and •OH. One group of investigators also pointed out similarities in neuropathological changes between schizophrenic patients and those with vitamin E deficiency (Miyakawa et al. 1972); the latter group clearly is linked to damage resulting from unchecked free-radical attack.

Tardive dyskinesia is a result of chronic use of antipsychotic drugs and includes a variety of choreoathetoid movements. Although there are a variety of potential mechanisms that could be the basis of the disorder, catecholamine-induced oxygen-radical damage to the brain is one proposed process that may be involved. A significant component of the condition may be peroxidized lipids, which would lead to destabilization of neuronal cell membranes (Zubenko and Cohen 1984). It also is possible that subjects with tardive dyskinesia may have inherently low radical-scavenging mechanisms in their brain, making the cells susceptible to free-radical attack (Cadet and Kohler 1994).

Conclusion

Within the last decade, free radicals as potential causative factors in neurodegenerative diseases and behavioral disorders have attracted increasing attention (Floyd 1990; Halliwell 1992; Reiter 1995b). During the same interval, discoveries related to melatonin as a neuroactive substance have increased in frequency (Reiter 1991b, 1995b). These observations, coupled with the findings that melatonin readily crosses the blood-brain barrier and gains access to subcellular compartments within neurons (Menendez-Pelaez and Reiter 1993; Menendez-Pelaez et al. 1993), in addition to the elucidation of melatonin as a potent antioxidant (Poeggeler et al. 1993; Reiter 1995b; Reiter et al. 1994a; Reiter et al. 1995), make a case for the possible involvement of melatonin in some neurodegenerative disorders. This involvement would seem more likely in cases where the frequency of the condition increases with advancing age (Poeggeler et al. 1993; Reiter et al. 1994a, 1994b) because the production and secretion of this important hormone falter badly late in life (Reiter 1992; Reiter 1995c). The groundwork certainly has been laid for experimental tests of the proposed relationships. It seems likely that melatonin eventually will be shown to be linked to some of the conditions mentioned in this chapter.

References

Acuña-Castroviejo D, Reiter RJ, Menendez-Pelaez A, et al: Characterization of high-affinity melatonin binding sites in purified cell nuclei of liver. J Pineal Res 16:100–112, 1994

Arendt J, Borbely AA, Franey C, et al: The effect of chronic small doses of melatonin given in the late afternoon on fatigue in man: a preliminary study. Neurosci Lett 5:317–321, 1984

Arendt J, Bojkowski C, Franey C, et al: Immunoassay of 6-hydroxymelatonin sulfate in human plasma and urine: abolition of the urinary 24-hour rhythm with atenolol. J Clin Endocrinol Metab 60:1166–1173, 1985

Arendt J, Aldhous M, English J, et al: Some effects of jet lag and their alleviation by melatonin. Ergonomics 30:1379–1383, 1987

Armstead WM, Mirro R, Leffler CW, et al: Cerebral superoxide anion generation during seizures in newborn pigs. J Cereb Blood Flow Metab 9:175–179, 1989

Beal MF: Energy, oxidative damage, and Alzheimer's disease: clues to the underlying puzzle. Neurobiol Aging 15 (suppl 2):171–174, 1994

Becker-Andre M, Wiesenberg I, Schaeren-Wiemers U, et al: Pineal hormone melatonin binds and activates an orphan of the nuclear receptor superfamily. J Biol Chem 269:28531–28534, 1994

Bellamy N: The jet lag phenomenon: etiology, pathogenesis, clinical features and management. Modern Medicine of Canada 41:717–732, 1986

Bowling AC, Schulz JB, Brown RH, et al: Superoxide dismutase activity, oxidative damage and mitochondrial energy metabolism in familial and sporadic amyotrophic lateral sclerosis. J Neurochem 61:2322–2325, 1993

Bozan NG, Birkle DL, Tang W, et al: The accumulation of free arachidonic acid, diacylglycerols, prostaglandins, lipoxygenase reaction products in the brain during experimental epilepsy. Adv Neurol 44:879–902, 1986

Brismar K, Hylander B, Eliasson K, et al: Melatonin secretion related to side-effects of beta-blockers from the central nervous system. Acta Medica Scandinavica 223:525–530, 1988

Bruce J, Tamarkin L, Riedel C, et al: Sequential cerebrospinal fluid and plasma sampling in humans: 24-hour melatonin measurements in normal subjects and after peripheral sympathectomy. J Clin Endocrinol Metab 72:819–823, 1991

Cadet JL, Kohler LA: Free radical mechanisms in schizophrenia and tardive dyskinesia. Neurosci Biobehav Rev 18:457–467, 1994

Carlberg C, Wiesenberg I: The orphan receptor family RZR/ROR, melatonin and 5-lipoxygenase: an unexpected relationship. J Pineal Res 18:171–178, 1995

Choi DW: Excitotoxic cell death. J Neurobiol 23:1261–1262, 1991

Colwell CS, Foster RG, Menaker M: NMDA receptor antagonists block the effects of light on circadian behavior in the mouse. Brain Res 554:105–110, 1991

Cotman CW: Report of Alzheimer's disease working group A. Neurobiol Aging 15 (suppl 2):517–522, 1994

Dahlitz M, Alvarez B, Vigeau J, et al: Delayed sleep phase syndrome response to melatonin. Lancet 337:1121–1124, 1991

Dawson D, Encel N: Melatonin and sleep in humans. J Pineal Res 15:1–12, 1993

Demisch C: Chemical pharmacology of melatonin regulation, in Melatonin: Biosynthesis, Physiological Effects, and Clinical Applications. Edited by Yu H-S, Reiter RJ. Boca Raton, FL, CRC Press, 1993

DeVries MJ, Cardozo BN, Van der Want J, et al: Glutamate immunoreactivity in terminals of the retinohypothalamic tract of the Norwegian rat. Brain Res 506:231–234, 1993

Dyrks T, Dyrks E, Hartmann T, et al: Amyloidogenicity of bA4 and bA4-bearing amyloid protein precursor fragments by metal-catalyzed oxidation. J Biol Chem 267:18210–18217, 1992

Fahn S, Cohen C: The oxidant stress hypothesis in Parkinson's disease: evidence supporting it. Ann Neurol 32:804–812, 1992

Fevre-Montange M, Van Cauter E, Pefatoff S, et al: Effects of "jet lag" on hormonal patterns, II: adaptation of melatonin circadian periodicity. J Clin Endocrinol Metab 52:642–649, 1981

Floyd RA: Role of oxygen free radicals in carcinogenesis and brain ischemia. FASEB J 4:2587–2597, 1990

Giarman NJ, Freedman DX, Picard-Ami L: Serotonin concentration of the pineal of man and monkey. Nature 186:480–482, 1960

Giusti P, Gusella M, Lipartiti M, et al: Melatonin protects primary cultures of cerebellar granular neurons from kainate but not from N-methyl-D-aspartate excitotoxicity. Exp Neurol 131:39–46, 1995

Graham D: Oxidative pathways for catecholamines in the genesis of neuromelanin and cytotoxic quinones. Mol Pharmacol 14:633–637, 1978

Gupta D: Pathophysiology of pineal function in health and disease. Pineal Research Reviews 6:261–300, 1988

Gupta D: The role of melatonin in human pathophysiology, in Melatonin: Biosynthesis, Physiological Effects, and Clinical Applications. Edited by Yu H-S, Reiter RJ. Boca Raton, FL, CRC Press, 1993

Haimov I, Laudon M, Zisapel N, et al: Sleep disorders and melatonin rhythms in elderly people (letter). BMJ 309:167, 1994

Halliwell B: Reactive oxygen species and the central nervous system. J Neurochem 59:1609–1623, 1992

Hardeland R, Reiter RJ, Poeggeler B, et al: The significance of the metabolism of the neurohormone melatonin: antioxidative protection and formation of bioactive substances. Neurosci Biobehav Rev 17:347–357, 1993

Heikilla RE, Sieber BA, Mansimo L, et al: Some features of the nigrostriatal dopaminergic neurotoxin 1-methyl-4-phenyl-1,2,3,6-tetrahydropyridine (MPTP) in the mouse. Mol Chem Neuropathol 10: 171–183, 1989

Iguchi H, Kato K, Ibayashi H: Age-dependent reduction in serum melatonin concentrations in healthy individuals. J Clin Endocrinol Metab
55:27–29, 1982

Kehrer JP: Free radicals, mediators of tissue injury and disease. Crit Rev
Toxicol 23:21–48, 1993

Kenneway DJ, Mathews DC, Seamark RP, et al: On the presence of
melatonin in pineal gland and plasma of foetal sheep. Journal of
Steroid Biochemistry 8:559–563, 1987

Kitagawa K, Matsumoto M, Oda T, et al: Free radical generation during
brief periods of ischemia may trigger delayed neuronal death. Neuroscience 35:551–558, 1990

Kneisley LW, Moskowitz MA, Lynch HJ: Cervical spinal cord lesions
disrupt the rhythm in human melatonin secretion. Journal of Neural
Transmission 13 (suppl):325–338, 1978

Le Vine SM: The role of reactive oxygen species in the pathogenesis of
multiple sclerosis. Med Hypotheses 39:271–274, 1992

Lewy AJ, Wehr TA, Goodwin FK, et al: Light suppresses melatonin secretion in humans. Science 210:1267–1269, 1980

Lewy AJ, Ahmed S, Jackson JM, et al: Melatonin shifts human circadian
rhythms according to a phase response curve. Chronobiol Int 9:380–
392, 1992

Madakoro S, Nakagawa H, Misaka K, et al: Melatonin rhythms in irregular shift workers. Japanese Journal of Psychiatry and Neurology
47:466–467, 1993

Maurizi CP: Could supplementary dietary tryptophan prevent sudden
infant death syndrome? Med Hypotheses 17:149–154, 1988

Mauviard F, Pevet P, Forlat P: 5-Methoxypsoralen enhances plasma
melatonin concentrations in the male rat: non-noradrenergic stimulation and lack of effect in pinealectomized animals. J Pineal Res 11:35–
41, 1991

McIntyre IM, Norman TR, Burrows GD, et al: Human melatonin suppression by light is intensity dependent. J Pineal Res 6:149–159, 1989

Melchiorri D, Reiter RJ, Sewerynek E, et al: Melatonin reduces kainate-
induced lipid peroxidation in homogenates of different brain regions.
FASEB J 9:1205–1210, 1995

Menendez-Pelaez A, Reiter RJ: Distribution of melatonin in mammalian
tissues: the relative importance of nuclear versus cytosolic receptors.
J Pineal Res 15:59–69, 1993

Menendez-Pelaez A, Poeggler B, Reiter RJ, et al: Nuclear localization of melatonin in different mammalian tissues: immunocytochemical and radioimmunoassay evidence. J Cell Biochem 53:373–382, 1993

Miyakawa T, Sumiyoshi S, Deshimura M, et al: Electron microscopic study of schizophrenia: mechanisms of pathologic changes. Acta Neuropathol (Berl) 20:67–77, 1972

Monteleone P, Forzeati D, Orazzo C, et al: Preliminary observations on the suppression of nocturnal melatonin levels by short-term administration of diazepam. J Pineal Res 6:253–258, 1989

Murphy TH, Miyamato M, Sastre A, et al: Glutamate toxicity in a neuronal cell line involves inhibition of cystine transport leading to oxidative stress. Neuron 2:1547–1558, 1989

Nair NPV, Hariharasubramanian M, Pilapil C, et al: Plasma melatonin, an index of brain aging in humans? Biol Psychiatry 21:141–150, 1986

Norlund JJ, Lerner AB: The effects of oral melatonin on skin color and the release of pituitary hormones. J Clin Endocrinol Metab 45:768–774, 1977

Olney JW, Gubareff T: Glutamate neurotoxicity and Huntington's chorea. Nature 271:557–559, 1978

Petrie K, Conaglen JV, Thompson L, et al: Effect of melatonin on jet lag after long haul flight. BMJ 298:705–707, 1989

Petrie K, Dawson AG, Thompson L, et al: A double-blind trial of melatonin as a treatment for jet lag in international cabin crew. Biol Psychiatry 33:526–530, 1993

Pieri C, Marra M, Moroni F, et al: Melatonin: a paroxyl radical scavenger more effective than vitamin E. Life Sci 55:271–276, 1994

Poeggeler B, Reiter RJ, Tan DX, et al: Melatonin, hydroxyl radical-mediated oxidative damage and aging: a hypothesis. J Pineal Res 14:151–168, 1993

Poeggeler B, Barlow-Walden LR, Reiter RJ, et al: Red light–induced suppression of melatonin synthesis is mediated by NMDA receptor activation in retinally normal and retinally degenerate rats. J Neurobiol 28:1–8, 1995

Polazidou E, Franey C, Arendt J, et al: Evidence for a functional role of alpha-1 adrenoceptors in the regulation of melatonin secretion in man. Psychoneuroendocrinology 14:131–135, 1989

Poyer JL, McCoy PB: Reduced triphosphopyridine nucleotide oxidase–catalyzed alterations of phospholipids. J Biol Chem 246:263–269, 1991

Pozo D, Reiter RJ, Calvo JR, et al: Physiological concentrations of melatonin inhibit nitric oxide synthase in rat cerebellum. Life Sci 55: PL455–PL460, 1994

Puig-Domingo M, Webb SM, Serrano J, et al: Melatonin-related hypogonadotrophic hypogonadism. N Engl J Med 357:1355–1356, 1992

Reiter RJ: Melatonin: the chemical expression of darkness. Mol Cell Endocrinol 79:C153–C158, 1991a

Reiter RJ: Pineal melatonin: cell biology of its synthesis and of its physiological interactions. Endocr Rev 12:151–180, 1991b

Reiter RJ: The aging pineal gland and its physiological consequences. Bioessays 14:169–175, 1992

Reiter RJ: Functional pleiotropy of the neurohormone melatonin: antioxidant protection and neuroendocrine regulation. Front Neuroendocrinol 16:383–415, 1995a

Reiter RJ: Oxidative processes and antioxidative defense mechanisms in the aging brain. FASEB J 9:526–533, 1995b

Reiter RJ: The pineal gland and melatonin in relation to aging: a summary of the theories and of the data. Exp Gerontol 30:199–212, 1995c

Reiter RJ, Blask ED, Talbot JA, et al: The nature and time course of seizures associated with surgical removal of the pineal gland from parathyroidectomized rats. Exp Neurol 38:376–379, 1973

Reiter RJ, Johnson LY, Steger RW, et al: Pineal biosynthetic activity and neuroendocrine physiology in the aging hamster and gerbil. Peptides 1 (suppl 1):69–77, 1980a

Reiter RJ, Richardson BA, Johnson LY, et al: Pineal melatonin rhythm: reduction in aging Syrian hamster. Science 210:1372–1373, 1980b

Reiter RJ, Craft CM, Johnson JR Jr, et al: Age-associated reduction in nocturnal melatonin levels in rats. Endocrinology 109:1295–1297, 1981

Reiter RJ, Tan DX, Poeggeler B, et al: Melatonin as a free radical scavenger: implications for aging and age related diseases. Ann N Y Acad Sci 719:1–12, 1994a

Reiter RJ, Poeggeler B, Chen LD, et al: Melatonin as a free radical scavenger: theoretical implications for neurodegenerative disorders in the aged. Acta Gerontologica 44:92–114, 1994b

Reiter RJ, Melchiorri D, Sewerynek E, et al: A review of the evidence supporting melatonin's role as an antioxidant. J Pineal Res 18:1–11, 1995

Reppert SM, Weaver DR, Ebisawa T: Cloning and characterization of a mammalian melatonin receptor that mediates reproductive and circadian responses. Neuron 13:1177–1185, 1994

Sack RL, Lewy AJ, Erb DL, et al: Human melatonin production decreases with age. J Pineal Res 3:379–388, 1986

Schulz JB, Henshaw DR, Sivek D, et al: Involvement of free radicals in excitotoxicity in vivo. J Neurochem 64:2239–2247, 1995

Sewerynek E, Melchiorri D, Chen LD, et al: Melatonin reduces both basal and lipopolysaccharide-induced lipid peroxidation in vitro. Free Radic Biol Med 19:903–909, 1995

Singh R, Pathak DN: Lipid peroxidation and glutathione peroxidase, glutathione reduction, superoxide dismutase, catalase and glucose-6-phosphate dehydrogenase activities in $FeCl_3$–induced epileptogenic foci in the rat brain. Epilepsia 31:15–26, 1990

Skene DJ, Vivien Roels B, Sparks LD, et al: Daily variation in the concentration of melatonin and 5-methoxytryptophol in the human pineal gland: effect of age and Alzheimer's disease. Brain Res 528:170–174, 1990

Sparks DL, Hunsaker JC III: The pineal gland in sudden infant death syndrome: preliminary observations. J Pineal Res 5:111–118, 1988

Stankov B, Reiter RJ: Melatonin receptors: current status, facts and hypotheses. Life Sci 46:971–982, 1990

Stokkan KA, Reiter RJ, Nanaka KO, et al: Food restriction retards aging of the pineal gland. Brain Res 545:66–72, 1991

Sturner WQ, Lunch HJ, Deng MH, et al: Circadian rhythm in SIDS: melatonin levels in body fluids (abstract). Abstracts of the International Association of Forensic Science 8:120, 1994

Subbarao S, Richardson JS, Ang L: Autopsy samples of Alzheimer's cortex show increased peroxidation in vitro. J Neurochem 55:342–345, 1990

Tan DX, Chen DX, Poeggeler B, et al: Melatonin: a potent, endogenous hydroxyl radical scavenger. Endocr J 1:57–60, 1993

Torbati D, Church DF, Keller JM, et al: Free radical generation in the brain precedes hyperbaric oxygen-induced convulsions. Free Radic Biol Med 13:101–114, 1992

Touitou Y, Fevre M, Langugvey M, et al: Age and mental health related circadian rhythms of plasma levels of melatonin, prolactin, luteinizing hormone and follicle stimulating hormone. J Endocrinol 9:467–475, 1981

Tzischensky O, Pal I, Epstein R, et al: The importance of time in melatonin administration in man. J Pineal Res 12:105–108, 1992

Vaughan GM: Melatonin in humans. Pineal Research Reviews 2:141–201, 1984

Waldhauser F, Ehrhart B, Forster E: Clinical aspects of melatonin action: impact on development, aging and puberty, involvement of melatonin in psychiatric disease and importance of neuroimmunoendocrine interactions. Experientia 49:671–681, 1993

Wetterberg L, Iselius L, Lindsten J: Genetic regulation of melatonin excretion in urine. Clin Genet 24:399–402, 1983

Wu W, Li L: Inhibition of nitric oxide synthase reduces motoneuron death due to spinal root avulsion. Neurosci Lett 153:121–124, 1993

Youdim MBH, Ben-Schachar D, Riederer P: The possible role of iron in the etiopathology of Parkinson's disease. Mov Disord 8:1–12, 1993

Zubenko G, Cohen BM: In vitro effects of psychotropic agents on the microviscosity of platelet membranes. Psychopharmacology (Berl) 84:289–292, 1984

Chapter 2

The Structure and Evolutionary Development of the Pineal Gland

Kunwar P. Bhatnagar, Ph.D.

O ur knowledge of the pineal gland has progressed considerably in the last quarter of this century in the areas of morphology, biochemistry, neurobiology, and pharmacology. Even though the pineal gland is a discrete entity in vertebrates, particularly humans, our knowledge of its function is just beginning to unfold.

In this chapter, I briefly review the evolutionary development of the pineal gland in vertebrates and concisely discuss the structure of the pineal gland in humans, with emphasis on recent developments. For a more detailed and comprehensive review of the anatomy and structure of the pineal gland, see Bhatnagar (1990, 1992), Eakin (1973), Karasek and Reiter (1992), Quay (1979), Reiter (1980, 1992), Reiter and Vaughan (1988), and Vollrath (1981, 1985).

The Vertebrate Pineal Gland

From an evolutionary perspective, the pineal gland (epiphysis cerebri) appears for the first time as a vertebrate brain embellishment in the lampreys (Cyclostomata). In the lamprey *Petromyzon*, fishes, amphibians, and lacertilian reptiles, the pineal is a fully functional photoreceptor organ (Ralph 1975). In these vertebrate groups, the pineal gland is accompanied by accessory pineal organs, such as the parapineal organ of Petromyzontidae, the frontal organ of anuran amphibians, and the parietal eye of lacertilians (Quay 1979), whereas in snakes, turtles, birds, and mammals, the parapineal organs are lacking and the direct photosensitivity of the pineal is replaced by a secretory phenomenon—melatonin synthesis from serotonin. Whereas in the lower vertebrates the pineal neurosensory cells send afferent fibers to the brain, in birds and mammals the principal pineal innervation is efferent, being autonomically sympathetic via the superior cervical ganglia (Bhatnagar 1990).

Pineal Correlative Phenomena in the Invertebrates

In vertebrates, the pineal gland is an integral component of the visual pathway. However, even in the invertebrate orders (i.e., in Arthropoda and Mollusca), the visual systems are made up of discrete visual elements. For example, the optic lobes of cockroaches are reported to be the sites of circadian pacemakers (Edmunds 1988, p. 1982). Circadian oscillation and photoreception have been reported for even small parts of the chicken pineal gland (Takahashi and Menaker 1984). It would seem possible, therefore, that circadian rhythmicity is an essential property of visual elements, be it within the eyes, the pineal, or the related optic brain.

Melatonin Secretion From Algae to Humans

Recent findings indicate that in the unicellular alga, *Gonyaulax polyedra* (a bioluminescent dinoflagellate), melatonin and serotonin are present and exhibit circadian rhythmicity (Balzer and Hardeland 1991; Balzer et al. 1993; Hardeland et al. 1993; Poeggeler et al. 1991). Also, melatonin has been identified in many of the edible plants (Dubbels et al. 1995) and in the multicellular alga *Pterygophora* (Fuhrberg et al. 1996).

Melatonin has been reported in *Drosophila melanogaster* (Finocchiaro et al. 1988), the compound eye of *Locusta migratoria* (Vivien-Roels et al. 1984), and planarian species (Yoshizawa et al. 1991). Because melatonin has now been reported in a variety of plant and animal species (both invertebrates and vertebrates) and in nonpineal tissues such as the retina, harderian glands, hypothalamus, gut, exorbital lacrimal glands, inner ear, peripheral mononuclear cells, platelets, and peripheral nerves (see review by Menen-dez-Pelaez and Reiter 1993), it can no longer be considered as a pineal-specific product. Reiter et al. (1993) report that melatonin is the most effective •OH free-radical scavenger, that it is "produced in all vertebrates and perhaps in all species between algae and humans" (pp. 108–109), and that its binding to nuclear compo-nents suggests genomic involvement.

The Structure of the Human Pineal Gland

Despite the available reports on the structure of the fetal (Møller 1974, 1976) and adult human pineal gland (Bhatnagar 1990, 1992; Hasegawa et al. 1990, 1991; Krstic 1976, 1986; Kurumado and Mori 1976; Tapp and Huxley 1972), our knowledge of its microanatomy and fine structure is far from complete. Most studies have had to use postmortem pineal gland tissue. Lack of fresh and optimally fixed tissues for such studies has handicapped our understanding of human pineal structure. The establishment of the National Can-cer Institute Cooperative Human Tissue Network with regional divisions is expected to bridge this gap. The following description of the human pineal gland structure is based upon the work of Bhatnagar (1990, 1992), along with the published reports referred to previously.

The human pineal gland is a part of the epithalamus. It is a small, flat, pine cone–shaped structure (Table 2–1) occupying the superior subarachnoid cistern in between the splenium of the corpus callosum and the superior colliculi (Figure 2–1). With a hollow and pedunculated base, it is attached to the roof of the third ventricle, which extends into the pineal stalk as the pineal recess of the third ventricle. Another recess of the third ventricle, the suprapineal recess, overlies the pineal. The pineal gland is spheroidal in the newborn; the adult shape and size are reached around the fourth year of life. From then on, no structural changes are known to occur in the pineal gland, other than the possible development of calcareous concretions and cysts or pathological formations. The weight and dimensions of the pineal are highly variable.

The pineal parenchyma is formed of pinealocytes. Glial cells (which are few), blood vessels, nerves, neurons, connective tissue septae forming follicles, and cords of pinealocytes are interspersed

Table 2–1. Biological data on human pineal gland

Characteristics	Data	Reference
Shape	Pine-cone shaped	Vollrath 1981
Pineal type	A	Vollrath 1979
Dimension[a] (height, maximum width)	8.8 mm, 5.2 mm	Bhatnagar 1990
Weight[a,b]	138.60 mg	Legait and Legait 1977
	109.25 mg	Bhatnagar 1990
Volume[a]	46.12 mm^3	Legait et al. 1976a, 1976b
Specific gravity (fresh, unfixed pineal)	1.197 ± 0.036 at 20°C	Bhatnagar et al. 1991
First appearance in development	33rd postovulatory day (6–8 mm crown-rump length embryo)	O'Rahilly 1968
Melatonin levels[c] nighttime/daytime	3.80 ± 0.3/0.85 ± 0.4 ng/mg protein	
Pineal size index[d]	176	Bhatnagar et al. 1990

[a]The usual shape of the human pineal gland is conical, and therefore there are only two dimensions, height and maximum width at the base. All dimensions are extremely variable, not only in humans but also in other species (Bhatnagar et al. 1986, 1990), so much so that there could hardly be an average dimension, weight, or volume for the pineal gland.
[b]Like dimension, human pineal gland weight also is highly variable. It is subject to the degree of calcification (Tapp and Huxley 1972) and cystic formations and is lower after decalcification.
[c]Different laboratories have reported different levels of melatonin in humans, based on whether it was pineal melatonin (from autopsy tissue; Schmid et al. 1993) or blood-derived plasma melatonin (Waldhauser et al. 1984a, 1984b). Melatonin production is reported to decline with age (Sack et al. 1986; Schmid et al. 1993) and during puberty (see review by Poeggeler et al. 1993, p. 165).
[d]Compare with the pineal size index of 4393 in the bat *Dobsonia* and with the pineal size index of 2156 in the seal *Phoca* (Bhatnagar et al. 1990).
Source.   Adapted from Bhatnagar 1990.

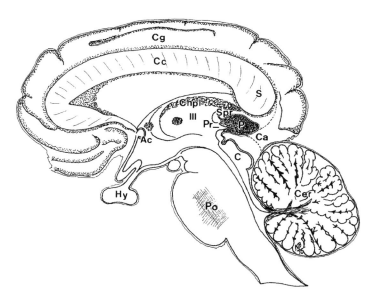

Figure 2–1. Schematic median view of the human brain stem emphasizing the pineal-brain relationships. Ac, anterior commissure; C, colliculi, superior and inferior; Ca, cisterna ambiens or the superior subarachnoid cistern; Cc, corpus callosum; Cer, cerebellum; Cg, cingulate gyrus; Chpl, choroid plexus of the third ventricle (III); Hy, hypophysis; P, pineal gland; Po, pons; Pr, pineal recess; S, splenium of corpus callosum; Spr, suprapineal recess.

throughout (Figure 2–2). Other constituents are the calcareous concretions, melanocytes, and other parenchymal elements.

In the ultrastructure of the pineal gland, juxtaposition of alternating dark and light pinealocytes are sometimes observed (Jouvet et al. 1994). Zonulae adherentes are long. Multipolar pinealocytes, many times with two prominent nucleoli, have been reported. Terminals of pinealocyte processes with club-shaped endings reach the perivascular space. The irregular round-to-oval nucleus has a number of invaginations. The Golgi complex is well developed and consists of several stacks of flattened sacs, vacuoles, and vesicles. These and other cytoplasmic organelles are polarized and consist of prominent microfilaments, 20- to 25-nm long microtubules especially abundant in pinealocyte processes,

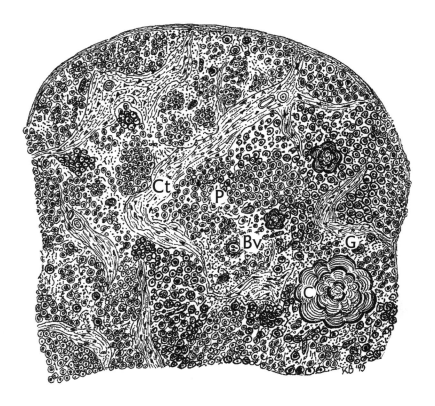

Figure 2–2. Light microscopic schematized illustration of a section through the human pineal. Bv, blood vessels; C, concretions or acervuli; Ct, connective tissue septa; G, glial cell; P, pineal parenchyma containing pinealocytes.

cilia with 9 + 0 configuration extending into the intercellular space, microtubular sheaves, clusters of centrioles, mitochondrial clusters, more rough endoplasmic reticulum than the smooth variety, and lipid droplets. Additional organelles include the coated vesicles, synaptic ribbons (mostly lying close to the plasma membrane) and ribbon fields, lipofuscin granules, clear vesicles, 80- to 120-nm dense-cored vesicles (which are rare), dark lysosomes, bundles of 5- to 8-nm packed filaments, and 10-nm paired twisted filaments (Figure 2–3).

The other cell type, which is by far smaller in number, is the glial cell, recognizable by its dense characteristic. Its nucleus contains chromatin aggregations. These various organelles in the cytoplasm are concentrated in the perinuclear region. Glial fibers occur throughout the cell body extending into the processes. The immunohistochemical presence of glial marker proteins (glial fibrillary acidic protein and protein S-100) in these cells has clearly established their astroglial nature. Most of these are considered to be fibrous astrocytes; however, some protoplasmic astrocytes are believed to be present also.

Other constituents of the human pineal gland are macrophages; melanocytes; lymphocytes; skeletal muscle fibers (Bhatnagar 1994); mast cells; concretions (acervuli); blood vessels, some showing fenestrae (Jouvet et al. 1994); connective tissue elements; and the thin pial capsule. Often, cysts develop within the pineal parenchyma. Nerve fibers and intrapineal neurons are some additional components of the human pineal gland.

Arterial supply to the pineal gland is through branches of the posterior cerebral arteries, the posterolateral central arteries, whereas the immense venous return is into the great cerebral vein (of Galen). Lymphatics are not reported in the pineal. The variability of interpretation of and confusion about pineal innervation remain unexplored. Intrapineal neurons, juxtapineal ganglia, nerve fibers, sympathetic and parasympathetic autonomic nerves, and pinealofugal and pinealopetal innervation have been described (Møller 1976). Pineal innervation is clearly deserving of serious attention.

Pineal Cysts

It is not uncommon to find cystic inclusions within the human pineal gland. Such cysts can escape detection in brain scans by computed tomography (CT) and can be confused with the quadrigeminal cistern (Mamourian and Towfighi 1986). Pineal cysts are observed in other animals also (Bhatnagar et al. 1986, 1990). Recently, Costanzo et al. (1993) found seven cases of pineal

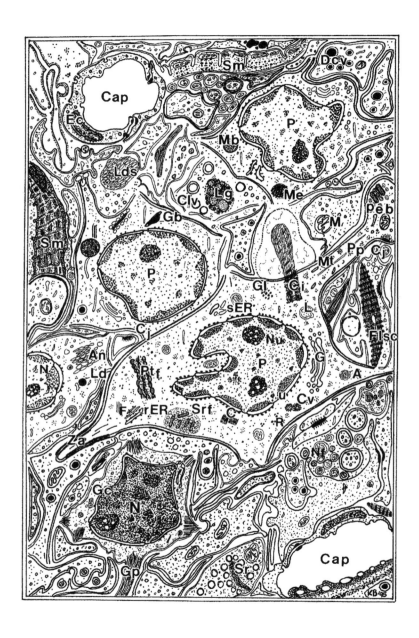

cysts in 400 consecutive magnetic resonance imaging (MRI) examinations of humans. They believe that cases of symptomatic pineal cysts have been overemphasized. Because of these cases, Costanzo and colleagues suggested that pineal cysts are always asymptomatic and are an incidental MRI finding.

Pineal Concretionary Deposits

Human pineal glands are endowed with calcareous concretions (acervuli, brain sand, corpora arenacea), as are the pineal glands of a few other animals such as gerbils, ungulates, rodents, monkeys, and certain birds (e.g., ducks and herons). In humans, the concretions can fill the pineal parenchyma so extensively as to nearly destroy it. Thus, in combination with pineal cysts, the parenchyma could be effectively compromised functionally. Detailed studies of the human pineal concretions have not been carried out for obvious reasons. Based upon experimental investigation of the gerbil pineal (Karasek and Reiter 1992; Welsh and Reiter 1978), the concretions develop within the pinealocyte vacuoles, grow, and reach

Figure 2–3. A schematic and idealized ultrastructural representation of human pineal parenchyma showing pinealocytes, glial cells, and adjacent intercellular components, based primarily on descriptions by Bhatnagar (1990, 1992), Hasegawa et al. (1990, 1991), and Jouvet et al. (1994). A, acervulus (early stage); An, annulate lamellae; C, centrioles; Cap, capillary; Ci, cilium; Cj, cell junction (intermediate type); Clv, clear vesicles; Cv, coated vesicles; Dcv, dense-cored vesicles; Ec, endothelial cell; F, filaments; Flsc, fibrous long-spacing collagen; G, Golgi complex; Gb, granular body; Gc, glial cell; Gl, glycogen; Gp, glial process with intermediate filaments; L, lysosome; Ld, lipid droplet; Lds, lamellar disc structure; Lg, lipofuscin granules; M, mitochondrion; Mb, multivesicular body; Me, melanin granules; Mt, microtubules; N, nucleus; Nf, nerve fibers; Nu, nucleolus; P, pinealocyte; Peb, pinealocyte end bulb; Pp, pinealocyte process; Ptf, paired twisted filaments; R, ribosomes; rER and sER, rough and smooth endoplasmic reticulum; Sm, striated muscle fibers (some in cross section); Sr and Srf, synaptic ribbons and synaptic ribbon fields; u, nuclear pore; Za, zonulae adherentes.

the extracellular space, where they are held permanently. No relationship with aging or any of the disease states has ever been established beyond a conjectural level. Compounding the matter further is the fact that pineal concretions are reported to be lacking in most other species. However, the pineal gland and the associated meninges have not been examined meticulously because such work is painstakingly difficult. Recently, pineal concretions have been reported in a bat, *Anoura caudifer* (Bhatnagar and Hoffman 1995).

Pineal Tumors

Using light and electron microscopy and immunohistochemical markers for glial fibrillary acidic protein (GFAP), protein S-100, neurofilaments, synaptophysin, and chromogranin A, Jouvet et al. (1994) studied human pineal parenchymal tumors and normal or cystic pineal glands. Synaptic ribbons were a consistent finding in both normal and tumoral pineals, but dense-cored vesicles were many only in the tumoral glands as compared with the normal glands. Synaptophysin, neurofilaments, and chromogranin A were present in the pineocytomas.

Conclusions

Continued structural investigation of the human pineal gland is essential for a more thorough understanding of its functions and of the target organs. Pathological specimens of the pineal obtained at autopsy are no longer adequate. Currently, this promising area of research involves the use of fetal pineal tissue for tissue culture, in situ hybridization, and other molecular biological techniques.

The measurement and role of melatonin, a hormone of the pineal gland, and/or its metabolite, α6-hydroxymelatonin sulfate (αMT6s), in various body fluids in both healthy subjects and those with disorders undertaken in studies during the last two decades have provided a beginning understanding of the function of melatonin, but far more in-depth studies are needed.

The emerging field of pinealology has become a fertile ground for collaborative and integrative studies among the anatomical sciences, cellular biology, endocrinology, oncology, gerontology, chronobiology, and psychiatry and the behavioral sciences.

References

Balzer I, Hardeland R: Photoperiodism and effects of indolamines in a unicellular alga, *Gonyaulax polyedra.* Science 253:795–797, 1991

Balzer I, Pöeggeler B, Hardeland R: Circadian rhythms of indolamines in a dinoflagellate, *Gonyaulax polyedra:* persistence of melatonin rhythm in constant darkness and relationship to 5-methoxytryptamine, in Excerpta Medica: Melatonin and the Pineal Gland: From Basic Science to Clinical Application. Edited by Touitou Y, Arendt J, Pèvet P. Amsterdam, Elsevier, 1993, pp 183–186

Bhatnagar KP: Comparative morphology of the pineal gland, in Biological Rhythms, Mood Disorders, Light Therapy, and the Pineal Gland. Edited by Shafii M, Shafii SL. Washington, DC, American Psychiatric Press, 1990, pp 1–37

Bhatnagar KP: The ultrastructure of mammalian pinealocytes: a systematic investigation. Microsc Res Tech 21:85–115, 1992

Bhatnagar KP: Skeletal muscle in the pineal gland of the bat, *Rhinopoma microphyllum:* an ultrastructural investigation. J Anat 184:171–176, 1994

Bhatnagar KP, Hoffman RA: Calcareous concretions in the pineal gland of the long-tongued bat, *Anoura caudifer* (abstract). Paper presented at the Tenth International Bat Research Conference, Boston, MA, August 1995

Bhatnagar KP, Frahm H, Stephan H: The pineal organ of bats: a comparative morphological and volumetric investigation. J Anat 147:143–161, 1986

Bhatnagar KP, Frahm H, Stephan H: The megachiropteran pineal organ: a comparative morphological and volumetric investigation with special emphasis on the remarkably large pineal of *Dobsonia praedatrix.* J Anat 168:143–166, 1990

Bhatnagar KP, Veling M, Ouseph PJ, et al: Determination of the specific gravity of human pineal. J Pineal Res 11:168–172, 1991

Costanzo AD, Tedeschi G, Salle FD, et al: Pineal cysts: an incidental MRI finding? J Neurol Neurosurg Psychiatry 56:207–208, 1993

Dubbels R, Reiter RJ, Klenke E, et al: Melatonin in edible plants identified by radioimmunoassay and by high performance liquid chromatography-mass spectrometry. J Pineal Res 18:28–31, 1995

Eakin RM: The Third Eye. Berkeley, University of California Press, 1973

Edmunds LN: Cellular and Molecular Bases of Biological Clocks: Models and Mechanisms for Circadian Timekeeping. Heidelberg, Germany, Springer, 1988

Finocchiaro L, Callebert J, Launay JM, et al: Melatonin biosynthesis in *Drosophila:* its nature and its effects. J Neurochem 50:382–387, 1988

Fuhrberg B, Balzer I, Hardeland R, et al: The vertebrate pineal hormone melatonin is produced by the brown algaa *Pterygophora californica* and mimics dark effects on growth rate in the light. Planta 200:125–131, 1996

Hardeland R, Reiter RJ, Poeggeler B, et al: The significance of the neurohormone melatonin: antioxidative protection and formation of bioactive substances. Neurosci Biobehav Rev 17:347–357, 1993

Hasegawa A, Ohtsubo K, Izumiyama N, et al: Ultrastructural study of the human pineal gland in aged patients including a centenarian. Acta Pathologica Jpn 40:30–40, 1990

Hasegawa A, Shimada H, Izumiyama N, et al: Paired twisted filaments in human pinealocytes. Acta Pathologica Jpn 41:265–269, 1991

Jouvet A, Fèvre-Montange M, Besancon R, et al: Structural and ultrastructural characteristics of human pineal gland, and pineal parenchymal tumors. Acta Neuropathol (Berl) 88:334–348, 1994

Karasek M, Reiter RJ: Morphofunctional aspects of the mammalian pineal gland. Microsc Res Tech 21:136–157, 1992

Krstic R: A combined scanning and transmission electron microscopic study and electron probe microanalysis of human pineal acervuli. Cell Tissue Res 174:129–137, 1976

Krstic R: Pineal calcification: its mechanism and significance. J Neural Transm (Suppl) 21:415–432, 1986

Kurumado K, Mori W: Synaptic ribbon in human pinealocyte. Acta Pathologica Jpn 26:381–384, 1976

Legait H, Legait E: Contribution á l'étude de la glande pinéale humaine: étude faite á l'aide de 747 glandes. Bull Assoc Anat (Nancy) 61:107–121, 1977

Legait H, Bauchot R, Stephan H, et al: Etude des corrélations liant le volume de l'épiphyse aux poids somatique et encéphalique chez les rongeurs, les insectivores, les chiroptéres, les prosimiens et les simiens. Mammalia 40:327–337, 1976a

Legait H, Bauchot R, Contet-Audonneau JL: Etude des corrélations liant les volumes des lobes hypophysaires et de l'épiphyse aud poids somatique et au poids encéphalique chez les chiroptéres. Bull Assoc Anat (Nancy) 60:175–188, 1976b

Mamourian AC, Towfighi J: Pineal cysts: magnetic resonance imaging. AJNR Am J Neuroradiol 7:1081–1086, 1986

Menendez-Pelaez A, Reiter RJ: Distribution of melatonin in mammalian tissues: the relative importance of nuclear versus cytosolic localization. J Pineal Res 15:59–69, 1993

Møller M: The ultrastructure of the human fetal pineal gland, I: cell types and blood vessels. Cell Tissue Res 152:13–30, 1974

Møller M: The ultrastructure of the human fetal pineal gland, II: innervation and cell junctions. Cell Tissue Res 169:7–21, 1976

O'Rahilly R: The development of the epiphysis cerebri and the subcommisural complex in staged human embryos (abstract). Anat Rec 160:488–489, 1968

Pöeggeler B, Balzer I, Hardeland R, et al: Pineal hormone melatonin oscillates also in the dinoflagellate *Gonyaulax polyedra*. Naturwissenschaften 78:268–269, 1991

Pöeggeler B, Reiter RJ, Tan D-X, et al: Melatonin, hydroxyl radical-mediated oxidative damage, and aging: a hypothesis. J Pineal Res 14:151–168, 1993

Quay WB: The parietal eye-pineal complex, in Biology of the Reptilia, Vol 9: Neurology A. Edited by Gans C, Northcutt RG, Ulinski P. London, Academic Press, 1979, pp 245–406

Ralph CL: The pineal gland and geographical distribution of animals. Int J Biometeorol 19: 289–303, 1975

Reiter RJ: The pineal gland: a regulator of regulators. Progress in Psychiatry and Physiological Psychology 9:109–131, 1980

Reiter RJ: The aging pineal gland and its physiological consequences. Bioessays 14:169–175, 1992

Reiter RJ, Vaughan MK: Pineal gland, in Endocrinology: People and Ideas, Edited by McCann SM. Bethesda, MD, American Physiological Society, 1988, pp 471

Reiter RJ, Pöeggeler B, Tan DX, et al: Antioxidant capacity of melatonin: a novel action not requiring a receptor. Neuroendocrinology Letters 15:103–116, 1993

Sack RL, Lewy AJ, Erb DL, et al: Human melatonin production decreases with age. J Pineal Res 3:379–388, 1986

Schmid HA, Requintina PJ, Oxenkrug GF, et al: Calcium, calcification, and melatonin biosynthesis in the human pineal gland: a postmortem study into age-related factors. J Pineal Res 16:178–183, 1993

Takahashi JS, Menaker M: Multiple redundant circadian oscillators within the isolated avian pineal gland. J Comp Physiol [A] 154:435–440, 1984

Tapp E, Huxley M: The histological appearance of the human pineal gland from puberty to old age. J Pathol 108:137–144, 1972

Vivien-Roels B, Pèvet P, Beck O, et al: Identification of melatonin in the compound eye of an insect, the locust (*Locusta migratoria*), by radioimmunoassay and gas chromatography-mass spectrometry. Neurosci Lett 49:153–157, 1984

Vollrath L: Comparative morphology of the vertebrate pineal complex, in The Pineal Gland of Vertebrates Including Man. Edited by Kappers JA, Pévet P. Prog Brain Res 52:25–38, 1979

Vollrath L: The pineal organ, in Handbuch der mikroskopischen Anatomie des Menschen, Vol vi/7. Edited by Oksche A, Vollrath L. Berlin, Springer, 1981

Vollrath L: Mammalian pinealocytes: ultrastructural aspects and innervation. Ciba Found Symp 117:9–22, 1985

Waldhauser F, Weissenbacher G, Zeitlhuber U, et al: Fall in nocturnal serum melatonin levels during prepuberty and pubescence. Lancet 1:262–265, 1984a

Waldhauser F, Lynch HJ, Wurtman RJ: Melatonin in human body fluids: clinical significance, in The Pineal Gland. Edited by Reiter RJ. New York, Raven, 1984b

Welsh MG, Reiter RJ: The pineal gland of the Mongolian gerbil, *Meriones unguiculatus,* I: an ultrastructural study. Cell Tissue Res 193:323–336, 1978

Yoshizawa Y, Wakabayashi K, Shinozawa T: Inhibition of planarian regeneration by melatonin. Hydrobiologica 227:31–40, 1991

Part II

Melatonin in Psychiatric Disorders in Adults

Chapter 3

Melatonin in Adult Depression

Lennart Wetterberg, M.D., Ph.D.

lready at the beginning of the twentieth century, Simpsom and Galbraith (1906) observed that some body rhythms, for instance, variations in body temperature (lower temperature at night), are influenced by the light-dark cycle. In the 1950s, Pittendrigh (1967) demonstrated that an inner biological clock governed temperature control. Certain anatomical structures in the mammalian brain, such as the suprachiasmatic nucleus (SCN) of the hypothalamus in the midbrain, serve as regulators of endogenous rhythms. SCN cells have been transplanted from one strain of hamsters with a short diurnal rhythm to another strain, with the result that the shorter rhythm from the host strain was transferred to the recipient (Ralph et al. 1990). This result shows that the SCN cells function as a biological clock in the regulation of circadian rhythms. Further investigations point to the importance of light for synchronizing circadian rhythms in general (Pittendrigh 1993).

Melatonin Production Regulated by Light and Darkness

Both light and darkness affect the production of the hormone melatonin in the pineal gland (Wetterberg 1978). The system that generates the diurnal rhythms of melatonin includes signal transmission of light impulses via the retina to the hypothalamus and via the upper cervical ganglion to the pineal gland (see Reiter, Chapter 1, in this volume). Formation of melatonin from the pineal gland is rhythmically regulated by alterations in light/darkness that affect noradrenaline concentrations through nerve pathways from the eye to the hypothalamus and SCN, via the thoracic spinal cord and upper cervical ganglion to the pineal gland. The nerve endings release noradrenaline in the β-adrenergic receptors that stimulate the transformation of adenosine triphosphate (ATP) to cyclic adenosine monophosphate (cAMP) and thereby increase the protein synthesis in the pineal gland. The activity of two enzymes, N-acetyltransferase (NAT) and hydroxyindole-O-methyltransferase (HIOMT), increases in darkness and makes possible the synthesis of melatonin from serotonin. Melatonin is immediately secreted from the pineal gland into the blood. Blood levels of melatonin reach their highest values during the night, at about 2 A.M.; during daytime and with exposure to bright light at night, melatonin formation decreases.

Melatonin Monitors the Internal Body Rhythms

The basis for measuring melatonin in depressive disorders is related to, among others, Wetterberg et al.'s (1979) report in which a patient had higher cortisol levels during depression than during recovery, with a concomitant decrease in the nocturnal serum melatonin level from 0.12 nmol/L to 0.06 nmol/L. Also, in this patient the peak level of melatonin occurred earlier (midnight) during the depressive episode than during recovery (4 A.M.). The potential use of melatonin as a biological marker in depression was obvious. Not only is melatonin dependent on both noradrenergic and serotonergic transmissions for its regulation, it also seems to be related to the hypothalamic-pituitary-adrenal (HPA) axis, which is affected in depressive states (elevated nocturnal cortisol levels and early escape in the dexamethasone suppression test [DST]). In adult patients with depression, a coupling between the rhythms of secretion of melatonin and of cortisol (adrenal cortical hormone), as well as possible rhythm disturbances of these two hormones, was reported by Wetterberg et al. (1979).

Additionally, melatonin is useful in indicating the phase and the amplitude of the biological clock mechanism. The variation in melatonin concentrations over a 24-hour period allows scientists to study the hypothesis of free-running rhythm failure in subtypes of depression and to test the phase-advance theory of affective illness introduced by Halberg et al. (1968). Free-running rhythm refers to the genetically determined internal rhythm that each healthy individual may display when isolated from all external time cues. Normally, the internal body rhythm is synchronized with the external clock (i.e., the light-dark cycle arising from the sun-earth rotation). A free-running rhythm may be longer or shorter than 24 hours; this rhythmic activity is the basis for the term *circadian*, meaning nearly 24 hours. The term *phase advance* refers to a behavioral or hormonal rhythm with an appearance earlier than its normal circadian pattern. The phase-advance theory of manic-depressive illness hypothesizes a pathological phase-advanced free-running rhythm, which is based on internal (e.g., body temperature rhythm versus sleep-wake cycle) and external (e.g., body temperature rhythm versus light-dark cycle) desynchronization of physiological functions. The phase-advance theory was evaluated by Kripke (1983), who proposed that depression may be the result of an internal desynchronization of circadian oscillators, with the strong oscillator being phase advanced in relation to a weak oscillator. The internal rhythm also could be phase delayed, as has been proposed in seasonal affective disorder (SAD) or "winter depression" (Lewy et al. 1987; Sack and Lewy 1988).

Temporal external desynchronization, such as in jet lag, can occur in some individuals during flights over time zones. Rapid time-zone changes may even precipitate mood disorders in predisposed persons, as Jauhar and Weller (1982) showed in a study at Heathrow Airport in London. Recently, Healy (1987) has convincingly argued for a "circadian rhythm dysfunction in affective disorders" linking "rhythm and blues." It is obvious that as a rhythm-regulating factor and a marker for rhythm disturbances, melatonin offers a valuable tool in research on mood disorders.

Diurnal Rhythm Disturbances and Depression

A disturbed diurnal rhythm, which could include sleep and appetite disturbances, early morning awakening, difficulty in concentration, and body temperature variations, is a common symptom in depression. Sleep deprivation is a nonpharmacological treatment mode for depression that has been investigated during recent decades. Complete 40-hour sleep deprivation (Roy-Byrne et al. 1984), partial sleep deprivation (Schilgen and Tolle 1980), and rapid eye movement (REM) (Vogel et al. 1980) have shown significant improvement in the symptoms of depression on a short-term basis. Sleep deprivation, however, has not been compared to placebo. Also, there have been difficulties in assessing whether the sleep deprivation effect is truly antidepressant or merely symptomatic. Hypothetically, the sleep deprivation effect operates by a chronobiological mechanism irrespective of whether the effect is antidepressant or symptomatic. This hypothesis is supported by the observations of changes in body temperature rhythm during this treatment (Pflug et al. 1981).

Acute exposure to light at night reduces the nocturnal decline of core body temperature and inhibits the secretion of the pineal hormone melatonin. Results show that the elevation of core body temperature induced by nocturnal exposure to bright light can be reversed completely by circumventing the decline of serum melatonin levels with concurrent oral administration of melatonin. Because melatonin acts as a mediator of the effect of light on core body temperature, there is a rationale for the use of oral melatonin as an aid in the reentrainment of the body temperature in desynchronized conditions (Cagnacci et al. 1993).

Melatonin, Seasonal Variations, and Depression

Seasonal variations in the incidence of depression and suicide in mood disorders are well documented (Eastwood and Peacocke 1976; Eastwood and Stiasny 1978; Rosenthal et al. 1983). Circannual rhythms in pineal function in animals have been reported over the last two decades (Griffiths et al. 1979; Illnerová and Vanecek 1980). Seasonal variation in pineal gland weights in human autopsy material has been described (Wetterberg 1978). Seasonal variations in melatonin production measured in 24-hour serum levels and in urine have been shown at least on some latitudes (Arendt et al. 1977; Wetterberg et al. 1981; Wirz-Justice and Arendt 1979). Based on these reports, it is probable that some forms of depression could be biochemically linked to a disturbance in melatonin production, secretion, or function. The close relationship between the pituitary, adrenal, thyroid, and gonadal systems and the pineal gland, and especially melatonin, may be reflected in corresponding neuropsychoendocrine dysfunctions of clinical importance. Serum and plasma melatonin determinations may thus be of interest in different disease states and diagnostic subgroups.

Factors Influencing Melatonin Production

It is clear that factors other than psychiatric diagnoses are of importance for melatonin levels. It has been reported that bright light (Lewy et al. 1980; Wetterberg 1978), age (Attanasio et al. 1985; Iguchi et al. 1982; Nair et al. 1986; Sharma et al. 1989; Thomas and Miles 1989; Waldhauser and Waldhauser 1988; Wetterberg 1979), body weight (Arendt et al. 1982; Ferrier et al. 1982), body height (Beck-Friis et al. 1984), use of glasses (Erikson et al. 1983), use of drugs (e.g., β-adrenergic receptor blocking agents [Beck-Friis et al. 1983; Hanssen et al. 1977; Moore et al. 1979], chlorpromazine [Smith et al. 1979], antidepressant drugs [for review, see Checkley and Palazidou 1988]), and genetic variation (Wetterberg et al. 1983) are among factors that to different degrees and under various circumstances may influence melatonin levels in humans.

In addition, melatonin antiserum may react with plasticizers, such as dimethyl phthalate, which may be part of various plastic materials and an ingredient of insect-repellent formulations (Wetterberg et al. 1984). When sampling tissues, it is important to avoid plasticizers in the collection tubes and pipettes. Furthermore, the plasticizers may interfere with melatonin function and affect various mechanisms that depend on intact melatonin receptors, as has been recently discussed in relation to environmental hazards of different plastic material (Ema et al. 1997).

Among these factors, age has been consistently connected with a concomitant reduction of melatonin levels. The influence of various drugs on melatonin metabolism is obvious, as well as the influence of possible differences in the assay methods used (see Reiter, Chapter 1, in this volume). In the evaluation of melatonin levels, after all of the previously mentioned factors are considered, there is support for a correlation between some subtypes of depression and melatonin concentrations.

Melatonin in Mood Disorders

Several studies involving extensive neuroendocrine testing (e.g., of melatonin and cortisol secretion) have been reported over the past decades. Views on using melatonin as a tool in diagnosing mental disorders were reviewed by Miles and Thomas (1988). Other recent overviews concerning melatonin and its physiological functions are found in three monographs by Yu and Reiter (1993), Wetterberg (1993), and Arendt (1995).

Specific findings relating serum melatonin to clinical variables in patients with mood disorders have been reported by Wetterberg et al. (1981), Beck-Friis (1983), and Beck-Friis et al. (1984, 1985a, 1985b). The conclusions in these studies are based on the examination of 87 individuals, including acutely ill patients with major depression according to the Research Diagnostic Criteria (RDC) of Spitzer et al. (1978), patients in clinical remission, and healthy control subjects. Brown et al. (1987), using the Hamilton factor scores (Rhoades and Overall 1983), reported correlation among clinical symptoms of depressed mood ($r = .43$, $P < .04$), reality disturbance ($r = .41$, $P < .04$), and a decrease of nocturnal serum melatonin, and a trend for correlation between sleep disturbance and melatonin ($r = .33$, $P < .09$), but no correlation for symptom clusters of somatization, diurnal variation, agitation/anxiety, weight loss, or cognitive or vegetative factors. The symptom clusters of depressed mood also included motor retardation, inability to work, suicide, indications of reality disturbance, guilt feelings, depersonalization, and paranoid symptoms such as suspiciousness, referential thinking, and delusions. In summary, nighttime melatonin levels may vary in different groups of depressed patients. Several studies have, however, found samples of patients with low nighttime levels of melatonin.

The Low-Melatonin Syndrome

The clinical finding of a subgroup of depressed patients with "low-melatonin syndrome" was introduced in 1983 by Beck-Friis, one of the investigators on our research team. Our study included 32 acutely depressed inpatients diagnosed with major depressive illness according to RDC and 33 healthy control subjects. Seventeen of the depressed patients had early escape of DST (serum cortisol not suppressed by dexamethasone) and 15 had normal DST. Twenty-six of these patients were restudied 1 month to 1 year later while in a state of partial or complete remission. Clinical ratings were made with the Comprehensive Psychopathological Rating Scale (CPRS; Åsberg et al. 1978).

We found that the depressed patients with early DST escape had significantly lower melatonin levels compared with depressed patients with a normal DST and the healthy control group. The patients' use of drugs in the study did not influence the statistical outcome (Beck-Friis et al. 1984). After adjustment for relevant influencing factors, the results of our study (Beck-Friis et al. 1984, 1985a) showed no statistical difference in nocturnal maximum serum melatonin levels (MT max) between the depressed patients (0.25 ± 0.03 nmol/L, mean $\pm$ SE) and the healthy control subjects (0.30 ± 0.03 nmol/L). However, when the depressed patients were divided into those with an abnormal response to the DST (DST+) and those with a normal response (DST−), a statistical difference was found. MT max in the DST+ depressed patients ($n = 17$) *was* 0.19 ± 0.03 nmol/L and in the DST− group ($n = 15$) was 0.30 ± 0.03 nmol/L. The statistical analysis of the hypothesis of equal MT max among the DST+, DST−, and control groups showed a significant difference in MT max among the groups ($P = .004$).

Furthermore, a significant negative regression ($P = .04$) was found in the DST+ group between the MT max level and the serum cortisol level at 8 A.M. after oral dexamethasone administration in those patients who did not suppress the cortisol below 200 nmol/L at 8 A.M. ($n = 8$). Their MT max level was 0.17 ± 0.05 nmol/L, compared with 0.20 ± 0.02 nmol/L in those patients in the DST+ group who did suppress cortisol below 200 nmol/L at 8 A.M. but not at 4 P.M. or 10 P.M. ($n = 9$).

When the depressed patients ($n = 26$) were restudied in clinical remission, the MT max levels did not change significantly (0.24 ± 0.03 nmol/L in relapse; 0.23 ± 0.04 nmol/L in remission, NS). The same was true for the DST+ and DST− groups. In the DST+ group, the cortisol levels and response in the DST normalized. This difference in melatonin and cortisol levels between relapse and remission led us to test the possibility of melatonin as a trait marker for certain types of depression. Therefore, we further studied the clinical features of these patients (Beck-Friis et al. 1985b).

Patients with no reported diurnal variation of depressive symptoms ($n = 7$) had significantly lower MT max levels (0.15 ± 0.05 nmol/L) than patients with reported diurnal variation ($n = 25$; 0.26 ± 0.03 nmol/L, $P = .047$). Patients with several (more than three) registered depressive periods in the summer (June, July, and August) ($n = 12$) had significantly lower mean MT max levels (0.17 ± 0.04 nmol/L) than patients with three or less corresponding periods ($n = 20$). When the number of months with registered depressions was divided by the number of registered depressive episodes, patients in the DST+ group had a significantly higher quotient (7.4 ± 1.0 nmol/L) than patients in the DST− group (4.1 ± 0.2 nmol/L; $P = .01$), indicating that patients with abnormal DST have longer depressive episodes. A trend toward higher number of patients with more than three registered depressive periods during the summer was found in the DST+ group compared with the DST− group ($P = .08$). Eight of 12 (67%) of the patients in the DST− group but only 3 of 16 (19%) of the patients in the DST+ group reported an increase of depressive symptoms during the spring ($P = .02$). Patients in the DST+ group seemed to have their depressive episodes more equally distributed during the year, in contrast to the patients in the DST− group, who tended to have their depressive episodes more frequently in spring and autumn (Beck-Friis et al. 1985b).

It was suggested that the following features constitute a low-melatonin syndrome: low nocturnal melatonin levels, an abnormal DST, a disturbed 24-hour rhythm of cortisol, and as the main clinical feature, a less pronounced daily and annual cyclic variation in depressive symptomatology. Clinically, this means that the depression is more or less unlinked to the influence of external temporal cues. In this study, there was a correlation between low nocturnal melatonin levels and the symptoms of lassitude, sadness, and inability to feel, as reported on the CPRS (Åsberg et al. 1978) clinical rating. Also, there was a correlation between low melatonin levels and cluster of conative and emotional retardation symptoms. Findings by Brown et al. (1987) also support the correlation between low melatonin levels and depressed mood and/or retardation symptoms. The different studies on depression and low melatonin previously have been reviewed in detail by Wetterberg et al. (1990).

In summary, all but three studies have not shown low melatonin in depressed patients. These three were by Jimerson et al. (1977), Stewart and Halbriech (1989), and Thompson et al. (1988). Jimerson et al. (1977) used a bioassay, which has not been used in other studies. The patients were diagnosed as moderately to severely depressed, but no clinical ratings were shown. No difference was observed in the nocturnal melatonin rhythm between patients and control subjects during one or two baseline days, a sleep-deprivation day, and a recovery day. Although Thompson et al. (1990) claimed in their study the strength of matched control subjects, the number of patients in the study ($n = 9$; 5 females) and the matching of age, body height, and weight between patients and control subjects do not seem sufficient, especially when testing patients according to their DST status. Furthermore, the selection and diagnoses of patients in this study seem mixed. Six patients were drug free for at least 1 year and three were chronically depressed patients, who had been drug free for at least 6 weeks, admitted for assessment for prefrontal lobotomy. Thus, the selection of the patients in this study differs from the selection of the patients in the Stockholm study (Beck-Friis 1983; Wetterberg et al. 1981). Patients with various mixtures of depression were included in the study by Stewart and Halbreich (1989). The authors mention that the high levels of daytime melatonin suggest a nonspecificity of the assay. In my opinion, these three studies do not convincingly refute the association between low melatonin and some types of depressive disorders.

The relation between low melatonin levels and disturbances in the HPA axis has been supported in many studies, but not all, and therefore needs further evaluation. Steiner and Brown (1985) and Brown et al. (1985) found melatonin levels to be decreased in depressed patients but found no association between low melatonin levels and suppression in the DST. Boyce (1985) found no clear association between melatonin secretion and the HPA axis. Lang and Sizonenko (1988) recently reviewed the literature on reported possible interactions between adrenal and pineal functions in mammals and found that no definite conclusions on this issue can be made as yet, but they suggested a possible age-dependent relationship. Demisch et al. (1988) suggested, in a study of dexamethasone administration in healthy subjects, that dexamethasone affects nocturnal production of melatonin by means of mechanisms within the pineal gland. Kennedy et al. (1989) reported on melatonin and cortisol levels in 33 female subjects of comparable age with eating disorders. They found significantly higher nocturnal levels of plasma cortisol in the patients compared with the control subjects; however, when patients were divided according to depression status, those with concurrent major depression had significantly lower nocturnal melatonin values than the nondepressed groups. The depressed patients in this study also had a significantly lower ratio of melatonin to cortisol.

When looking at the relationship between low-melatonin syndrome and the diagnosis of melancholia in DSM-III-R (American Psychiatric Association 1987), the rigidity of the diagnostic criteria should be taken into consideration. Rigidity of the criteria may explain the lack of a correlation between low melatonin and melancholia in some studies. In DSM-III-R, the diagnosis of major depressive disorder with melancholic features is made by inclusion criteria, such as early morning awakening and symptoms worse in the morning. However, Rafaelsen and Mellerup (1979) showed that the diurnal symptom variation disappeared during the most severe states of melancholia but reappeared when the patients had started responding to treatment. Thus, the diurnal rhythm disturbances in melancholia are dynamic and not static.

Furthermore, in one Swedish study (von Knorring et al. 1977), early awakening and increased dysphoric mood in the early morning were not specific for "depressive syndrome" but were typically also seen in other diagnostic groups (e.g., anxiety disorders and neurotic depressions). Rhythmic variations of melancholic symptoms therefore seem to relate more closely to health than to the most severe state of melancholia.

In a chronobiological sense, health can be defined as the individual's maintained ability to make rhythms well functioning (i.e., to adapt external and internal biological rhythms). Melatonin and a normal pineal function seem to be involved in this adaptation. In depressed patients, low melatonin levels therefore hypothetically may impair this adaptation with a subsequent locked rhythmic capacity manifested in persistence of dysphoric mood and prolonged depressive episodes. The finding in our study that patients with low-melatonin syndrome could have longer depressive periods than patients with higher melatonin levels also may indicate that the low-melatonin patient group receives inadequate therapy.

Melatonin levels could serve as a marker for noradrenergic tone in the brain. If low melatonin concentrations reflect a deficiency of noradrenaline at receptor sites, the possibility that the low-melatonin syndrome might respond to noradrenergic antidepressive pharmacotherapy should be tested. A dysfunction in the serotonergic system also theoretically could lead to a low-melatonin syndrome. The diagnostic categories in DSM-IV (American Psychiatric Association 1994), with specifiers for melancholic features, atypical features, and seasonal pattern, allow for symptomatic classifications of major depressive disorders and will be helpful in further diagnostics using several biological markers, one of which is melatonin.

On the functional level, low-melatonin syndrome in depression may be interpreted as a loss of rhythm amplitude, which could be a sign of dysfunction between the pineal gland and the SCN in the hypothalamus (Klein et al. 1991).

The low nocturnal melatonin levels in these depressed patients are likely genetically determined (Wetterberg et al. 1983). The early findings by Reppert et al. (1988) of melatonin receptors in the "biological clock" (i.e., nuclei suprachiasmatic) are in line with such a hypothesis. A new frontier in the knowledge about melatonin recently opened when the Reppert group reported on two specific types of melatonin receptors, cloned and located to specific areas on the human genome. Melatonin$_{1a}$ receptors are mapped to chromosome 4q35.1 and may be involved in genetically based circadian and neuroendocrine disorders (Slaugenhaupt et al. 1995). Melatonin$_{1b}$ receptors, which were localized to chromosome 11q21-22 (Reppert et al. 1995), may mediate action of melatonin on the retinal level and participate in some of the atypical mood disorders responding to light treatment.

The genetically predisposed pineal rhythm function and the melatonin levels may be influenced by environmental factors in critical periods of life (e.g., impaired parent-child relationship, early psychic traumas, or other stressful factors in the first few years of life) when the fundamentals of self-esteem and self-respect are laid down. Psychological injuries and traumas during such critical periods could hypothetically influence the ground for self-esteem, according to the concepts of the narcissistic development formulated by Kohut (1971) and Kernberg (1975), and the soma (e.g., the endocrine system). Such a hypothesis is supported by the findings of Yuwiler (1985), who reported that steroid treatment in newborn rats reduces the normal catecholamine-induced increase in pineal NAT activity, indicating that stress in the neonatal period can alter pineal function. These animal studies support some of the psychoanalytic theories about the relationship between stress exposure and psychic trauma in early childhood and adult psychopathology. Breier et al. (1988) recently reported a significant correlation between early parental loss, development of adult psychopathology, and endocrine changes in the HPA axis with elevated levels of cortisol and adrenocorticotropic hormone

(ACTH). In the study by Beck-Friis et al. (1985b), depressed adult patients but not healthy subjects who lost one parent, whether by death or divorce, before age 17 years had very low levels of nocturnal melatonin and differed from patients with no reported parental loss. If this holds true, in Western societies, many individuals who live in a single-parent household may be at risk for melatonin deficiency and the potential health risks that it entails.

The question arises whether low melatonin is a state or trait marker for depression (Miles and Thomas 1988; Sack and Lewy 1988). Relating melatonin and pineal function to the "rhythm-generating system" low melatonin in depressive states, as expressed in the low-melatonin syndrome, can be seen as a trait marker for the clinical time course of the depressive state. However, in other subtypes of mood disorders not related to melatonin (e.g., in patients with bipolar disorders and, hypothetically, especially in "rapid cyclers" [DSM-IV], or patients with rapid and sudden mood swings), changes in the melatonin secretion amplitude also may be state dependent.

Melatonin Decreases by Age

Age and melatonin have been addressed separately in a comparative study among healthy control subjects and two groups of patients, one with depression and one with alcoholism (Wetterberg et al. 1992). Two healthy control populations, separated by 8,000 miles and 24 degrees of latitude, had similar mean values for overnight urinary melatonin concentrations. These values were significantly higher than 6-month values for depressed subjects and abstinent alcoholic subjects, whereas means for the two clinical populations were similar. Age and urinary melatonin concentrations in the control and clinical populations were inversely related, but the slopes of the linear regression equations were 10 times steeper for the control groups than for the clinical populations. Differences in age and sex distribution accounted for some of the differences, although control subjects differed from the clinical populations, even after sex and age were factored out. The disparate slopes for age and melatonin concentrations may contribute to some of the conflicting findings of studies comparing populations of different ages. The total melatonin content in the samples from alcoholic subjects, but not the depressed subjects, was lower than that for control subjects. The difference in melatonin concentration between control subjects and patients was not accounted for by difference in duration of urinary collection period, hours of sleep, or body weight.

Melatonin, Cortisol, and Monoamine Oxidase in Platelets as Markers for Depression: A Multidimensional Analysis

New diagnostic trends emphasize the importance of reliable biological markers to differentiate subtypes of depressive disorders. This differentiation will enable clinicians to choose the appropriate therapy for the individual patient and/or to better predict the patient's response to different biological therapies, such as pharmacotherapy, light therapy, or electroconvulsive therapy.

Multidimensional analysis of several biological factors may reveal hidden subgroups, as has been demonstrated recently in a study examining monoamine oxidase (MAO) and cortisol together with melatonin in depressed patients (Wahlund et al. 1995). In the follow-up study, a total of 28 acutely ill inpatients fulfilling RDC for major affective disorder were investigated and compared with 20 apparently healthy subjects. The patients were followed for 10 years and the diagnoses evaluated according to the *International Classification of Diseases,* Ninth Revision, Clinical Modification (ICD-9-CM; World Health Organization 1980). ICD-9-CM 296 includes 296B, 296D, 296E, and 296X (i.e., unipolar affective psychosis; bipolar affective psychosis with melancholia; bipolar affective psychosis, mixed form; and nonspecific affective psychosis, respectively). ICD-9-CM 300 represents 300E (i.e., neurotic depression). Platelet MAO activity was assayed, as well as serum melatonin and cortisol, at the beginning of the study. DST also was performed, with the oral administration of 1 mg dexamethasone at 10 P.M. Serum samples were drawn at 8 A.M., 4 P.M., and 10 P.M. the following day. Maximum post-DST cortisol levels (Cpdx) were used for calculation. Discrimination of subgroups of depressed patients and separation of control subjects from patients were evaluated using biochemical variables with exploratory data analysis, principal component analysis (PCA), and discriminant analysis.

The multivariate data analysis was performed in several steps. The total sample was analyzed across the three dimensions (3-D) by means of rotating the three standardized and scaled biochemical variables in a 3-D computer program. The data set consisted of two main nonspherical clusters. To visualize the 3-D findings, PCA and multidimensional scaling (MDS) were performed. PCA was performed on melatonin, platelet MAO activity, and Cpdx, and the first two standardized principal components captured 83% of total variance.

The results showed the Cpdx was a powerful discriminator between patients with affective psychosis and patients with neurotic depression. Using all three variables (i.e., platelet MAO activity, peak nocturnal melatonin, and Cpdx), it was possible to separate ICD-9-CM categories 296 and 300 with a higher accuracy of 90% sensitivity and 89% specificity. Thus, the two clinical subgroups of depressed patients compared with control subjects showed diverse patterns in the three variables, indicating a biological difference between the clinical groups. Melatonin may thus be combined with other biological markers to improve the diagnostic power of different clinical subgroups. The use of melatonin in combination with such markers may prove useful in predicting prognosis, as well as in choosing the right treatment for the individual patient with different subtypes of major depression.

Melatonin and Light Treatment

Although its mechanism of action remains to be explained, light therapy appears to be a safe and useful treatment for patients with depression (Avery et al. 1990; James et al. 1985; Kjellman et al.

1993; Kripke et al. 1992; Lewy et al. 1982; Rosenthal et al. 1984; Sack et al. 1990; Terman et al. 1989; Thalén et al. 1995a, 1995b, 1995c; Wirz-Justice et al. 1993).

We recently have reported that patients with a nonseasonal pattern of depression have less efficient treatment outcome compared with patients with a seasonal pattern of depression (Kjellman et al. 1993; Thalén et al. 1995a, 1995b, 1995c). Ninety patients with a major depressive disorder were classified according to seasonal or nonseasonal pattern. They were clinically evaluated before and after light treatment in the morning or in the evening. The results of this study suggest a specific nonplacebo effect of light treatment in patients with a seasonal pattern of depression. In our current study, we have been using matched groups of patients with seasonal or nonseasonal depression receiving light treatment either in the morning or in the evening.

The amplitude and the circadian phase hypotheses of light treatment in depression were tested using melatonin as a marker of circadian rhythm. According to the amplitude hypothesis, the amount of melatonin produced will increase with light treatment due to an increase in β-adrenergic receptor activity. We also tested the two main hypotheses about the relationship between timing of light and therapeutic outcome to elucidate which one was the most compatible with our results. Some researchers maintain that timing of light is not critical (James et al. 1985), whereas others have reported that bright light is more effective in the treatment of depression when light is administered in the morning (Lewy et al. 1985, 1987). Lewy et al. (1987) considered that most patients with seasonal depression have a phase delay of their biological rhythms, mainly revealed by the delayed sleep-wake cycle and verified by the dim-light melatonin onset.

The phase position of the nightly serum melatonin profile was established before light treatment in depressed patients. The timing of the treatment was given without previous knowledge about the internal circadian phase position in the individual patient. If the phase-shift hypothesis of depression is correct, patients with a phase-delayed sleep-wake cycle and delayed internal rhythms manifested by a delayed melatonin phase position should accordingly benefit from morning light and not by light treatment in the evening. Patients with a phase-advanced sleep-wake cycle and advanced internal rhythms manifested by an advanced melatonin phase should, according to the same hypothesis, benefit from evening light and not by light treatment in the morning.

To explore the theory of melatonin as an internal amplitude and rhythm marker, we studied patients with either seasonal or non-seasonal patterns of depression and addressed the following questions:

1. Is there a difference in melatonin amplitude and phase position between patients with seasonal and nonseasonal patterns of depression a) before and after light treatment and b) when treatment is given in the morning or in the evening?
2. Will the melatonin phase position predict a preferential treatment response to morning or evening light?
3. Is a low circadian amplitude of melatonin related to less favorable therapeutic response?
4. Is the degree of suppression and the rebound of serum melatonin by light exposure at night (10–11 P.M.) correlated to the therapeutic outcome of light treatment?

The study included 63 patients (51 females and 12 males) with a major depressive episode (Thalén et al. 1995b). The mean age was 50 ± 2 (SE) years for females (range, 31–70 years) and 50 ± 3 years for males (range, 36–68 years). The study was performed from the autumn of 1988 to the spring of 1992 in Stockholm, Sweden, at latitude 590 N. The patients were referred by physicians or consulted the light treatment unit directly. All depressed patients were diagnosed as having a major depressive episode according to DSM-III-R.

From an original sample of 127 patients (99 with a seasonal pattern and 28 with a nonseasonal pattern of depression), two subgroups were selected and matched as follows: For each non-seasonal patient who had completed the study, two seasonal patients were matched with respect to time of light treatment, degree of depression rated as total scores of the Hamilton Depression Rating Scale (HDRS; Hamilton 1967), and age. The matched group consisted of 42 patients with a seasonal pattern of depression and 21 patients with a nonseasonal pattern of depression. The mean age of patients with a seasonal and a nonseasonal pattern was similar: for seasonal, 50 years, and for nonseasonal, 51 years. Of the patients with a seasonal pattern, 33 were unipolar, 1 bipolar I, and 8 bipolar II. The corresponding figures for patients with a nonseasonal pattern were 17, 3, and 1, respectively. Among patients treated in the morning, 32 were unipolar, 1 bipolar I, and 6 bipolar II. The corresponding figures for evening treatment were 18, 3, and 3, respectively. The assignment to treatment in the morning ($n = 39$) or in the evening ($n = 24$) was based on global clinical assessment of the sleep-wake cycle in the recent medical history. Patients who went to bed early and/or had an early awakening were selected for evening light treatment, and the remaining patients received light treatment in the morning. Patients with abuse of alcohol or drugs, severe psychiatric disease such as schizophrenia and dementia, and serious somatic disease were excluded.

Melatonin Measured Before and After Light Treatment

The study was designed as follows: On day 1, a diagnostic interview according to DSM-III-R took place. During the night at the following nine time points, 8 P.M., 10 P.M., 10:30 P.M., 11 P.M., midnight, 2 A.M., 4 A.M., 6 A.M., and 8 A.M., blood samples were drawn from an indwelling catheter for assaying serum melatonin concentration before light treatment (basal melatonin levels before treatment = B1). The set of repeated measurement of serum melatonin levels during one night from 8 P.M. to 8 A.M. is called the hormone profile. The patients slept in darkness between 11 P.M. and 6 A.M. Two days later, clinical ratings were performed by two physicians independently, using the first 17 items with diurnal variation added to the HDRS (Hamilton 1967). In the night before treatment, a light test was performed. The patients were exposed to bright light for 1 hour between 10 P.M. and 11 P.M. (referred to as light test 1 = T1), and blood samples were drawn for melatonin at the same time points as on day 1. After 10 days of light treatment, the same protocol was applied as before light treatment, measuring serum melatonin during one night (day 15). The results of the melatonin measures after treatment are referred to as basal levels 2 (B2). After 10 days of light treatment, the clinical ratings with HDRS (Hamilton 1967) were repeated by two physicians independently.

Melatonin as a Marker of Circadian Phase Position in Relation to Light

Light Treatment and Light Test

The light treatment was applied in a light treatment room with white ceiling, walls, and floor. The reflection from 24 fluorescent tubes in the ceiling gave indirect light with a luminance of 350 candela/m^2, giving an approximate illuminance of 1,500 lux 0.8 m above the floor. The patients were clad in white clothes to minimize light absorption and to give maximal reflection.

The light source was full-spectrum light with one of two different light temperatures, 4,000 kelvin (kelvin A, $n = 13$) and 6,500 kelvin (kelvin B, $n = 50$), with no significant subgroup differences in assignment. The time of light treatment was either 6–8 A.M. (morning light) or 6–8 P.M. (evening light) for 10 consecutive days. A light test to measure degree of suppression of serum melatonin concentration and a possible rebound of serum melatonin was performed with bright light between 10 P.M. and 11 P.M., using the light tubes of 6,500 kelvin with a luminance of 350 candela/m^2 as the light source. The light test was performed with the same light source as during the light treatment.

Laboratory Measurements and Statistical Methods

The serum samples were analyzed for melatonin by the radioimmunoassay (RIA) method of Wetterberg et al. (1978). The lower limit of detection was 0.01 nmol/L. The intra-assay coefficient of variation (CV) for samples 0.1–0.15 nmol/L was 12.3%, > 0.15 nmol/L 7.4%, and < 0.10 nmol/L 28% ($n = 100$). The interassay CV for serum melatonin levels > 0.15 nmol/L was 4.8% ($n = 60$).

For each individual, the area under the profile time curve (AUC) for melatonin was calculated by means of the trapezoidal rule. AUC is an index of melatonin production and, because the time points are not equidistant, AUC is a more consistent estimate of the average hormone level than the arithmetic mean value. AUC was highly correlated to the maximum nightly value of the melatonin profile (before treatment, $r = 0.95$, $P < .001$; after treatment, $r = 0.96$, $P < .001$).

As an estimate of the "mean appearance time," the first-order time moment ("time center of gravity" = TC) of the profile time curve was calculated, also using a trapezoidal rule (linear interpolation between time points). TC appeared to be a variable independent of AUC (before treatment, $r = -0.003$, $P = 0.98$; changes after treatment, $r = 0.017$, $P = 0.17$).

Serum Melatonin Amplitude and Phase Position: 10 P.M. to 8 A.M.

For the whole group of 63 patients, light treatment given either in the morning or in the evening decreased melatonin significantly ($P < .01$). When corrections for age and height were made, there was no significant difference in serum melatonin (AUC) between patients with seasonal and nonseasonal patterns of depression treated with morning light either before (AUC B1) or after (AUC B2) light treatment.

Melatonin phase position (TC) before light treatment was not significantly related to month of treatment, diagnosis, or time of light treatment, and there were no factor interactions. After 10 days of light treatment, patients treated with morning light significantly advanced their phase and patients treated with evening light significantly delayed their phase ($P < .001$). Patients treated with light in the morning had significantly later TC than patients treated with evening light.

Suppression of Melatonin by Bright Light: 10 P.M. to 11 P.M.

Melatonin Suppression During the Light Test

The degree of AUC reduction of melatonin, due to the light test in the time interval 10 P.M.–11 P.M., was significantly positively related to the AUC value before the test ($P < .001$). Both in the time intervals 10 P.M.–11 P.M. and 10 P.M.–4 A.M., the melatonin AUC showed a significantly greater reduction in patients selected for evening treatment compared with patients receiving morning treatment ($P < .005$ and $P < .02$, respectively).

Melatonin and Therapeutic Outcome

Absolute changes in HDRS (Hamilton 1967) were not significantly correlated to B1 levels of melatonin (TC and AUC) or changes (B2 to B1) of melatonin (TC and AUC) as a result of light treatment. The subgroup defined by the highest and lowest quartile of melatonin AUC did not differ with respect to absolute changes in HDRS.

The factors expected to influence the melatonin phase position (TC) due to light treatment are its value before treatment (phase advance or phase delay) and time of light treatment (morning or evening). A line halfway between the two regression lines crosses the TC axis at 6.13 hours, which means that half of the melatonin production was reached. This point at 2:13 A.M. constitutes an operational break point discriminating between phase advance and phase delay before light treatment. Twenty-one patients had a phase advance and 42 patients a phase delay. Of the 21 patients with a phase advance, 8 were treated with morning light and 13 with evening light. The corresponding numbers for 42 patients with a phase delay were 31 treated with morning light and 11 treated with evening light. Patients with a seasonal pattern of depression improved significantly more than patients with a non-seasonal pattern when the four groups (advance morning, delay morning, advance evening, delay evening) were related to treatment efficacy (HDRS [Hamilton 1967] $P < .01$). There was no significant dependence on the factor phase advance/delay or any significant interaction between the two factors with respect to therapeutic outcome. No correlation was found between changes in AUC or the rebound effect of serum melatonin levels and therapeutic outcome.

Outcome of 10 Days of Light Treatment: Clinical Ratings

After 10 days of light treatment, the patients with a seasonal pattern of depression improved significantly more than patients with a nonseasonal pattern (HDRS [Hamilton 1967] relative changes $P < .001$). The mean relative improvement in HDRS was more than 50% in the 42 patients with a seasonal pattern and less than 21% in the 21 patients with a nonseasonal pattern. There was no significant diagnosis and time of light treatment interaction or any significant differences in improvement between patients with or without antidepressant medication or patients treated in the morning or in the evening.

Serum melatonin production expressed as AUC was significantly negatively correlated to age (−0.039 [pmol/L] × [hours/year]; $P < .02$). The patients selected for morning light treatment were significantly younger than those selected for evening light treatment (morning, 46 ± 2 years; evening, 55 ± 2 years; $P < .002$). The age of the patients was not significantly correlated to the absolute or relative clinical improvement according to the clinical ratings in HDRS (Hamilton 1967). An analysis of regression between the variables age and melatonin AUC showed no significant differences between patients with a seasonal and nonseasonal pattern of depression.

The seasonal patients reported carbohydrate craving significantly more often than nonseasonal patients (22 of 37 versus 4 of 16; $P < .05$). Melatonin AUC was higher in patients with a carbohydrate craving both before and after treatment due to higher serum melatonin in the nonseasonal patients compared with seasonal patients.

Patients with a nonseasonal pattern of depression had more often been hospitalized than patients with a seasonal pattern (12 of 17 versus 11 of 40; $P < .01$). There were no significant differences between seasonal and nonseasonal patients with respect to reported earlier treatment of depression, sick leave, psychotherapy, appetite, hospitalized patients versus patients on leave, weight changes, consulting a physician, medication on admission, or changes in appetite.

The proportion of uni-/bipolarity was not significantly different between patients with a seasonal or nonseasonal pattern of depression or between patients treated with morning or evening light. There were no significant differences in the phase (TC) or amount of melatonin (AUC) between patients with a unipolar, bipolar I, or bipolar II disorder and no differences in serum melatonin as a result of the light test. However, all four patients with a bipolar I diagnosis showed a reduction of their serum melatonin.

There are some specific questions that could be answered about possible differential effects of light on serum melatonin between depressed patients with and without a seasonal pattern. There is no difference in melatonin amplitude between patients with a seasonal and nonseasonal pattern of depression, either before or after light treatment or when treatment was given, in the morning or in the evening. The melatonin phase position did not predict a preferential treatment response to morning or evening light. A low circadian amplitude of melatonin did not correlate to a less favorable therapeutic response. The degree of light suppression or rebound of serum melatonin in relation to light exposure at night from 10 P.M. to 11 P.M. was not significantly related to the therapeutic outcome of light treatment.

General Effects of Light Treatment on Melatonin: Hypothetical Explanations

There are, however, some interesting results related to the questions about the general effects of bright light on serum melatonin amplitude and phase position. The amplitude hypothesis formulated as an increase in the β-adrenergic receptor activity at the pinealocytes would result in an increase in melatonin formation. In the whole group of depressed patients, light treatment instead caused a significantly lowered secretion of melatonin.

Salinas et al. (1992) also found that bright light of 3,000 lux lowered melatonin, but dim light of 300 lux gave a rebound of melatonin. Our finding of lowered melatonin following light treatment supports the argument against the amplitude hypothesis, which states that an increase in melatonin following light treatment should indicate an increase in receptor sensitivity related to the melatonin rhythm-generating system. Because we now find an overall significant decrease in melatonin AUC, even in patients with clinical improvement in their depressive symptoms, this finding may lead us to test the further hypothesis that light treatment has similar effects on central neurotransmitter activities as the serotonin-specific reuptake inhibitor fluoxetine, which also decreases melatonin (Childs et al. 1995) levels, in contrast to fluvoxamine and tricyclic antidepressants (Skene et al. 1994).

Light is likely to act via the retinal-hypothalamic-pineal pathway and lower melatonin levels by effects on the pinealocytes. Continuing the reasoning that the therapeutic effect of light is similar to fluoxetine, light might decrease β-adrenergic function. Fluoxetine alone did not produce β-adrenergic receptor down-regulation but significantly reduced cAMP accumulation after 2 weeks of treatment (Baron et al. 1988). Melatonin also might be lowered by stimulation of an α_2-adrenergic receptor agonist (Palazidou et al. 1989).

Furthermore, light treatment may change receptor sensitivity at the hypothalamic level. There is some evidence of dysregulation in serotonergic neurotransmission in seasonally depressed patients that normalizes following light treatment (Jacobsen et al. 1994). The SCN mediates the reduction in melatonin followed by acute exposure to light at night, which may be modulated by serotonergic receptor activity (Thompson et al. 1990). It is possible that light treatment down-regulates the SCN output and, as a consequence, the production of melatonin. The findings of similarities between light treatment and the effects of fluoxetine but not of other serotonin-specific reuptake inhibitors may be a useful discovery in the further elucidation of the antidepressant effects of light treatment.

The effects of light on melatonin have been studied by Terman et al. (1988) and Lewy et al. (1985), with both groups reporting phase-advancing effects of morning light in patients with seasonal depression. Lewy et al. (1985, 1987) reported that the changes of melatonin phase were of therapeutic importance, noting that a phase advancement of the melatonin rise in the evening after treatment has a better clinical effect.

Lemmer et al. (1994) showed a significant phase advance in the circadian rhythm of melatonin when bright light was given to young healthy individuals in the morning but not when given in the evening. The two oscillators hypothesis indicates a different regulatory mechanism for melatonin onset in the evening and for melatonin offset in the morning. It appears that in both animals and humans, the evening melatonin production onset does not necessarily phase-shift in parallel with the morning offset (Ill-nerová et al. 1993). If the finding of Lemmer et al. (1994) is correct, that healthy individuals do not shift their melatonin phase when light is given in the evening or in the morning, this would indicate a disturbance or instability of the evening melatonin onset oscillator in depression. Rao et al. (1992), on the other hand, found no significant effects of morning light treatment on melatonin rhythms in patients with a nonseasonal pattern of depression. Winton et al. (1989) found that the clinical effect of light treatment in depressed patients was dissociated from the effect on the nightly melatonin rhythm. The same research group also found a normal circadian rhythm of melatonin in patients with SAD (Checkley et al. 1993). An interesting finding was a difference in cerebral blood flow between depressed patients and control subjects in response to artificial light, indicating the possibility of a general lowered cerebral metabolism in depression, which might be normalized by light treatment (Murphy et al. 1993). This hypothesis needs to be tested in further studies. Wirz-Justice et al. (1993) found that morning and evening light were equally effective as an antidepressant but did not determine a more exact change of circadian phase position because serum melatonin was estimated from the excretion of a urinary melatonin metabolite.

The light regulation of the pineal hormone melatonin as a serotonin-related neurotransmitter has received a new momentum of interest because it has been shown that a single pulse of light is capable of inducing the circadian phase–dependent gene expression in neurons (Takahashi 1993). A genetic predisposition for high responsiveness to light may occur in patients with seasonal depression (Nurnberger et al. 1988). The biological correlate to this responsiveness may involve melatonin production, which has been shown to be under genetic control (Wetterberg et al. 1983).

The Need for Future Research

The altered gene expression induced by light and its effect on melatonin production may account for a specific effect that may mediate the antidepressant effect of phototherapy. The pineal hormone melatonin also regulates seasonal reproductive function and modulates several circadian rhythms in many mammals. The recent cloning and characterization of a high-affinity receptor for melatonin from humans is the next step in identifying one of the hypothetical vulnerability factors of seasonal depression (Reppert et al. 1994). The receptor genes encode several proteins that are members of a group within the G-protein–coupled receptor family. In situ hybridization studies of melatonin receptor messenger RNA in mammals reveal signals in the hypophyseal tissue and the hypothalamic SCN. The high-affinity melatonin receptor is likely to mediate the circadian actions of melatonin in humans.

Only complete results with more patients followed for longer periods and taking the response of several other hormones into account are useful for determining the possible predictive value of different melatonin measures. An illustration of this type of multidimensional study is presented in the previous discussions. The recent discoveries about melatonin receptors will give new momentum to the studies of melatonin amplitude and phase position during light treatment in depressed patients to elucidate interaction with other possible biological correlates.

The secretion of melatonin is strongly influenced by environmental factors such as the light-dark cycle and also is dependent on neurotransmitter regulation of serotonin and noradrenaline. Chronobiological aspects of mood disorders, such as mood swings and sleep problems, also may be at least partly related to disturbances in the function of the pineal gland and the secretion of melatonin.

Some patients with depressive disorders may exhibit the low-melatonin syndrome. In these patients, a diminished rhythmic functioning is manifested in the clinical symptoms and in longer depressive phases. Identification of these patients may make it possible to provide more specific pharmacotherapy when the biochemical disturbances underlying this syndrome are better understood.

Patients with low-melatonin syndrome appear to differ clinically and biochemically from patients who have depressive disorders with normal or high nocturnal melatonin levels, who seem to be more apt to relapse seasonally. This latter group includes patients with SAD, "winter depression." Depressed patients with low-melatonin syndrome, and—even more so—patients with nonseasonal depression, seem to respond to a lesser degree to light therapy.

However, when using melatonin as a diagnostic marker in clinical practice for identifying subgroups of depressive disorders, clinicians must further understand and carefully consider several factors influencing nocturnal melatonin secretion because melatonin levels in humans are influenced by genetic and environmental factors. The further study of melatonin offers a natural pathway between the soma and psyche for exploration of the psychoneuroendocrinological aspects of mood disorders.

Melatonin as a Potential Therapeutic Agent

In the fall of 1995, melatonin suddenly appeared in health stores all over the United States and was claimed to cure everything from cancer and aging to insomnia and jet lag. The open sale to the public caused a shortage of melatonin on the market (Bonn 1996). In some countries, melatonin is only available by a physician's prescription or not at all until proper toxicological studies, as well as double-blind controlled investigations of its effect and side effects, have been elucidated. There are people who suffer from melatonin deficiency (e.g., following removal of the pineal gland), and there is a clinical need for a body-rhythm regulator. Melatonin supplementation also has been used successfully in people without their own production (Petterborg et al. 1991). Melatonin also may correct rhythm disturbances (e.g., in blind children with a non-24-hour sleep-wake cycle [Palm et al. 1991]). Melatonin is thus a potent rhythm-regulatory hormone and, in many countries, is classified as a medicine. Only proper clinical studies will confirm when melatonin as a rhythm-regulating hormone by itself or together with other drugs may be useful in the treatment of subgroups of mood disorders (e.g., the low-melatonin syndrome). The potential positive effects of melatonin to coordinate and restore disturbed biological rhythm are now being studied; it is hoped that its true diagnostic and therapeutic niche will be defined. Also, the recent findings of at least two distinct melatonin receptors, 1a and 1b, signaling different biological messages (e.g., one regulating the sleep-wake cycle and one the reproductive functions) will be helpful in further research to find the proper dose, the proper time of administration, and the proper application of melatonin.

References

American Psychiatric Association: Diagnostic and Statistical Manual of Mental Disorders, 3rd Edition, Revised. Washington, DC, American Psychiatric Association, 1987

American Psychiatric Association: Diagnostic and Statistical Manual of Mental Disorders, 4th Edition. Washington, DC, American Psychiatric Association, 1994

Arendt J: Melatonin and the mammalian pineal gland. London, Chapman & Hall, 1995

Arendt J, Wirz-Justice A, Bradtke J: Annual rhythm of serum melatonin in man. Neurosci Lett 7:327–330, 1977

Arendt J, Hampton S, English J, et al: 24-hour profiles of melatonin, cortisol, insulin, C-peptide and GIP following a meal and subsequent fasting. Clin Endocrinol (Oxf) 16:89–95, 1982

Attanasio A, Borrelli P, Gupta D: Circadian rhythms in serum melatonin from infancy to adolescence. J Clin Endocrinol Metab 61:388–390, 1985

Åsberg M, Montgomery SA, Perris C, et al: A comprehensive psycho-pathological rating scale. Acta Psychiatr Scand Suppl 271:5–27, 1978

Avery DH, Khan A, Dager SR, et al: Bright light treatment of winter depression: morning versus evening light. Acta Psychiatr Scand 82:335–338, 1990

Baron BM, Ogden AM, Siegel BW, et al: Rapid down regulation of beta-adrenergic adrenoreceptors by co-administration of desimipramine and fluoxetine. Eur J Pharmacol 154:125–134, 1988

Beck-Friis J: Melatonin in depressive disorders: a methodological and clinical study of the pineal-hypothalamic-pituitary-adrenal cortex system. Doctoral dissertation. Karolinska Institute, Stockholm, Sweden, 1983

Beck-Friis J, Hanssen T, Kjellman BF, et al: Serum melatonin and cortisol in human subjects after the administration of dexamethasone and propranolol. Psychopharmacol Bull 19:646–648, 1983

Beck-Friis J, von Rosen D, Kjellman BF, et al: Melatonin in relation to body measures, sex, age, season and the use of drugs in patients with major affective disorders and healthy subjects. Psychoneuroendocrinology 9:261–277, 1984

Beck-Friis J, Ljunggren JG, Thorén M, et al: Melatonin, cortisol and ACTH in patients with major depressive disorders and healthy humans with special reference to the outcome of the dexamethasone suppression test. Psychoneuroendocrinology 10:173–186, 1985a

Beck-Friis J, Kjellman BF, Aperia B, et al: Serum melatonin in relation to clinical variables in patients with major depressive disorders and hypothesis of a low melatonin syndrome. Acta Psychiatr Scand 71:319–330, 1985b

Bonn D: Melatonin's multifarious marvels: miracle or myth (editoral)? Lancet 347:184, 1996

Boyce PM: 6-sulphatoxy melatonin in melancholia. Am J Psychiatry 142:125–127, 1985

Breier A, Kelsoe JR, Kirwin PD, et al: Early parental loss and development of adult psychopathology. Arch Gen Psychiatry 45:987–993, 1988

Brown RP, Kocsis JH, Caroff S, et al: Differences in nocturnal melatonin secretion between melancholic depressed patients and control subjects. Am J Psychiatry 142:811–816, 1985

Brown RP, Kocsis JH, Caroff S, et al: Depressed mood and reality disturbance correlate with decreased nocturnal melatonin in depressed patients. Acta Psychiatr Scand 76:272–275, 1987

Cagnacci A, Soldani R, Yen SSC: The effect of light on core body temperature is mediated by melatonin in women. J Clin Endocrinol Metab 76:1036–1038, 1993

Checkley SA, Palazidou E: Melatonin and antidepressant drugs: clinical pharmacology, in Melatonin: Clinical Perspectives. Edited by Miles A, Philbrick DRS, Thompson S. New York, Oxford University Press, 1988, pp 190–204

Checkley SA, Murphy DG, Abbas M, et al: Melatonin rhythms in seasonal affective disorder. Br J Psychiatry 163:332–337, 1993

Childs PA, Rodin I, Martin NJ, et al: Effects of fluoxetine on melatonin in patients with seasonal affective disorder and matched controls. Br J Psychiatry 166:196–198, 1995

Demisch L, Demisch K, Nickelsen T: Influence of dexamethasone on nocturnal melatonin production in healthy adult subjects. J Pineal Res 5:317–322, 1988

Eastwood MR, Peacocke J: Seasonal pattern of suicide, depression and electroconvulsive therapy. Br J Psychiatry 129:472–475, 1976

Eastwood MR, Stiasny S: Psychiatric disorder, hospital admission and season. Arch Gen Psychiatry 35:769–771, 1978

Ema M, Harazona A, Miyawaki E, et al: Embryolethality following maternal exposure to dibutyl phthalate during early pregnancy in rats. Bull Environ Contam Toxicol 58:636–643, 1997

Erikson C, Küller R, Wetterberg L: Nonvisual effects of light (abstract). Neuroendocrinology Letters 5:412, 1983

Ferrier IN, Arendt J, Johnstone EC, et al: Reduced nocturnal melatonin secretion in chronic schizophrenia: relationship to body weight. Clin Endocrinol (Oxf) 17:181–187, 1982

Griffiths D, Seamark RFA, Bryden MM: Summer and winter cycles in plasma melatonin levels in the elephant seal. Australian Journal of Biological Science 32:581–586, 1979

Halberg F, Vestergaard P, Sakai M: Rhythmometry on urinary 17-ketosteroid excretion by healthy men and women and patients with chronic schizophrenia; possible chronopathology in depressive illness. Arch Anat Histol Embryol 51:299–311, 1968

Hamilton M: Development of a rating scale for primary depressive illness. Br J Clin Psychol 6:278–296, 1967

Hanssen T, Heyden T, Sundberg I, et al: Effect of propranolol on serum melatonin. Lancet 2:309–310, 1977

Healy D: Rhythm and blues: neurochemical, neuropharmacological and neuropsychological implications of a hypothesis of a circadian rhythm dysfunction in affective disorders. Psychopharmacology (Berl) 93:271–285, 1987

Iguchi H, Kato KI, Ibayashi H: Age-dependent reduction in serum melatonin concentrations in healthy human subjects. J Clin Endocrinol Metab 55:27–29, 1982

Illnerová H, Vanecek J: Pineal rhythm in *N*-acetyltransferase activity in rats under different artificial photoperiods and natural daylight in the course of a year. Neuroendocrinology 31:321–326, 1980

Illnerová H, Samkova L, Buresova M: Light entrainment of rat and human circadian melatonin rhythms, in Light and Biological Rhythms in Man. Edited by Wetterberg L. New York, Pergamon, 1993, pp 161–171

Jacobsen FM, Muller EA, Rosenthal NE, et al: Behavioral responses to intravenous meta-chlorophenylpiperazine in patients with seasonal affective disorder and control subjects before and after phototherapy. Psychiatry Res 52:181–197, 1994

James SP, Wehr TA, Sack DA, et al: Treatment of seasonal affective disorder with light in the evening. Br J Psychiatry 147:424–428, 1985

Jauhar P, Weller MPI: Psychiatric morbidity and time zone changes: a study from Heathrow Airport. Br J Psychiatry 140:231–235, 1982

Jimerson DC, Lynch HJ, Post RM, et al: Urinary melatonin rhythms during sleep deprivation in depressed patients and normals. Life Sci 20:1501–1508, 1977

Kennedy SH, Garfinkel PE, Parienti V, et al: Changes in melatonin levels but not cortisol levels are associated with depression in patients with eating disorders. Arch Gen Psychiatry 46:73–78, 1989

Kernberg O: Borderline conditions and pathological narcissism. New York, Jason Aronson, 1975

Kjellman BF, Thalén B-E, Wetterberg L: Light treatment of depressive states: Swedish experiences at latitude 597 north, in Light and Biological Rhythms in Man. Edited by Wetterberg L. New York, Pergamon, 1993, pp 351–370

Klein DC, Moore RY, Reppert SM (eds): Suprachiasmatic Nucleus: The Mind's Clock. New York, Oxford University Press, 1991

Kohut H: The Analysis of Self. New York, International Universities Press, 1971

Kripke DF: Phase-advance theories for affective illness, in Circadian Rhythms in Psychiatry. Edited by Wehr TA, Goodwin FK. Pacific Grove, CA, Boxwood Press, 1983, pp 41–69

Kripke DF, Mullaney DJ, Klauber MR, et al: Controlled trial of bright light for nonseasonal major depressive disorders. Biol Psychiatry 31:119–134, 1992

Lang U, Sizonenko PC: Melatonin and human adrenocortical function, in Melatonin: Clinical Perspectives. Edited by Miles A, Philbrick DRS, Thompson C. New York, Oxford University Press, 1988, pp 79–91

Lemmer B, Brühl T, Witte K, et al: Effects of bright light on circadian patterns of cyclic adenosine monophosphate, melatonin and cortisol in healthy subjects. Eur J Endocrinol 130:472–477, 1994

Lewy AJ, Wehr TA, Goodwin FK, et al: Light suppresses melatonin secretion in humans. Science 210:1267–1269, 1980

Lewy AJ, Herbert KA, Rosenthal NE, et al: Bright artificial light: treatment of a manic depressive patient with a seasonal mood cycle. Am J Psychiatry 139:1496–1498, 1982

Lewy AJ, Sack RL, Singer CM: Bright light, melatonin and biological rhythms: implications for the affective disorders. Psychopharmacol Bull 21:3368–3372, 1985

Lewy AJ, Sack RL, Miller LS, et al: Antidepressant and circadian phase-shifting effects of light. Science 235:352–354, 1987

Miles A, Thomas DR: Melatonin: a diagnostic marker in laboratory medicine, in Melatonin: Clinical Perspectives. Edited by Miles A, Philbrick DRS, Thompson C. New York, Oxford University Press, 1988, pp 253–279

Moore DC, Paunier L, Sizonenko PC: Effects of adrenergic stimulation and blockade on melatonin secretion in the human, in The Pineal Gland of the Vertebrates Including Man. Edited by Ariens Kappers J, Pevét P. Amsterdam, Elsevier North-Holland, 1979, pp 517–521

Murphy DG, Murphy DM, Abbas M, et al: Seasonal affective disorder: response to light as measured by electroencephalogram, melatonin suppression, and cerebral blood flow. Br J Psychiatry 163:327–331; 335–337, 1993

Nair NVP, Hariharasubramanian N, Pilapil C, et al: Plasma melatonin: an index of brain aging in humans. Biol Psychiatry 21:141–150, 1986

Nurnberger JI, Berritini W, Tamarkin L, et al: Supersensitivity to melatonin suppression by light in young people at high risk for affective disorder. Neuropsychopharmacology 1:217–233, 1988

Palazidou E, Papadopoulos A, Sitsen A, et al: An alpha$_2$ adrenoreceptor antagonist, Org 3770, enhances nocturnal melatonin secretion in man. Psychopharmacology (Berl) 97:115–117, 1989

Palm L, Blennow G, Wetterberg L: Correction of non-24-hour sleep/wake cycle by melatonin in a blind retarded boy. Ann Neurol 39:336–339, 1991

Petterborg LJ, Thalén BE, Kjellman B, et al: Effect of melatonin replacement on serum hormone rhythms in a patient lacking endogenous melatonin. Brain Res Bull 27:181–185, 1991

Pflug B, Johnsson A, Ekse AT: Manic-depressive states and daily temperature: some circadian studies. Acta Psychiatr Scand 63:277–289, 1981

Pittendrigh CS: Circadian systems, I: the driving oscillation and its assay in Drosophila pseudoobscura. Proc Natl Acad Sci U S A 58:1762–1767, 1967

Pittendrigh CS: Temporal organization: reflections of a Darwinian clockwatcher. Annu Rev Physiol 55:16–54, 1993

Rafaelsen OJ, Mellerup ET: Circadian rhythms in depressive disorders. Depressive Disorders Feb 21:409–417, 1979

Ralph MR, Foster RG, Davis FC, et al: Transplanted suprachiasmatic nucleus determines circadian period. Science 247:975–978, 1990

Rao ML, Muller-Oerlinghauser B, Mackert A, et al: Blood serotonin, serum, melatonin and light therapy in healthy subjects and in patients with nonseasonal depression. Acta Psychiatr Scand 86:127–132, 1992

Reppert SM, Weaver DR, Rivkess SA, et al: Putative melatonin receptors in a human biological clock. Science 142:78–81, 1988

Reppert SM, Weaver DR, Ebisawa T: Cloning and characterization of a mammalian melatonin receptor that mediates reproductive and circadian responses. Neuron 13:1177–1185, 1994

Reppert SM, Godson C, Mahle CD, et al: Molecular characterization of a second melatonin receptor expressed in human retina and brain: the Mel_{1b} melatonin receptor. Proc Natl Acad Sci U S A 92:8734–8738, 1995

Rhoades HM, Overall JE: The Hamilton Depression Scale: factor scoring and profile classification. Psychopharmacol Bull 19:91–96, 1983

Rosenthal NE, Sack DA, Wehr TA: Seasonal variation in affective disorders, in Circadian Rhythms in Psychiatry. Edited by Wehr TA, Goodwin FK. Pacific Grove, CA, Boxwood Press, 1983, pp 185–201

Rosenthal NE, Sack DA, Gillin JC, et al: Seasonal affective disorder: a description of the syndrome and preliminary findings with light therapy. Arch Gen Psychiatry 41:72–80, 1984

Roy-Byrne PP, Joffe RT, Uhde TW, et al: Approaches to the evaluation and treatment of rapid-cycling affective illness. Br J Psychiatry 145:543–550, 1984

Sack RL, Lewy AJ: Melatonin and major affective disorders, in Melatonin: Clinical Perspectives. Edited by Miles A, Philbrick DRS, Thompson C. New York, Oxford University Press, 1988, pp 205–227

Sack RL, Lewy AJ, White DM, et al: Morning vs evening light treatment for winter depression. Arch Gen Psychiatry 47:343–351, 1990

Salinas EO, Hakim-Kreis CM, Piketty ML, et al: Hypersecretion of melatonin following diurnal exposure to bright light in seasonal affective disorder: preliminary results. Biol Psychiatry 32:387–398, 1992

Schilgen B, Tolle R: Partial sleep deprivation as therapy for depression. Arch Gen Psychiatry 37:267–271, 1980

Sharma M, Palacios-Bois J, Schwartz G, et al: Circadian rhythms of melatonin and cortisol in aging. Biol Psychiatry 25:305–319, 1989

Simpsom S, Galbraith JJ: Observations on the normal temperature of the monkey and its diurnal variation, and on the effect of changes in the daily routine on the variation. Transactions of the Royal Society of Edinburgh, Earth Sciences 45:5, 1906

Skene DJ, Bojkowski CJ, Arendt J: Comparison of the effects of acute fluvoxamine and desipramine administration on melatonin and cortisol production in humans. Br J Clin Pharmacol 37:181–186, 1994

Slaugenhaupt SA, Roca AL, Liebert CB, et al: Mapping of the gene for the Mel_{1a}-melatonin receptor to human chromosome 4 (MTNRIA) and mouse chromosome 8 (Mtnr1a). Genomics 27:355–357, 1995

Smith JA, Barnes JL, Mee TJ: The effect of neuroleptic drugs on serum and cerebrospinal fluid melatonin concentration in psychiatric subjects. J Pharm Pharmacol 31:246–248, 1979

Spitzer RL, Endicott J, Robins E: Research Diagnostic Criteria: rationale and reliability. Arch Gen Psychiatry 35:773–782, 1978

Steiner M, Brown GM: Melatonin-cortisol ratio and the dexamethasone suppression test in newly admitted psychiatry inpatients, in Advances in the Biosciences, Vol 53: The Pineal Gland: Endocrine Aspects. Edited by Brown GM, Wainwright SD. Oxford, England, Pergamon, 1985, pp 347–353

Stewart JW, Halbreich U: Plasma melatonin levels in depressed patients before and after treatment with antidepressant medication. Biol Psychiatry 25:33–38, 1989

Takahashi JS: Biological rhythms: from gene expression to behavior, in Light and Biological Rhythms in Man. Edited by Wetterberg L. New York, Pergamon, 1993, pp 3–20

Terman M, Terman JS, Quitkin FM, et al: Response of melatonin cycle to phototherapy for seasonal affective disorder. J Neural Transm 72:147–165, 1988

Terman M, Terman JS, Quitkin FM, et al: Light therapy for seasonal affective disorder: a review of efficacy. Neuropsychopharmacology 2:1–22, 1989

Thalén B-E, Kjellman BF, Mørkrid LS, et al: Light treatment in seasonal and nonseasonal depression. Acta Psychiatr Scand 91:352–360, 1995a

Thalén B-E, Kjellman BF, Mørkrid LS, et al: Melatonin in light treatment in seasonal and nonseasonal depression. Acta Psychiatr Scand 92:274–284, 1995b

Thalén B-E, Kjellman BF, Mørkrid LS, et al: Seasonal and nonseasonal depression: a comparison of clinical characteristics in Swedish patients. Eur Arch Psychiatry Clin Neurosci 245:101–108, 1995c

Thomas DR, Miles A: Melatonin secretion and age (letter). Biol Psychiatry 25:364–367, 1989

Thompson C, Franey C, Arendt J, et al: A comparison of melatonin secretion in normal subjects and depressed patients. Br J Psychiatry 152:260–266, 1988

Thompson C, Stinson D, Smith A: Seasonal affective disorder and seasonal-dependent abnormalities of melatonin depression by light. Lancet 336:703–706, 1990

Vogel GW, Vogel F, McAbee RS, et al: Improvement of depression by REM sleep deprivation: new findings and a theory. Arch Gen Psychiatry 37:247–253, 1980 von Knorring L, Perris C, Strandman E: Diurnal variation in intensity of symptoms in patients of different diagnostic groups. Archiv fur Psychiatrie und Nervenkrankheiten 244:295–312, 1977

Wahlund B, Sääf J, Wetterberg L: Classification of patients with affective disorders using platelet monoamine oxidase activity, serum melatonin and post dexamethasone cortisol. Acta Psychiatr Scand 91:313–321, 1995

Waldhauser F, Waldhauser M: Melatonin and aging, in Melatonin: Clinical Perspectives. Edited by Miles A, Philbrick DRS, Thompson C. New York, Oxford University Press, 1988, pp 174–189

Wetterberg L: Melatonin in humans: physiological and clinical studies. J Neural Transm Suppl 13:289–310, 1978

Wetterberg L: Clinical importance of melatonin. Prog Brain Res 52:539–547, 1979

Wetterberg L (ed): Light and Biological Rhythms in Man. London, Pergamon, 1993

Wetterberg L, Eriksson O, Friberg Y, et al: A simplified radioimmunoassay for melatonin and its application to biological fluids: preliminary observation on the half-life of plasma melatonin in man. Clin Chim Acta 86:169–177, 1978

Wetterberg L, Beck-Friis J, Aperia B, et al: Melatonin/cortisol ratio in depression (letter). Lancet 2:1361, 1979

Wetterberg L, Aperia B, Beck-Friis J, et al: Pineal-hypothalamic-pituitary function in patients with depressive illness, in Steroid Hormone Regulation of the Brain. Edited by Fuxe K, Gustafsson JA, Wetterberg L. Oxford, England, Pergamon, 1981, pp 397–403

Wetterberg L, Iselius L, Lindsten J: Genetic regulation of melatonin excretion in urine. Clin Genet 24:403–406, 1983

Wetterberg L, Sääf J, Norén B, et al: Interference with the radio-immunoassay of melatonin by dimethyl phthalate (letter). Journal of Steroid Biochemistry 20:63, 1984

Wetterberg L, Beck-Friis J, Kjellman BF: Melatonin as a marker for a subgroup of depression in adults, in Biological Rhythms, Mood Disorders, Light Therapy, and the Pineal Gland. Edited by Shafii M, Shafii SL. Washington, DC, American Psychiatric Press, 1990, pp 69–95

Wetterberg L, Aperia B, Gorelik DA, et al: Age, alcoholism and depression are associated with low levels of urinary melatonin. J Psychiatry Neurosci 17:215–224, 1992

Winton F, Corn T, Huson LW, et al: Effects of light treatment upon mood and melatonin in patients with seasonal affective disorders. Psychol Med 19:585–590, 1989

Wirz-Justice A, Arendt J: Diurnal, menstrual cycle and seasonal indole rhythms in man and their modification in affective disorders, in Biological Psychiatry Today. Edited by Obiols J, Ballús C, Gonzáles Monclús E, et al. Amsterdam, Elsevier North-Holland, 1979, pp 294–302

Wirz-Justice A, Graw P, Kräuchi K, et al: Light therapy in seasonal affective disorder is independent of time of day or circadian phase. Arch Gen Psychiatry 50:929–937, 1993

World Health Organization: International Classification of Diseases, 9th Revision, Clinical Modification. Geneva, World Health Organization, 1980

Yu H-S, Reiter RJ: Melatonin, Biosynthesis, Physiological Effects, and Clinical Applications. London, CRC Press, 1993

Yuwiler A: Neonatal steroid treatment reduces catecholamine-induced increases in pineal serotonin N-acetyltransferase activity. J Neurochem 44:1185–1193, 1985

Chapter 4

Melatonin in Circadian Phase Sleep and Mood Disorders

Alfred J. Lewy, M.D., Ph.D., Robert L. Sack, M.D.,
Neil L. Cutler, B.A., Vance K. Bauer, M.A., and
Rod J. Hughes, Ph.D.

A ppropriately timed bright light exposure is the treatment of choice for winter depression (WD), which is commonly referred to as seasonal affective disorder, or SAD. Other types of depressed patients, particularly those who have a concomitant chronobiological sleep disorder, also benefit to some extent from appropriately timed bright light exposure. Treatment principles are the same for all patients who have circadian (i.e., 24-hour) phase disorders. These disorders include advanced and delayed sleep phase syndromes, jet lag, and maladaptation to shift work. An individual thought to have a phase-advanced type of disorder (characterized by circadian rhythms that are shifted abnormally early) should be treated with bright light in the evening and/or melatonin in the morning to provide a corrective phase delay. An individual thought to have a phase-delayed type of disorder should be treated with bright light in the morning and/or melatonin in the afternoon or evening to provide a corrective phase advance.

We thank the nursing staff of the Oregon Health Sciences University Clinical Research Center (OHSU GCRC) and acknowledge the assistance of Clifford M. Singer, Angela J. McArthur, Mary T. Moffit, Mary L. Blood, Rick S. Boney, Neil R. Anderson, Sovann D. Pen, Aaron A. Clemons, Joanne M. Otto, Rhonda E. Ross, and Joe Johnson. Supported by Public Health Service research grants MH40161, MH00703, MH01005, PO1 AG10794, and M01 RR00334 (OHSU GCRC).

Not all patients with mood disorders have illnesses with a chronobiological component. However, to the extent that the illness is chronobiological, appropriately timed bright light exposure should be therapeutic. In these patients, bright light treatment might serve as a useful, although ancillary, function secondary to pharmacotherapy or psychotherapy; avoiding one more medication (even for sleep) is nonetheless desirable.

History

Before 1980, scientists in the field of pineal physiology thought that human melatonin production was not affected by light exposure (Vaughan et al. 1979), although the relationship between the light/dark cycle and biological rhythms was well established in animals, and all other species studied to date showed suppressed nighttime melatonin production in response to light (Binkley et al. 1975; Klein and Weller 1972; Minneman et al. 1974; Perlow et al. 1980; Rollag and Niswender 1976; Tamarkin et al. 1979; Wurtman et al. 1963). It was known in animals that photic information conveyed by the retinohypothalamic tract to the suprachiasmatic nuclei results in suppression of nighttime melatonin production. Klein (1979) speculated that humans lacked the neural pathways accounting for the regulation of melatonin production so carefully delineated in other species, perhaps as a result of an evolutionary independence of circadian rhythms from the effect of environmental lighting unique to humans (Richter 1977). At that time, human chronobiologists concurred that the light/dark cycle was relatively unimportant as compared with social cues, for example, for the cuing of human circadian rhythms (Wever 1979).

Apparently, a paradigm shift followed our discovery (Lewy et al. 1980) that humans require substantially brighter light than do other animals to suppress nighttime melatonin production (Figure 4–1). That human nighttime melatonin production is suppressed by exposure to bright (rather than ordinary room) light suggested that human circadian rhythms are synchronized by the 24-hour natural light/dark cycle and that seasonal rhythms are cued by the

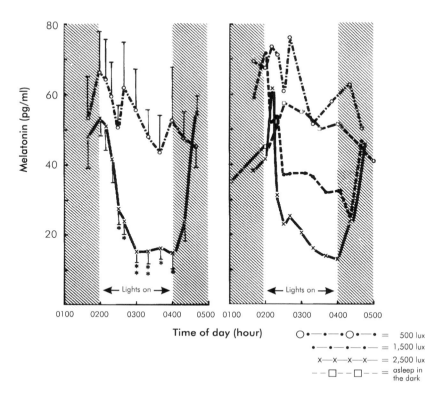

Figure 4–1. Effect of light on melatonin secretion. *(left)* Each point represents the mean concentration of melatonin ($\pm$ SE) for six subjects. A paired *t*-test, comparing exposure to 500 lux with exposure to 2,500 lux, was performed for each data point. A two-way analysis of variance with repeated measures and the Newman-Keuls statistic for the comparison of means showed significant differences between 02.50 and 04.00 ($^*P <$ .05; $^{**}P <$ .01). *(right)* Effect of different light intensities on melatonin secretion. The averaged values for two subjects are shown.

Source. Reprinted from Lewy AJ, Wehr TA, Goodwin FK, et al.: "Light Suppresses Melatonin Secretion in Humans." *Science* 210:1267–1269, 1980. Copyright 1987 American Association for the Advancement of Science. Used with permission.

change in natural day length throughout the year, relatively unperturbed by the use of ordinary-intensity indoor light. For example, the use of ordinary-intensity room light to extend day length during the winter might not provide the equivalent of a summer photoperiod; similarly, exposure to ordinary-intensity light during the middle of the night may not be bright enough to reset circadian rhythms in humans. Our findings also suggested that bright artificial light (e.g., five times brighter than ordinary-intensity room light) could be substituted for sunlight to manipulate these rhythms, experimentally and perhaps therapeutically.

One of the first disorders treated with bright light was WD. We had been unaware of this disorder until a patient named Herb Kern contacted us (Kern and Lewy 1990; Wehr and Rosenthal 1989, 1990). Kern was a research engineer who had concluded that his 13-year history of manic and depressive mood swings was linked to the change in daylight throughout the year. Over the years, physicians, including psychiatrists, were unable to offer him more than the usual drug regimens, which he could not tolerate because of a hypersensitivity to side effects. Finally, he contacted us after reading about a new technique we had published for measuring melatonin in human plasma (Lewy and Markey 1978).

After listening to Kern's observations, we decided to treat him with bright light during his next WD. We did not think that bright light would be antidepressant per se, but we thought we might be able to use it to mimic a spring day, the time of year when Kern normally switched out of his depression. Because day length conveys the time of the year for many other species, we decided to expose Kern in the short days of winter to 2,000 lux light between 6 A.M. and 9 A.M. and between 4 P.M. and 7 P.M. After 4 days, he began to switch out of his depression (Lewy et al. 1982). His successful treatment led to the first controlled study of winter depressive patients (Rosenthal et al. 1984), which utilized a double-blind crossover design with dim light exposure as a placebo control, but also encouraged a number of other researchers to identify more patients with WD (reviewed by Tam et al. 1995).

Our discovery also launched a number of other investigations into the use of bright light to manipulate circadian rhythms in humans. Wever et al. (1983) tested bright light cycles under conditions of temporal isolation. At about the same time, we showed that scheduled exposure to bright light could be used to treat chronobiological sleep disorders and also to speed adaptation to alleviate jet lag (Daan and Lewy 1984; Lewy et al. 1983). In addition, we found that shifting the (bright) light/dark cycle could shift circadian rhythms even while holding the sleep-wake cycle constant (Lewy et al. 1984; Lewy et al. 1985a). Specifically, we showed that bright light exposure in the morning advances circadian rhythms, shifting them to an earlier time, whereas bright light exposure in the evening delays circadian rhythms, shifting them to a later time. These findings have been expanded to describe four complete phase-response curves (PRCs) to bright light (Czeisler et al. 1989; Honma and Honma 1988; Minors et al. 1991; Wever 1989) that, in general, agree with each other and with the hypothesized PRC to bright light that we originally proposed (Lewy et al. 1983).

Treatment of Jet Lag

Treatment of jet lag is based on our hypothesized PRC to bright light (Figure 4–2). Accordingly, we have proposed a set of recommendations regarding when to obtain outdoor sunlight exposure and in some cases when to remain indoors, depending on which direction is traveled and how many time zones are crossed (Daan and Lewy 1984).

In summary, those who travel eastward through less than six time zones should go outside for a few hours just after dawn, whereas those who travel westward should do this for a few hours just before dusk. When travelers fly through more than six time zones, outdoor light should be obtained in the middle of the first day they arrive. Eastward travelers should avoid outdoor light in the morning on that day (Figure 4–3) and go outdoors progressively later on ensuing days; conversely, westward travelers should avoid late afternoon light and go outdoors progressively later. Travelers should follow these instructions for the first few days after they have arrived at their destination. When outdoors, they should not look directly at the sun, which would harm the eyes. Simply being outdoors, even on a cloudy day, will provide sufficiently bright light to achieve the desired chronobiological effect.

The "middle-of-the-night" portion of the PRC can be used to

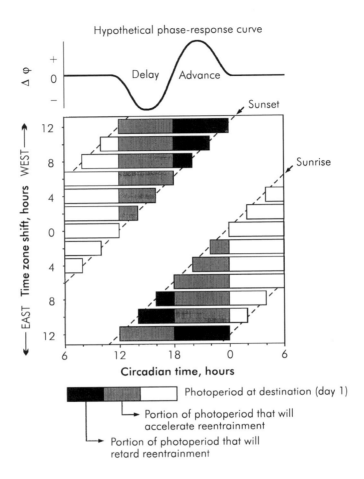

Figure 4–2.   Our hypothetical phase-response curve to light and the proposed times for when bright light exposure should occur and when bright light exposure should be avoided the first few days after trans-meridional flight. For example, after a 2-hour west-to-east trip, bright light exposure should begin at dawn. After a 10-hour west-to-east trip, however, bright light exposure should be *avoided* until 4 hours after sunrise.

Source.   Adapted from Daan and Lewy 1984.

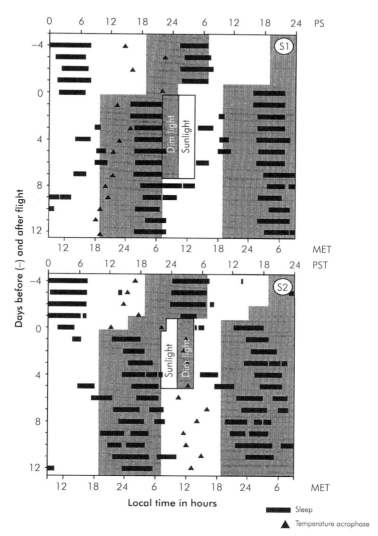

Figure 4–3. Two subjects flew from Portland, Oregon, to Amsterdam. *(top)* Subject 1, receiving bright light exposure to the phase-advance portion of the phase-response curve, entrained by the sixth day after west-to-east travel across nine time zones. *(bottom)* Subject 2, receiving bright light exposure to the phase-delay portion of the phase-response curve, had still not entrained by the 12th day. Symbols: *bars* = sleep; *triangle* = oral temperature maxima.
Source. Adapted from Daan and Lewy 1984.

treat problems associated with jet lag and shift work. For example, it may be effective to use bright artificial light at this time for a few days before embarkation. However, sleep deprivation will occur. Because of this deprivation, with the exception of shift workers, patients with chronobiological sleep and mood disorders will probably utilize primarily the morning or evening portions of the light PRC.

More recently, jet lag has been treated with melatonin (Arendt et al. 1987; Armstrong et al. 1986; Claustrat et al. 1992; Deacon and Arendt 1996; Petrie et al. 1989, 1993; Samel et al. 1991; Skene et al. 1989). Melatonin has proved useful as a treatment for jet lag, both as a soporific and perhaps as a phase-resetting agent. Melatonin's soporific effects appear to be dose-dependent: the higher the dose, the more likely this soporific effect, although not everyone becomes sleepy when using melatonin. A few individuals, however, are extremely sensitive to this "side effect."

The phase-shifting response to melatonin even at low physiological doses, however, is universal. We have shown that even 0.5 mg of melatonin can shift circadian rhythms according to a PRC (Lewy et al. 1992) (Figure 4–4). The melatonin PRC is 12 hours out of phase with the light PRC. This fact has significant implications for the function of endogenous melatonin in humans (Figure 4–5) and is of critical importance when scheduling melatonin treatment in order to achieve either phase delays or phase advances.

According to the melatonin PRC, melatonin should be administered in the night or morning to cause a phase delay. To cause a phase advance, melatonin should be administered in the afternoon or evening. Melatonin administration, although still considered experimental, has obvious practical advantages over light treatment for the treatment of jet lag and perhaps other circadian phase disorders.

Treatment of Chronobiological Sleep Disorders

There are essentially two types of circadian phase sleep disorders, advanced sleep phase syndrome (ASPS) and delayed sleep phase syndrome (DSPS). Treatment of these chronobiological sleep disorders with light is relatively straightforward (Lewy 1987; Terman et al. 1995).

ASPS is described in people who sleep between 9 P.M. and 4 A.M. They have difficulty staying awake in the evening and have early morning awakening. People with ASPS respond to 1 or 2 hours of

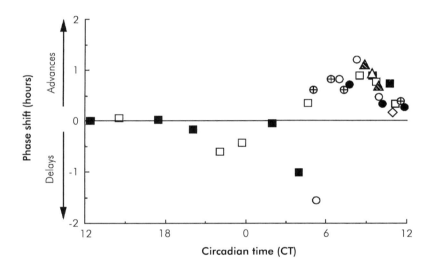

Figure 4–4. Phase shifts of the dim light melatonin onset (DLMO) as a function of circadian time (CT) of exogenous melatonin administration for nine subjects (a total of 30 trials), providing the first evidence for a human melatonin phase-response curve. Each subject is represented by a different symbol. Exogenous melatonin (0.5 mg) was administered at various times with respect to the time of endogenous melatonin production (CT 14 = baseline DLMO for each trial). The time of administration appears as CT by convention and, because of interindividual variability in sleep-wake cycles, perceived light-dark cycles and internal CT. On average, CT 0 = 07.00 clock time.

Source. Reprinted from Lewy AJ, Ahmed S, Jackson JML, et al.: "Melatonin Shifts Circadian Rhythms According to a Phase-Response Curve." *Chronobiology International* 9:380–392, 1992. Used with permission.

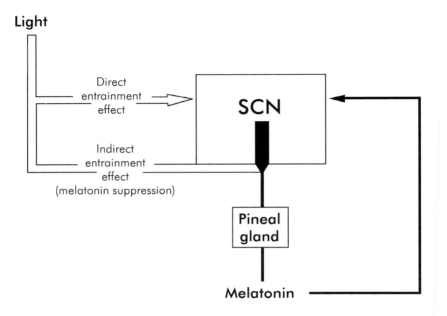

Figure 4–5. Schematic diagram of some of the relationships among nighttime melatonin production by the pineal gland, the light-dark cycle, and an endogenous circadian pacemaker (ECP) thought to be located in the hypothalamic suprachiasmatic nuclei (SCN). Acting on the SCN as described by the melatonin phase-response curve (Figure 4–4) at any given time of the day or night, melatonin causes phase shifts opposite to those that light would cause *(indicated by the opposing arrows).* However, the suppressant effect of light pares the margins of the nighttime melatonin profile *(tapered arrow)* and reduces endogenous melatonin's stimulation of the melatonin phase-response curve at the day-night transitions. This second (indirect) pathway for entrainment by light is particularly significant during shifts of the light-dark cycle. Our diagram is not meant to be complete; for example, there may be a clock in the eye that may be influenced by the light-dark cycle, the SCN, and endogenous melatonin production.

Source. Reprinted from Lewy AJ, Ahmed S, Jackson JML, et al.: "Melatonin Shifts Circadian Rhythms According to a Phase-Response Curve." *Chronobiology International* 9:380–392, 1992. Used with permission.

bright light exposure scheduled between 8 P.M. and 11 P.M. (Lewy et al. 1985b). However, they must usually continue bright light exposure "as needed" (at least once every few days) or they will slip back into their phase-advanced state.

Patients with DSPS have difficulty falling asleep before 1 A.M. or 2 A.M. (Weitzman et al. 1981). These patients respond to 1 or 2 hours of bright light exposure scheduled in the morning (Lewy et al. 1983). They are able to gradually advance their sleep time (usually at the rate of 15 minutes earlier each day) provided they are exposed to bright light immediately upon awakening. This regimen may be difficult for some patients; they should be reassured that they will eventually be able to fall asleep earlier and therefore will not suffer much sleep deprivation. The rate of advancing should be tailored to each patient individually. For maintenance therapy (once they are sleeping at the desired time), DSPS patients will need at least 15 minutes of bright light exposure every few days as soon as they awaken.

Treatment of Shift-Work Maladaptation

Shift workers account for more than 20% of the United States work force. They generally do not reset their endogenous circadian rhythms to the appropriate schedule (Colquhoun et al. 1968, 1969; Folkard et al. 1978; Knauth et al. 1980; van Loon 1963). These individuals have a higher incidence of substance abuse and psychiatric and behavioral problems, as well as gastrointestinal, cardiovascular, and menstrual disorders (Gordon et al. 1986). Shift workers use more alcohol, stimulants, sedatives, and tobacco than day workers; suffer from more stress-related symptoms, such as fatigue, apathy, palpitations, nervousness, and muscle pain; and also have a higher incidence of divorce (Cole et al. 1990; Gordon et al. 1986; Moore-Ede and Richardson 1985). It is likely that circadian desynchrony underlies many of these problems.

To correct circadian desynchrony, shift workers have been treated by exposure to bright light according to the light PRC (Czeisler et al. 1990; Eastman 1987, 1990a, 1991). Avoiding bright light in the morning is also thought to help these individuals adapt to night work (Eastman 1993). As with the other circadian phase disorders, more research is necessary to optimize treatment parameters.

Melatonin administration can help promote circadian adaptation to shift work (Folkard et al. 1993; Sack et al. 1994, 1995). Shift workers who take 0.5 mg of melatonin scheduled according to the melatonin PRC can speed their adaptation to either work or off-work schedules. For convenience, they usually take melatonin just before bedtime (which is often the correct circadian time, particularly for the first day of the new schedule). They should be advised about the possible soporific side effect of even low doses whenever melatonin is taken during the day.

Treatment of Chronobiological Mood Disorders

As previously mentioned, there are essentially two types of circadian phase mood disorders, the phase-advanced type and the phase-delayed type. However, it was not immediately clear how to best treat mood disorders with light. Most investigators agree that WD can be successfully treated with bright light and that two pulses of bright light exposure per day are not essential. Unlike most melancholic patents with major depression who often have early morning awakening, WD patients usually have trouble getting up in the morning. Their difficulty awakening in the morning suggested to us that WD patients might have abnormally phase-delayed circadian rhythms and should respond best to bright light exposure in the morning (Lewy et al. 1987b). Just as patients with major melancholic depression who had early morning awakening were thought to have phase-advanced circadian rhythms (Kripke 1983; Sack et al. 1994; Wehr et al. 1979), we thought that WD patients were abnormally phase delayed because they seemed to have the opposite circadian rhythm problem.

We have two lines of evidence that WD patients are phase delayed. First, when compared with healthy control subjects, WD patients have delayed melatonin and temperature circadian rhythms when depressed in the winter (Avery et al. 1990c; Wirz-

Justice et al. 1995). The dim light melatonin onset (DLMO), a highly useful marker for circadian phase position (Lewy and Sack 1989), is delayed in WD patients, compared with healthy control subjects, when they are depressed in the winter—even after a week of standardized sleep and light/dark conditions (Lewy et al. 1987b; Sack et al. 1990) (Figure 4–6).

Second, and perhaps a more significant line of evidence, is that morning bright light exposure is more antidepressant compared with evening light (Avery et al. 1990a; Lewy et al. 1987a; Sack et al. 1990; Terman et al. 1989b). Depression ratings are also significantly lower after morning light exposure when compared with baseline conditions (Figure 4–7). Although patients become more depressed when switched from morning light to evening light, depression ratings after evening light are less than after baseline condition and in some studies are lower than after a placebo control (Terman and Terman 1996). However, it has not been shown that evening light is more effective than a "credible" placebo control, that is, one that is expected to be as antidepressant as light treatment. According to the phase-shift hypothesis (PSH), morning light is antidepressant at least partly because of its phase-advancing effect.

Bright light exposure upon awakening also can be achieved in another way. We have been able to treat patients with WD by delaying their sleep. From a practical point of view, many patients with WD can be advised to sleep past dawn and to go outside as soon as they get up. Indeed, Wirz-Justice et al. (1996) found that the "natural" light treatment of a morning walk is beneficial to individuals with WD. Oren et al. (1994) have found that the earlier this exposure to natural light occurs, the greater the antidepressant effect. Morning walks might obviate the need for purchasing a light fixture if the patient's schedule is sufficiently flexible.

Recently, there is interest in the use of dawn simulators, in which light intensity is gradually increased. Even at steady state, the intensity is less than that normally used for light treatment, particularly since the eyes are closed during most the of the exposure, which is expected to reduce light intensity by 70%. The PSH explains these results. The light PRC has a very sensitive phase-ad-

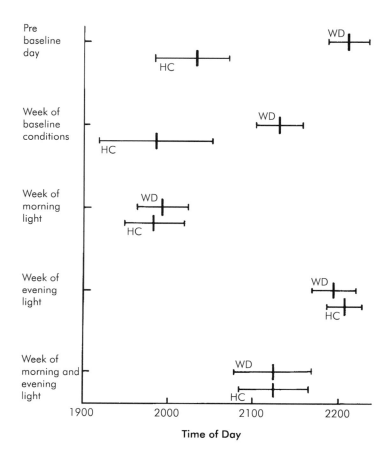

Figure 4–6. Average melatonin onset times (± SEM) for healthy control subjects (HC) and patients with winter depression (WD) (n = 6–8, except n = 4 for the prebaseline melatonin values). An analysis of variance for repeated measures indicated a significant difference between treatments for both patients (P = .001) and healthy control subjects (P = .009). Significant paired t-tests for the patients were baseline versus A.M. (P = .001), baseline versus P.M. (P = .012), and A.M. versus P.M. (P = 0.001). Significant paired t-tests for the healthy control subjects were baseline versus A.M. + P.M. (P = .039), A.M. versus P.M. (P = .004), and A.M. versus A.M. + P.M. (P = .003). Melatonin onset times of the WD patients were delayed compared with those of the healthy control subjects at both prebaseline (P = .02) and baseline (P = .05) (student's t-test).

Source. Reprinted from Lewy AJ, Sack RL, Miller S, et al.: "Antidepressant and Circadian Phase-Shifting Effects of Light." *Science* 235:352–354, 1987. Copyright 1987 American Association for the Advancement of Science. Used with permission.

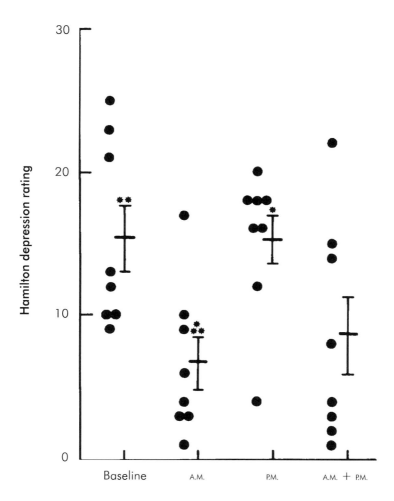

Figure 4–7. Individual and average 21-item Hamilton depression ratings (± SEM) for 8 patients with winter depression for each of the 4 weeks of the study. An analysis of variance for repeated measures indicated a significant (*P* = .026) difference between treatments. Only the paired *t*-tests comparing the week of morning (A.M.) light and the baseline week (**P* = .004) and comparing the week of A.M. light and the week of evening (P.M.) light (*P* = .045) were significant. Average depression ratings (± SEM) for the seven healthy control subjects were 3.0 ± 0.9 at baseline, 2.4 ± 0.3 (A.M. light), 6.1 ± 1.6 (P.M. light), and 4.3 ± 0.9 (A.M. + P.M. light).

Source.   Reprinted from Lewy AJ, Sack RL, Miller S, et al.: "Antidepressant and Circadian Phase-Shifting Effects of Light." *Science* 235:352–354, 1987. Copyright 1987 American Association for the Advancement of Science. Used with permission.

vance zone at the time dawn simulation is scheduled, usually a few hours before awakening. Preliminary results suggest that dawn simulation is antidepressant in WD and causes phase advances (Avery et al. 1992b, 1994; Terman et al. 1989a). If dawn simulation studies continue to be effective, this mode of treatment may become the standard for WD. It provides light exposure at a convenient time, mainly while patients are sleeping; patients generally do not awaken until the light intensity reaches some threshold.

Another recent modification of the standard light box fixture is the light visor. Developed to provide more convenient light exposure, the visor seems to be no more antidepressant than placebo (Joffe et al. 1993; Rosenthal et al. 1993), probably because its configuration does not provide sufficient bright light exposure to the eye.

Most investigators now agree that morning is the most effective time of the day for light treatment of WD. There is complete agreement that morning bright light shifts circadian rhythms earlier and that evening bright light shifts them later. However, there is still some disagreement about whether or not the antidepressant effect of light is based on this mechanism. Critics of the PSH explain the superiority of morning light over evening light as being due to an overall increase in sensitivity to light in the morning (Tassi and Pins 1997). Even if such a rhythm exists, it does not explain why patients become more depressed when switched from morning light to evening light, given that decreasing the duration of morning light by 70% is capable of maintaining an antidepressant response once it has been initiated (Lewy et al. 1987b). Currently, one of the most controversial issues is whether or not the modest antidepressant effect of evening light seen in some patients is anything more than a placebo effect (Eastman 1989, 1990b).

Treatment of chronobiological mood disorders requires appropriate "phase typing." Although many depressed patients may not have a phase disturbance and therefore may not be helped by bright light exposure, most WD patients appear to be abnormally phase delayed and are most helped by bright light scheduled for 1 or 2 hours immediately upon awakening. At first, sleep time may have to be advanced earlier to accommodate morning light exposure; it should then be held constant. Within 1 or 2 weeks, the antidepressant response should be maximal, after which the duration of light exposure can be reduced. Nonresponders should be switched to evening light (7 P.M.—9 P.M.) because they may be of the much smaller subgroup that has abnormally phase-advanced circadian rhythms. It is not clear how well other types of depressed patients respond to light treatment. More research needs to be done in this area.

The suppressant response to light appears to be dose or fluence dependent (Bojkowski et al. 1987; Brainard et al. 1988; Lewy et al. 1980, 1981; McIntyre et al. 1989); that is, the decline in melatonin levels resulting from exposure to light is a function of an individual's light sensitivity. Fluence dependency of melatonin suppression suggests that the phase-shifting effect of light is also fluence dependent as recently shown in humans (Boivin et al. 1996).

Although some investigators have shown that morning light, which provides a corrective phase advance, is most antidepressant for WD patients (Avery et al. 1990a, 1990b, 1991; Lewy et al. 1987a; Rafferty et al. 1990; Sack et al. 1990; Terman et al. 1989b), others have shown no difference between morning light and light exposure scheduled at other times of the day (Lafer et al. 1994; Thalén et al. 1995; Wirz-Justice et al. 1993). The large placebo effect of light probably makes demonstrating the superiority of morning light difficult in some studies. It remains controversial as to whether parallel-group or crossover studies are methodologically superior (Avery et al. 1990b; Blehar and Lewy 1990; Wirz-Justice and Anderson 1990). One argument favoring the crossover design is that nonspecific effects should be the same for each time of day and that patients can sample and compare both times of light exposure and arrive at a more informed opinion, perhaps less influenced by the placebo component, which might be quite large (Eastman 1989, 1990b).

Conclusions

In summary, there are two types of circadian phase disorders, the phase-advanced type and the phase-delayed type. Based on the

light PRC, 1 or 2 hours of bright (2,500 lux) light should be scheduled in the evening to treat the former and in the morning to treat
the latter. Once sleep time has normalized, it should be held
constant. Most patients with WD are phase delayed and should be
treated with bright light scheduled in the morning. At a physiological dose (< 0.5 mg), melatonin can be used to treat circadian
phase disorders, based on the melatonin PRC. More research is
needed to optimize treatment parameters for both light exposure
and melatonin delivery.

References

Arendt J, Aldhous M, English J, et al: Some effects of jet-lag and their
    alleviation by melatonin. Ergonomics 30:1379–1393, 1987
Armstrong SM, Cassone VM, Chesworth MJ, et al: Synchronization of
    mammalian circadian rhythms by melatonin. J Neural Transm Suppl
    21:375–394, 1986
Avery DH, Khan A, Dager SR, et al: Bright light treatment of winter
    depression: morning versus evening light. Acta Psychiatr Scand
    82:335–338, 1990a
Avery DH, Khan A, Dager S, et al: Is morning light exposure superior to
    evening light in treating seasonal affective disorder? Psychopharma-
    col Bull 26:521–524, 1990b
Avery DH, Dahl K, Savage M, et al: The temperature rhythm is phase-de-
    layed in winter depression (abstract). Biol Psychiatry 27:99A, 1990c
Avery DH, Khan A, Dager S, et al: Morning or evening bright light
    treatment of winter depression? the significance of hypersomnia. Biol
    Psychiatry 29:117–126, 1991
Avery DH, Bolte MA, Millet M: Bright dawn simulation compared with
    bright morning light in the treatment of winter depression. Acta
    Psychiatr Scand 85:430–434, 1992a
Avery DH, Bolte MA, Cohen S, et al: Gradual versus rapid dawn simula-
    tion treatment of winter depression. J Clin Psychiatry 53:359–363,
    1992b
Avery DH, Bolte MA, Dager SR, et al: Dawn simulation treatment of
    winter depression: a controlled study. Am J Psychiatry 150:113–117,
    1993

Avery DH, Bolte MP, Wolfson JK, et al: Dawn simulation compared with a dim red signal in the treatment of winter depression. Biol Psychiatry 36:181–188, 1994

Binkley S, MacBride SE, Klein DC, et al: Regulation of pineal rhythms in chickens: refractory period and nonvisual light perception. Endocrinology 96:848–853, 1975

Blehar MC, Lewy AJ: Seasonal mood disorders: consensus and controversy. Psychopharmacol Bull 26:465–494, 1990

Boivin DB, Duffey JF, Kronauer RE, et al: Dose-response relationships for resetting of human circadian clock by light. Nature 379:540–541, 1996

Bojkowski CJ, Aldhous ME, English J, et al: Suppression of nocturnal plasma melatonin and 6-sulphatoxymelatonin by bright and dim light in man. Horm Metab Res 19:437–440, 1987

Brainard GC, Lewy AJ, Menaker M, et al: Dose-response relationship between light irradiance and the suppression of plasma melatonin in human volunteers. Brain Res 454:212–218, 1988

Claustrat B, Brun J, David M, et al: Melatonin and jet lag: confirmatory result using a simplified protocol. Biol Psychiatry 32:705–711, 1992

Cole RJ, Loving RT, Kripke DF: Psychiatric aspects of shiftwork, in Occupational Medicine: Shiftwork. Edited by Scott AJ. Philadelphia, Hanley & Belfus, 1990, pp 301–314

Colquhoun WP, Blake MJF, Edwards RS: Experimental studies of shiftwork, II: stabilized 8-hour shift systems. Ergonomics 11:527–546, 1968

Colquhoun WP, Blake MJF, Edwards RS: Experimental studies of shiftwork, III: stabilized 12-hour shift systems. Ergonomics 12:865–882, 1969

Czeisler CA, Kronauer RE, Allan JS, et al: Bright light induction of strong (type O) resetting of the human circadian pacemaker. Science 244:1328–1333, 1989

Czeisler CA, Johnson MP, Duffy JF, et al: Exposure to bright light and darkness to treat physiologic maladaptation to night work. N Engl J Med 322:1253–1259, 1990

Daan S, Lewy AJ: Scheduled exposure to daylight: a potential strategy to reduce "jet lag" following transmeridian flight. Psychopharmacol Bull 20:566–568, 1984

Deacon S, Arendt J: Adapting to phase shifts, II: effects of melatonin and conflicting light treatment. Physiol Behav 59:675–682, 1996

Eastman CI: Bright light in work-sleep schedules for shift workers: application of circadian rhythm principles, in Temporal Disorder in Human Oscillatory Systems. Edited by Rensing L, an der Heiden U, Mackey MC. New York, Springer-Verlag, 1987, pp 176–185

Eastman CI: The placebo problem in phototherapy for winter SAD. Society for Light Treatment and Biological Rhythms Abstracts 1:36, 1989

Eastman CI: Circadian rhythms and bright light: recommendations for shift work. Work and Stress 4:245–260, 1990a

Eastman CI: What the placebo literature can tell us about phototherapy for SAD. Psychopharmacol Bull 26:495–504, 1990b

Eastman CI: Bright light on the night shift: circadian rhythms can advance or delay (abstract). Sleep Research 20:453, 1991

Eastman CI: Dark goggles during daylight and high intensity light during night shifts for circadian adaptation to simulated shift work (abstract). Sleep Research 22:402, 1993

Folkard S, Monk T, Lobban M: Short and long term adjustment of circadian rhythms in "permanent" night nurses. Ergonomics 21:785–799, 1978

Folkard S, Arendt J, Clark M: Can melatonin improve shift workers' tolerance of the night shift? Some preliminary findings. Chronobiol Int 10:315–320, 1993

Gordon NP, Cleary PD, Parlan CE, et al: The prevalence and health impact of shiftwork. Am J Public Health 76:1225–1228, 1986

Honma K, Honma S: A human phase response curve for bright light pulses. Japanese Journal of Psychiatry 42:167–168, 1988

Joffe RT, Moul DE, Lam RW, et al: Light visor treatment for seasonal affective disorder: a multicenter study. Psychiatry Res 46:29–39, 1993

Kern HE, Lewy AJ: Corrections and additions to the history of light therapy and seasonal affective disorder (letter). Arch Gen Psychiatry 47:90–91, 1990

Klein DC: Circadian rhythms in the pineal gland, in Comprehensive Endocrinology. Edited by Krieger DT. New York, Raven, 1979, pp 203–223

Klein DC, Weller JL: Rapid light-induced decrease in pineal N-acetyltransferase activity. Science 177:532–533, 1972

Knauth P, Rutenfranz J, Shultz H, et al: Experimental shift work studies of permanent night, and rapidly rotating, shift systems, II: behavior of various characteristics of sleep. Int Arch Occup Environ Health 46:111–125, 1980

Kripke DF: Phase-advance theories for affective illness, in Circadian Rhythms in Psychiatry. Edited by Wehr TA, Goodwin FK. Pacific Grove, CA, Boxwood Press, 1983, pp 41–69

Lafer B, Sachs GS, Labbate LA, et al: Phototherapy for seasonal affective disorder: a blind comparison of three different schedules. Am J Psychiatry 151:1081–1083, 1994

Lewy AJ: Treating chronobiologic sleep and mood disorders with bright light. Psychiatric Annals 17:664–669, 1987

Lewy AJ, Markey SP: Analysis of melatonin in human plasma by gas chromatography negative chemical ionization mass spectrometry. Science 201:741–743, 1978

Lewy AJ, Sack RL: The dim light melatonin onset (DLMO) as a marker for circadian phase position. Chronobiol Int 6:93–102, 1989

Lewy AJ, Wehr TA, Goodwin FK, et al: Light suppresses melatonin secretion in humans. Science 210:1267–1269, 1980

Lewy AJ, Wehr TA, Goodwin FK, et al: Manic-depressive patients may be supersensitive to light. Lancet 1:383–384, 1981

Lewy AJ, Kern HA, Rosenthal NE, et al: Bright artificial light treatment of a manic-depressive patient with a seasonal mood cycle. Am J Psychiatry 139:1496–1498, 1982

Lewy AJ, Sack RL, Fredrickson RH, et al: The use of bright light in the treatment of chronobiologic sleep and mood disorders: the phase-response curve. Psychopharmacol Bull 19:523–525, 1983

Lewy AJ, Sack RL, Singer CM: Assessment and treatment of chronobiologic disorders using plasma melatonin levels and bright light exposure: the clock-gate model and the phase response curve. Psychopharmacol Bull 20:561–565, 1984

Lewy AJ, Sack RL, Singer CM: Immediate and delayed effects of bright light on human melatonin production: shifting "dawn" and "dusk" shifts the dim light melatonin onset (DLMO). Ann N Y Acad Sci 453:253–259, 1985a

Lewy AJ, Sack RL, Singer CM: Melatonin, light and chronobiological disorders, in Photoperiodism, Melatonin and the Pineal. Edited by Evered D, Clark S. London, Pitman, 1985b, pp 231–252

Lewy AJ, Sack RL, Miller S, et al: Antidepressant and circadian phase-shifting effects of light. Science 235:352–354, 1987a

Lewy AJ, Sack RL, Singer CM, et al: The phase shift hypothesis for bright light's therapeutic mechanism of action: theoretical considerations and experimental evidence. Psychopharmacol Bull 23:349–353, 1987b

Lewy AJ, Ahmed S, Jackson JML, et al: Melatonin shifts circadian rhythms according to a phase-response curve. Chronobiol Int 9:380–392, 1992

McIntyre IM, Norman TR, Burrows GD, et al: Human melatonin suppression by light is intensity dependent. J Pineal Res 6:149–156, 1989

Minneman KP, Lynch H, Wurtman RJ: Relationship between environmental light intensity and retina-mediated suppression of rat pineal serotonin-N-acetyltransferase. Life Sci 15:1791–1796, 1974

Minors DS, Waterhouse JM, Wirz-Justice A: A human phase-response curve to light. Neurosci Lett 133:36–40, 1991

Moore-Ede MC, Richardson GS: Medical implications of shift work. Annu Rev Med 36:607–617, 1985

Oren DA, Moul DE, Schwartz PJ, et al: Exposure to ambient light in patients with winter seasonal affective disorder. Am J Psychiatry 151:591–593, 1994

Perlow MJ, Reppert SM, Tamarkin L, et al: Photic regulation of the melatonin rhythm: monkey and man are not the same. Brain Res 182:211–216, 1980

Petrie K, Conaglen JC, Thompson L, et al: Effect of melatonin on jet lag after long haul flights. BMJ 298:705–707, 1989

Petrie K, Dawson AG, Thompson L, et al: A double-blind trial of melatonin as a treatment for jet lag in international cabin crew. Biol Psychiatry 33:526–530, 1993

Rafferty B, Terman M, Terman JS, et al: Does morning light therapy prevent evening light effect? (abstract). Society for Light Treatment and Biological Rhythms Abstracts 2:18, 1990

Richter CP: Discovery of fire by man: its effect on his 24-hour clock and intellectual and cultural evolution. Johns Hopkins Medical Journal 141:47–61, 1977

Rollag MD, Niswender GD: Radioimmunoassay of serum concentrations of melatonin in sheep exposed to different lighting regimens. Endocrinology 98:482–489, 1976

Rosenthal NE, Sack DA, Gillin JC, et al: Seasonal affective disorder: a description of the syndrome and preliminary findings with light therapy. Arch Gen Psychiatry 41:72–80, 1984

Rosenthal NE, Moul DE, Hellekson CJ, et al: A multicenter study of the light visor for seasonal affective disorder: no difference in efficacy found between two different intensities. Neuropsychopharmacology 8:151–160, 1993

Sack RL, Lewy AJ, White DM, et al: Morning versus evening light treatment for winter depression: evidence that the therapeutic effects of light are mediated by circadian phase shifts. Arch Gen Psychiatry 47:343–351, 1990

Sack RL, Blood ML, Lewy AJ: Melatonin administration promotes circadian adaptation to night-shift work (abstract). Sleep Research 23:509, 1994

Sack RL, Blood ML, Lewy AJ: Melatonin administration to night-shift workers: an update (abstract). Sleep Research 24:539, 1995

Samel A, Wegmann HM, Vejvoda M, et al: Influence of melatonin treatment on human circadian rhythmicity before and after a simulated 9-hr time shift. J Biol Rhythms 6:235–248, 1991

Skene DJ, Aldhous ME, Arendt J: Melatonin, jet-lag and the sleep-wake cycle, in Sleep '88. Edited by Horne JA. New York, Gustav Fischer Verlag, 1989, pp 39–41

Tam EM, Lam RW, Levitt AJ: Treatment of seasonal affective disorder: a review. Can J Psychiatry 40:457–466, 1995

Tamarkin L, Reppert SM, Klein DC: Regulation of pineal melatonin in the Syrian hamster. Endocrinology 104:385–389, 1979

Tassi P, Pins D: Diurnal rhythmicity for visual sensitivity in humans? Chronobiol Int 14:35–48, 1997

Terman M, Terman JS: A multi-year controlled trial of bright light and negative ions. Society for Light Treatment and Biological Rhythms Abstracts 8:1, 1996

Terman M, Schlager D, Fairhurst S, et al: Dawn and dusk simulation as a therapeutic intervention. Biol Psychiatry 25:966–970, 1989a

Terman M, Terman JS, Quitkin FM, et al: Light therapy for seasonal affective disorder: a review of efficacy. Neuropsychopharmacology 2:1–22, 1989b

Terman M, Lewy AJ, Dijk DJ, et al: Light treatment for sleep disorders: consensus report, IV: sleep phase and duration disturbances. J Biol Rhythms 10:135–150, 1995

Thalén B-E, Kjellman BF, Mørkrid L, et al: Light treatment in seasonal and nonseasonal depression. Acta Psychiatr Scand 91:352–360, 1995

van Loon JH: Diurnal body temperature curves in shift workers. Ergonomics 6:267–273, 1963

Vaughan GM, Bell R, de la Peña A: Nocturnal plasma melatonin in humans: episodic pattern and influence of light. Neurosci Lett 14:81–84, 1979

Wehr TA, Rosenthal NE: In reply to: light therapy and the seasonal affective disorder (letter). Arch Gen Psychiatry 46:194–195, 1989

Wehr TA, Rosenthal NE: Reply to: corrections and additions to the history of light therapy and seasonal affective disorder (letter). Arch Gen Psychiatry 47:91, 1990

Wehr TA, Wirz-Justice A, Goodwin FK, et al: Phase advance of the circadian sleep-wake cycle as an antidepressant. Science 206:710–713, 1979

Weitzman ED, Czeisler CA, Coleman RM, et al: Delayed sleep phase syndrome: a chronobiological disorder with sleep-onset insomnia. Arch Gen Psychiatry 38:737–746, 1981

Wever RA: The Circadian System of Man: Results of Experiments Under Temporal Isolation. New York, Springer-Verlag, 1979

Wever RA: Light effects on human circadian rhythms: a review of recent Andechs experiments. J Biol Rhythms 4:161–186, 1989

Wever RA, Polasek J, Wildgruber C: Bright light affects human circadian rhythms. Pflugers Arch 396:85–87, 1983

Wirz-Justice A, Anderson J: Morning light exposure for the treatment of winter depression: the one true light therapy? Psychopharmacol Bull 26:511–520, 1990

Wirz-Justice A, Graw P, Kräuchi K, et al: Light therapy in seasonal affective disorder is independent of time of day or circadian phase. Arch Gen Psychiatry 50:929–937, 1993

Wirz-Justice A, Kräuchi K, Brunner DP, et al: Circadian rhythms and sleep regulation in seasonal affective disorder. Acta Neuropsychiatrica 7:41–43, 1995

Wirz-Justice A, Graw P, Kräuchi K, et al: Natural light treatment of seasonal affective disorder. J Affect Disord 37:109–120, 1996

Wurtman RJ, Axelrod J, Phillips LS: Melatonin synthesis in the pineal gland: control by light. Science 142:1071–1073, 1963

Chapter 5

Melatonin and Circadian Rhythms in Bipolar Mood Disorder

Aimee Mayeda, M.D., and
John I. Nurnberger Jr., M.D., Ph.D.

B ipolar mood disorder is marked by recurrent cycles of mania, depression, and normal mood. The cyclic nature of mood changes has prompted some investigators to suggest that mood disorders may be caused by disturbed circadian rhythms (Wehr et al. 1983). Several other clinical features of mood disorders lend support to this idea. Patients in both the manic and depressive states typically manifest profound disturbances in body functions that normally have circadian rhythms, including sleep, motor activity, appetite, and endocrine function.

Melatonin is secreted in a precise circadian rhythm. It appears to play a role in regulating other physiological rhythms in mammals (see Reiter, Chapter 1, and Bhatnagar, Chapter 2, in this volume). Investigations of disturbances in melatonin secretion in bipolar illness may shed light on the nature of this illness and its relationship to circadian rhythm disturbances.

Bipolar Disorder and Circadian Rhythm Disturbance

Many studies demonstrate disruptions of circadian rhythms in manic-depressive patients (Wehr et al. 1983). Depressive symptoms themselves frequently demonstrate a circadian rhythm, most severe in the early morning and almost absent in the evening. These findings suggest several hypotheses about the role circadian

105

rhythm disturbances play in bipolar illness, including internal desynchronization, phase advance, and genetic vulnerability.

Internal Desynchronization in Bipolar Illness

Bunney et al. (1972) and Sitaram et al. (1978) noted that bipolar patients showed a marked reduction in sleep on the night before they switched from depression into mania. Wehr and Goodwin (1980) noted that at the beginning of a manic episode, 9 of 10 manic-depressive patients had one or more 48-hour rest-activity cycles. Patients remained awake with no subjective sense of drowsiness for one to four alternate nights. The investigators were intrigued by the similarities between the rest-activity cycles of these patients and those of healthy subjects deprived of environmental time cues (zeitgebers) such as dawn, dusk, and social schedules.

Under normal conditions, the various circadian rhythms in the body are synchronized with each other and with the external dark-light cycle (Aschoff 1965). When healthy humans are deprived of zeitgebers, their rest-activity cycles and temperature cycles remain synchronized with a period near 25 hours for the first few weeks. For some subjects, however, the period of the rest-activity cycles lengthens to around 45 hours, whereas the period of the temperature cycle, which also appears to be coordinated with the cycles of rapid eye movement (REM) sleep and cortisol secretion, remains 25 hours. The result is "internal desynchronization." The two rhythms go in and out of phase, generating repeating 25-hour cycles occasionally interrupted by a 48-hour cycle. During the switch from short to long cycles, the subject may remain awake for 30 hours or more with no subjective drowsiness (Wever 1979).

Investigators have noted internal desynchronization in persons traveling across time zones and in shift workers (Arendt and Marks 1982). Jet lag or shift work can cause sleep disturbances with features of endogenous depression, such as weight loss, anorexia, irritability, and lack of energy (Akerstedt and Gillberg 1981; Arendt and Marks 1982). It is not clear why some workers adjust to changing shifts without difficulty, whereas others never adjust.

The similarity between the 48-hour cycles of bipolar patients at the beginning of a manic episode and those cycles in healthy subjects with internal desynchronization suggested that bipolar patients were internally desynchronized. Kripke et al. (1978) and others hypothesized that depression or mania results from beat phenomena generated when the two rhythms are in and out of phase.

Sleep-deprivation studies provided some support for the theory that internal desynchronization causes changes in mood states. Forty of 45 patients with major depression showed remission of depressive symptoms after sleep deprivation, with complete re-mission in 16 patients after a single night of sleep deprivation. Results were similar in a group of 12 bipolar patients (Pflug 1976). Wehr et al. (1982) asked nine rapid-cycling bipolar patients to simulate the 48-hour cycle of internal desynchronization by re-maining awake for 40 hours. Eight of the nine patients switched out of depression and seven developed mania or hypomania. In a number of patients, recovery sleep failed to reverse the hypo-manic state. Kripke et al. (1978) found further evidence consistent with this theory. They saw temperature rhythms in several bipolar patients in a normal environment advance earlier each day. This suggested that the period of their temperature rhythm was less than 24 hours. In some of these patients, lithium lengthened the period of the temperature rhythm, suggesting that lithium may prevent manic or depressed episodes by preventing internal desynchronization.

Some bipolar patients appear to have internal desynchroniza-tion, and at the time of a mood switch, their sleep-wake cycle mimics that of healthy subjects with internal desynchronization. However, evidence is lacking that temperature and sleep-wake cycles are desynchronized at the time of a mood switch. Wehr et al. (1985) saw no evidence for desynchronization of the two rhythms in a bipolar patient cycling rapidly between depression and mania. It is also not clear why internal desynchronization causes severe mood changes of mania and depression in bipolar patients but not in healthy subjects.

Phase Shift in Bipolar Disorder

Early morning awakening is a prominent feature of depression in some unipolar and bipolar patients. This finding has suggested to several investigators that the phase of the temperature-REM cycle was shifted earlier relative to the rest-activity cycle in these individuals. Wehr and Goodwin (1981) reviewed the evidence for phase advance in depression and found advances in several measures, including REM sleep, temperature, cortisol, and neurotransmitter metabolites.

Several studies have found similar phase advances in bipolar patients (Sack et al. 1987). Wehr et al. (1980) noted that patients who were either manic or depressed had a 3- to 6-hour advance in the peak of 3-methoxy-4-hydroxyphenylglycol (MHPG) secretion. Hartmann (1968) found a phase change in REM latency, the period from the time sleep begins until the time REM begins. In five of six bipolar patients, REM latency was state dependent: slightly increased in patients in the manic state and slightly decreased in patients in the depressed state. Four of seven bipolar patients spontaneously advanced their times of awakening as a depressive episode ended (Wehr et al. 1979).

Wehr et al. (1979) hypothesized that if the phase advance of the temperature-REM cycle relative to the rest-activity cycle was causing mood disorders, then changing sleep patterns to realign the phase of these cycles would restore normal mood. Several groups advanced the sleep period 5–6 hours in bipolar patients by altering their normal sleep period from 11 P.M.–7 A.M. to 5 P.M.–1 A.M. Many patients had remission of their depressive episodes, and the remissions lasted 1 week or more (see review in Sack et al. 1985, 1987). Partial sleep deprivation in the second half of the night was as effective an antidepressant as total sleep deprivation (Schilgen and Tolle 1980), whereas partial sleep deprivation in the first half of the night appeared to have little effect (see review in Sack et al. 1985). Partial sleep deprivation in the second half of the night is similar to phase advance of the sleep cycle in that both procedures cause a 5- to 6-hour advance in the time of awakening.

These studies suggest that bipolar patients have a phase advance of some cycles during the depressed state and perhaps a phase delay in manic states. Lewy et al. (1985) hypothesized that bipolar patients have increased sensitivity to light in the morning and that this caused the observed phase advance of circadian rhythms. However, most of the studies of phase advance have focused on unipolar patients. Phase advance of circadian cycles in bipolar patients in both the depressed and manic states needs further study.

Genetic Factors

Bipolar patients may have a genetic predisposition for disrupted circadian rhythms or increased susceptibility to mood disorder should circadian rhythm disruption occur. Internal desynchronization rarely precipitates severe affective changes such as mania or depression in healthy subjects. Ehlers et al. (1988) suggested that life events disrupt daily routines, causing circadian rhythm disruption, but whether this disruption leads to major depression depends on vulnerability factors such as genetic susceptibility.

There is evidence for a genetic diathesis, or predisposition, for bipolar disorder. On average, 25% of first-degree relatives of bipolar patients will have unipolar or bipolar illness at some point in their lives (see review in Nurnberger et al. 1994). Several putative major genes for bipolar mood disorder have been described in different sets of families: one linked to DNA markers on chromosome 18 (Berettini et al. 1994), one linked to DNA markers on chromosome 21 (Gurling et al. 1995; Straub et al. 1994), continuing evidence for a locus at p15 of chromosome 11 (Egeland et al. 1987; Kelsoe et al. 1989; Leboyer et al. 1990; Pauls et al. 1995), and one linked to markers on the X chromosome near Xq26 (Pekkarinen et al. 1995).

The nature of the genetic diathesis for bipolar disorder is unclear, but it may well include an abnormality in circadian rhythm regulation. Mutation studies have demonstrated that genetic factors determine circadian rhythms. "Clock mutants" have been identified in *Drosophila* and *Neurospora,* leading to the cloning of *frq, per,* and *tim* genes, which appear to play critical roles in circadian timing (Rosbash and Hall 1989; Sehgal et al. 1992, 1995). Ralph and Menaker (1988) found evidence that a mutation at a single autosomal locus caused a period of 20 hours in mutant golden hamsters. Autosomal mutations that cause changes in circadian period in mice include the *clock* locus on chromosome 5 (Vitaterna et al. 1994) and a region near the Mos locus on chromosome 4 (Nolan et al. 1995).

Studies in genetically defined mice have found evidence that multiple minor genes called quantitative trait loci (QTL) together determine features of circadian rhythms, including both period and response to light (Hofstetter et al. 1995; Mayeda et al. 1996). These studies have identified regions of the mouse chromosome that may determine the response of the mouse circadian system to light. It is of interest that lithium appears to modify circadian rhythms of motor activity and their light-responsiveness in C57BL/6J and DBA/2J mice (A. Mayeda and J. Hofstetter, unpublished data, 1997).

Genetic factors also influence melatonin secretion. Wetterberg et al. (1983) studied urinary melatonin in a group of 107 humans from 23 nuclear families. Complex segregation analysis showed that melatonin production may be regulated by an additive major gene (see Wetterberg, Chapter 3, in this volume).

Susceptibility to rhythm disruption also appears to have a genetic component. Ralph and Menaker (1988) noted that although wild-type hamsters cannot entrain if their endogenous and entraining cycle periods differ by more than an hour, many clock mutants could entrain to cycles different by 2 hours or more from their internal clock.

The nature of the genetic diathesis for bipolar disorder is unclear; it may involve an increased susceptibility to disruption of circadian rhythms. Animal data suggest that a predisposition to disrupted rhythms can be inherited. In addition, bipolar patients may have a genetic susceptibility to mood changes when circadian rhythms are disrupted. Certain shift workers seem to be more vulnerable than others to mood changes associated with circadian rhythm disruption. Bipolar patients may be especially vulnerable. Wehr et al. (1982) noted that rapid-cycling bipolar patients are more sensitive to the antidepressant effects of sleep deprivation than unipolar depressed patients. Kripke et al. (1978) suggested that bipolar patients have a genetic predisposition that causes desynchronization to be exacerbated once it occurs (Healy 1987; Healy and Waterhouse 1995).

Melatonin Secretion in Bipolar Illness

Most of the studies that have examined melatonin levels in patients with mood disorders have focused on patients with unipolar depression (see Wetterberg, Chapter 3; Lewy et al., Chapter 4; and Shafii and Shafii, Chapter 7, in this volume). Interindividual variation in melatonin secretion and single-time-point melatonin measurements complicated analysis of these studies. A low level of melatonin at a single time point can result from either a phase shift or a change in amplitude. Thompson et al. (1988) noted that many published studies had not tested for possible covariates that might affect melatonin secretion, such as age, sex, menstrual status, season of testing, height, and weight. However, more recent studies have considered these covariates (see Wetterberg, Chapter 3; Brown et al., Chapter 6; and Shafii and Shafii, Chapter 7, in this volume).

Psychoactive drugs also cause changes in melatonin secretion. Lithium treatment in rats causes a decrease in amplitude and a phase shift in melatonin secretion (Seggie and Werstiuk 1985; Yocca et al. 1983). Lithium administration tended to reduce the overnight melatonin secretion in bipolar patients compared with control subjects; however, the difference was not statistically significant (Grof et al. 1985). Antidepressant drugs have both increased and decreased melatonin secretion in humans (Miles and Philbrick 1988).

Investigations of melatonin secretion in bipolar disorder have included measurement of melatonin levels, phase shift of the melatonin secretion curve, and light suppression of melatonin secretion.

Melatonin Amplitude in Patients With Mood Disorder

In studies that focused on the amplitude of melatonin levels in bipolar patients, Beck-Friis et al. (1985b) studied 12 euthymic bipolar patients along with 12 euthymic unipolar patients, 30 acutely ill unipolar depressive patients, and 33 control subjects. The euthymic bipolar patients had significantly lower maximum melatonin levels than the control subjects. Euthymic unipolar depressive patients and acutely ill unipolar patients with abnormal dexamethasone suppression tests also showed low maximal melatonin levels. The authors hypothesized that low melatonin levels were a trait marker for the subgroup of depressed patients with abnormalities of the hypothalamic-pituitary-adrenal axis (see Wetterberg, Chapter 3, in this volume). Souetre et al. (1989) found reduced amplitude of melatonin in 11 depressed bipolar patients and normalization of amplitude with recovery. Lewy et al. (1979) found increased melatonin secretion during both day and night in four manic bipolar patients: 24-hour melatonin secretion was twice that of unmatched control subjects. Three of four had diminished melatonin secretion when they were depressed. From this finding, Lewy et al. (1985) hypothesized that the amplitude of melatonin secretion is state dependent and reflects central nervous system (CNS) β-adrenergic function. Kennedy et al. (1989) found a twofold increase in melatonin in a single manic bipolar patient compared with her melatonin levels in euthymia and depression. However, Leibenluft et al. (1993) found no consistent differences in melatonin amplitude in the hypomanic compared with the depressed state in nine patients with rapid-cycling bipolar disorder. The hypothesis of Lewy et al. (1985) is consistent with the studies of melatonin secretion amplitude in unipolar depressive patients, in whom the trend for decreased melatonin in depressed patients is striking. In 9 of 11 patient groups studied, depressed patients have lower than normal amplitude of melatonin secretion (Beck-Friis et al. 1985b; Boyce 1985; Branchey et al. 1982; Brown et al. 1985; Claustrat et al. 1984; Mendlewicz et al. 1979; Nair et al. 1984; Wetterberg 1983; Wirz-Justice and Arendt 1979). Two studies showed no difference (Jimerson et al. 1977;

Thompson et al. 1988) (see also Wetterberg, Chapter 3, and Shafii and Shafii, Chapter 7, in this volume).

Taken together, these data suggest that the amplitude of melatonin secretion is state dependent in bipolar patients, as Lewy et al. (1985) hypothesized. However, more data, especially on patients in the manic state, are needed to confirm this hypothesis.

Phase Shift in the Melatonin Cycle

Current evidence suggests that phase of melatonin secretion may vary systematically with mood changes in bipolar disorder. In a group of nine patients with rapid-cycling bipolar disorder, Leibenluft et al. (1993) found that the onset of nocturnal melatonin secretion was about 90 minutes earlier in the hypomanic compared with the depressed state. Lewy et al. (1979) found that the phase of maximum melatonin secretion was advanced in four manic patients relative to control subjects. They also noted that one subject had her peak melatonin secretion during the day, 180° out of phase with control subjects. During this time, her activity-rest cycle was completely disorganized, and she napped sporadically both day and night. When her melatonin secretion pattern was in phase with the light-dark cycle, her activity-rest cycle was relatively normal. However, Kennedy et al. (1989) did not find evidence of phase shift in either the melatonin or cortisol rhythm in a bipolar patient studied in manic, depressed, and euthymic conditions.

Leibenluft et al. (1995) examined the effect of bright light treatment on mood in nine patients with rapid-cycling bipolar disorder. Bright light can shift the phase of melatonin rhythms, with morning light shifting rhythms earlier and evening light shifting rhythms later (Minors et al. 1991). Bright light in the morning should thus advance the melatonin rhythms to the phase position found in hypomania. In fact, morning bright light caused several of the patients to cycle more dramatically. Midday bright light, however, appeared to stabilize mood in three of five patients. One explanation for this stabilization may be that midday bright light increases the amplitude of nocturnal melatonin secretion, thus making the rhythm less susceptible to phase shifts.

A subsequent study examined the effects of oral melatonin on rapid-cycling bipolar patients. Preliminary results suggest that 5–10 mg of melatonin given orally at 10 P.M. stabilizes mood (E. Leibenluft, personal communication, June 1996). The investigators hypothesize that nocturnal oral melatonin, like midday bright light, stabilizes the phase of the melatonin rhythm in these patients. These two studies suggest that circadian interventions may in the future be useful treatments for bipolar disorder.

Nocturnal Light-Suppression Studies

When humans are exposed to light during the night, melatonin secretion decreases within 30–60 minutes. The brighter the light, the greater the observed decline in plasma melatonin levels (Lewy et al. 1980). The intensity of ordinary room light is usually 200–300 lux and rarely over 500 lux, whereas the intensity of sunlight on a sunny afternoon is 100,000 lux (Lewy 1983). Several studies suggest that manic-depressive patients and their relatives have increased sensitivity to the melatonin-suppressing effects of light.

Lewy et al. (1981) reported that four bipolar patients had 50% suppression of plasma melatonin levels when exposed to 500 lux of light at 2 A.M. and almost complete suppression of melatonin when exposed to 1,500 lux. In six healthy, sex-matched control subjects, there was no suppression of melatonin when they were exposed to 500 lux and only 40% suppression in two control subjects who were exposed to 1,500 lux. Two of the bipolar patients were manic and two were depressed at the time of the study (Lewy et al. 1985).

In follow-up studies, 15 euthymic bipolar patients and 26 control subjects were evaluated (Lewy et al. 1985; Nurnberger et al. 1988), and supersensitivity to light in well-state bipolar patients was demonstrated. Five hundred lux of light decreased melatonin levels 62% on average for the 11 patients and 18% for the 24 control subjects in the first study (Lewy et al. 1985). Taken together with the earlier data from acutely ill bipolar patients, this finding suggested that augmented melatonin suppression was a trait marker for bipolar disorder.

A study of high-risk offspring of bipolar patients (Nurnberger et al. 1988) showed parallels between suppression of melatonin by

500 lux of light and risk of mood disorder. Patients with two ill parents had on average 73% suppression of melatonin, whereas patients with one ill parent had 57% suppression and control subjects had 45% suppression. The risk of mood disorder paralleled the percentage of melatonin suppression in five groups of subjects: psychiatrically screened control subjects, unscreened control subjects, patients with one parent ill, patients with two parents ill, and bipolar patients.

However, the findings of Lewy et al. (1985) were not replicated in a study of 15 drug-free euthymic bipolar patients (Whalley et al. 1991), nor were they replicated in acutely ill bipolar patients studied by Lam et al. (1990). There were some differences in methodology and subject population in these latter studies, but they did cast doubt on the generalizability of the finding.

At Indiana University, we have further examined light suppression in humans. First, we developed a sensitive and cost-efficient radioimmunoassay employing a column separation of plasma in combination with an antibody from Guildhay (Lahiri et al. 1993, 1994). Then we replicated light-suppression findings in healthy control subjects, showing a clear dose-response effect but no significant effects of posture or sleep (A. R. Mayeda et al., unpublished observations, 1996). We also demonstrated a lack of correlation between the effect of light and the effect of propranolol, suggesting that other factors besides β-adrenergic blockade are responsible for the light-suppression response. Our clinical procedures employed an indirect lighting design that minimizes the effect of behavioral variation (subjects are effectively exposed to a hemisphere of 500 lux light). We measured melatonin secretion in subjects on a dark night and a light-exposure night to control for circadian effects on melatonin secretion.

In this paradigm, control subjects showed suppression comparable to the range in our previous studies (Lewy et al. 1985; Nurnberger et al. 1988). Unipolar patients in the well state and off medications were not different from control subjects. Bipolar patients as a group did not show a significant increase in light suppression. However, the most severely ill bipolar I patients (in the well state and off medications) showed a trend to increased suppression (J. I. Nurnberger et al., unpublished observations, 1997). It is also notable that the subgroup of bipolar patients off lithium for more than 5 weeks ($N = 10$) showed significantly greater suppression than those off lithium for shorter periods ($N = 11$).

Taken together, the available data suggest reasons for continuing interest in light-suppression studies in bipolar illness. Behavioral variation among subjects exposed to light may be an important factor to control in studies of psychiatric populations. Recent studies suggest that diet and exercise may also be pertinent (Van Reeth et al. 1994; Zimmermann et al. 1993). The influence of lithium and other medications may be more potent than previously realized. Yet there is continuing reason to suspect that at least a subgroup of bipolar patients has circadian rhythm abnormalities manifest as an increased melatonin response to light. We are now attempting to identify the subgroup of patients most susceptible to circadian rhythm disruption in ongoing clinical studies.

The nature of the hypothesized vulnerability leading to hypersensitivity to light requires further clarification. The inhibitory effects of light on the suprachiasmatic nucleus (SCN) may be mediated by nicotinic cholinergic mechanisms; the hypersensitivity of these receptors in bipolar patients is possible. The projections from the superior cervical ganglion to the pineal gland, which stimulate melatonin production, are β-adrenergic; α-adrenergic receptors are also critical at the level of the pineal. GABA-ergic and glutamatergic influences on this pathway also have now been identified (see Reiter, Chapter 1, in this volume).

Buchsbaum et al. (1973) demonstrated greater rates of increased amplitude of average evoked responses to increasing intensities of light (augmentation) in bipolar patients, whether in the depressed or manic phase. Although another mechanism may mediate this phenomenon, these data indicate bipolar patients have increased sensitivity to light, which mediates increased melatonin suppression.

Summary

Patients with bipolar mood disorder have abnormalities of their circadian rhythms—the physiological and behavioral variations that recur daily and coordinate internal physiological events with the environment. At the beginning of a manic episode, certain patients have one or more 48-hour sleep-wake cycles (Wehr and Goodwin 1980), and some have temperature cycles that advance earlier every day (Kripke et al. 1978).

Experimentally manipulating the circadian rhythms of bipolar patients can cause mood changes. A number of rapid-cycling bipolar patients deprived of sleep for one night switched out of depression and developed mania (Wehr et al. 1982). Advancing the sleep period has been an effective antidepressant in bipolar patients (Sack et al. 1987).

Melatonin secretion and bipolar mood disorder seem to be subject to genetic control. A genetic predisposition for bipolar mood disorder may involve increased susceptibility to circadian rhythm disruption or susceptibility to changes in mood after rhythm disruption. This susceptibility may involve increased sensitivity to light in some subgroups of patients (Lewy et al. 1985; J. I. Nurnberger et al., unpublished observations, 1997). Melatonin secretion continues to be a useful tool for investigating the genetic vulnerability to bipolar disorder.

Melatonin secretion is under circadian control but is abnormal in some bipolar patients. Peak melatonin may be state dependent: decreased in depressed and euthymic states and increased in mania (Beck-Friis et al. 1985a; Lewy et al. 1979). The phase of melatonin secretion may be abnormal in bipolar patients (Leibenluft et al. 1993; Lewy et al. 1979). Both midday bright light and nocturnal oral melatonin appear to stabilize mood in patients with rapid-cycling bipolar disorder, possibly by stabilizing the phase of the melatonin rhythm (E. Leibenluft, personal communication, June 1996; Leibenluft et al. 1993). Circadian interventions may become useful treatments for bipolar disorder.

References

Akerstedt T, Gillberg M: Sleep disturbances and shift work. Advances in Bioscience 3:127–137, 1981

Arendt J, Marks V: Physiologic changes underlying jet lag. British Medical Journal (Clinical Research Edition) 284:144–146, 1982

Aschoff J: Circadian rhythms in man. Science 148:1427–1432, 1965

Beck-Friis J, Kjellman BF, Ljungren J-G, et al: The pineal gland and melatonin in affective disorders, in Advances in the Biosciences, Vol 53: The Pineal Gland: Endocrine Aspects. Edited by Brown GM, Wainwright SD. Oxford, England, Pergamon, 1985a

Beck-Friis J, Kjellman BF, Aperia B, et al: Serum melatonin in relation to clinical variables in patients with major depressive disorder and a hypothesis of a low melatonin syndrome. Acta Psychiatr Scand 71:319–330, 1985b

Berettini WH, Ferraro TN, Goldin LR, et al: Chromosome 18 DNA markers and manic-depressive illness: evidence for a susceptibility gene. Proc Natl Acad Sci U S A 91:5918–5921, 1994

Boyce PM: 6-Sulphatoxymelatonin in melancholia. Am J Psychiatry 142:125–127, 1985

Branchey L, Weinberg U, Branchey M, et al: Simultaneous study of 24-hour patterns of melatonin and cortisol secretion in depressed patients. Neuropsychobiology 8:225–232, 1982

Brown R, Kocsis JH, Caroff S, et al: Differences in nocturnal melatonin secretion between melancholic depressed patients and control subjects. Am J Psychiatry 142:811–816, 1985

Bunney WE, Murphy DL, Goodwin FK, et al: The "switch process" in manic-depressive illness. Arch Gen Psychiatry 27:295–302, 1972

Buchsbaum M, Landau S, Murphy D, et al: Average evoked response in bipolar and unipolar affective disorders: relationship to sex, age of onset, and monoamine oxidase. Biol Psychiatry 7:199–212, 1973

Claustrat B, Chazot G, Brun J, et al: A chronological study of melatonin and cortisol secretion in depressed subjects: plasma melatonin, a biochemical marker in major depression. Biol Psychiatry 19:1215–1228, 1984

Egeland JA, Gerhard DS, Pauls DL, et al: Bipolar affective disorders linked to DNA markers on chromosome 11. Nature 315:783–787, 1987

Ehlers CL, Frank E, Kupfer DJ: Social zeitgebers and biological rhythms. Arch Gen Psychiatry 45:948–952, 1988

Grof E, Grof P, Brown GM, et al: Investigations of melatonin secretion in man. Prog Neuropsychopharmacol Biol Psychiatry 9:609–612, 1985

Gurling H, Smyth C, Kalsi G, et al: Linkage findings in bipolar disorder (letter). Nat Genet 10:8–9, 1995

Hartmann E: Longitudinal studies of sleep and dream patterns in manic-depressive patients. Arch Gen Psychiatry 19:312–329, 1968

Healy D: Rhythm and blues: neurochemical, neuropharmacological and neuropsychological implications of a hypothesis of circadian rhythm dysfunction in the affective disorders. Psychopharmacology (Berl) 93:271–285, 1987

Healy D, Waterhouse JM: The circadian system and the therapeutics of the affective disorders. Pharmacol Ther 65:241–263, 1995

Hofstetter JR, Mayeda AR, Possidente B, et al: Quantitative trait loci (QTL) for circadian rhythms of locomotor activity in mice. Behav Genet 25:545–556, 1995

Jimerson DC, Lynch HJ, Post RM, et al: Urinary melatonin rhythms during sleep deprivation in depressed patients and normals. Life Sci 20:1501–1508, 1977

Kelsoe JR, Ginns EI, Egeland JA, et al: Re-evaluation of the linkage relationship between chromosome 11p loci and the gene for bipolar affective disorder in Old Order Amish. Nature 342:238–243, 1989

Kennedy SH, Tighe S, McVey G, et al: Melatonin and cortisol switches during mania, depression, and euthymia in a drug-free bipolar patient. J Nerv Ment Dis 177:300–303, 1989

Kripke DF, Mullaney DJ, Atkinson M, et al: Circadian rhythm disorders in manic-depressives. Biol Psychiatry 13:335–350, 1978

Lahiri DK, Davis D, Adkins M, et al: Factors that influence radioimmunoassay of human plasma melatonin: a modified column procedure to eliminate interference. Biochemical Medicine and Metabolic Biology 49:36–50, 1993

Lahiri DK, Davis D, Nurnberger JI Jr: Melatonin-like immunoreactivity in the presence of different chemicals as determined by the radioimmunoassay. Biochemical Medicine and Metabolic Biology 51:51–54, 1994

Lam RW, Berkowitz AL, Berga SL, et al: Melatonin suppression in bipolar and unipolar mood disorders. Psychiatry Res 33:129–143, 1990

Leboyer M, Malafosse A, Boularand S, et al: Tyrosine hydroxylase polymorphisms associated with manic-depressive illness (letter). Lancet 335:1219, 1990

Leibenluft E, Schwartz PJ, Turner EH, et al: State-dependent changes in pineal and thyroid axis function in patients with rapid-cycling bipolar disorder, in Proceedings of the 32nd Annual Meeting of the American College of Neuropsychopharmacology, 1993, p 184

Leibenluft E, Turner EH, Feldman-Naim S, et al: Light therapy in patients with rapid cycling bipolar disorder: preliminary results. Psychopharmacol Bull 31:705–710, 1995

Lewy AJ: Biochemistry and regulation of mammalian melatonin production, in The Pineal Gland. Edited by Relkin R. New York, Elsevier, 1983, pp 77–128

Lewy AJ, Wehr TA, Gold PW, et al: Plasma melatonin in manic-depressive illness, in Catecholamines: Basic and Clinical Frontiers, Vol 2. Edited by Usdin E, Kopin IJ, Barchas J. New York, Pergamon, 1979

Lewy AJ, Wehr TA, Goodwin FK, et al: Light suppresses melatonin secretion in humans. Science 210:1267–1269, 1980

Lewy AJ, Wehr TA, Goodwin FK, et al: Manic-depressive patients may be supersensitive to light. Lancet 1:383–384, 1981

Lewy AJ, Nurnberger JI, Wehr TA, et al: Supersensitivity to light: possible trait marker for manic-depressive illness. Am J Psychiatry 142:725–727, 1985

Mayeda AR, Hofstetter JR, Belknap JK, et al: Hypothesized quantitative trait loci (QTL) for circadian period of locomotor activity in CXB RI strains of mice. Behav Genet 26:505–511, 1996

Mendlewicz J, Linkowski P, Branchey L, et al: Abnormal 24 hour pattern of melatonin secretion in depression (letter). Lancet 2:1362, 1979

Miles A, Philbrick DRS: Melatonin and psychiatry. Biol Psychiatry 23:405–425, 1988

Minors D, Waterhouse JM, Wirz-Justice A: A human phase-response curve to light. Neurosci Lett 133:36–40, 1991

Nair NPV, Hariharasubramanian N, Pilapil C: Circadian rhythm of plasma melatonin in endogenous depression. Prog Neuropsychopharmacol Biol Psychiatry 8:715–718, 1984

Nolan PM, Sollars PJ, Bohne BA, et al: Heterozygosity mapping of partially congenic lines: mapping of a semidominant neurological mutation, Wheels (Wh1), on mouse chromosome 4. Genetics 140:245–254, 1995

Nurnberger JI Jr, Berrettini W, Tamarkin L, et al: Supersensitivity to melatonin suppression by light in young people at high risk for affective disorder. Neuropsychopharmacology 1:217–223, 1988

Nurnberger JI Jr, Goldin LR, Gershon ES: Genetics of psychiatric disorders, in The Medical Basis of Psychiatry. Edited by Winokur G, Clayton PJ. Philadelphia, WB Saunders, 1994

Pauls DL, Ott J, Paul SM, et al: Linkage analyses of chromosome 18 markers do not identify a major susceptibility locus for bipolar affective disorder in the Old Order Amish. Am J Hum Genet 57:636–643, 1995

Pekkarinen P, Terwilliger J, Bredbacka P-E, et al: Evidence of a predisposing locus to bipolar disorder on Xq24-q27.1 in an extended Finnish pedigree. Genome Res 5:105–115, 1995

Pflug B: The effect of sleep deprivation on depressed patients. Acta Psychiatr Scand 53:148–158, 1976

Ralph MR, Menaker M: A mutation of the circadian system in golden hamsters. Science 241:1225–1227, 1988

Rosbach M, Hall JC: The molecular biology of circadian rhythms. Neuron 3:387–398, 1989

Sack DA, Nurnberger JI, Rosenthal NE, et al: Potentiation of antidepressant medications by phase advance of the sleep-wake cycle. Am J Psychiatry 142:606–608, 1985

Sack DA, Rosenthal NE, Parry BL, et al: Biological rhythms in psychiatry, in Psychopharmacology, The Third Generation of Progress. Edited by Meltzer HY. New York, Raven, 1987, pp 669–685

Schilgen B, Tolle R: Partial sleep deprivation as therapy for depression. Arch Gen Psychiatry 37:267–271, 1980

Seggie J, Werstiuk ES: Lithium and melatonin rhythms: implications for depression, in Advances in the Biosciences, Vol 53: The Pineal Gland: Endocrine Aspects. Edited by Brown GM, Wainwright SD. Oxford, England, Pergamon, 1985, pp 333–338

Sehgal A, Man B, Price JL: New clock mutations in *Drosophila*. Ann N Y Acad Sci 618:1–10, 1992

Sehgal A, Rothenfluh-Hilfiker A, Hunter-Ensor M, et al: Rhythmic expression of *timeless:* a basis for promoting circadian cycles in *period* gene autoregulation. Science 270:808–810, 1995

Sitaram N, Gillin JC, Bunney WE: The switch process in manic-depressive illness. Acta Psychiatr Scand 58:267–278, 1978

Souetre E, Salvati E, Belugou JL, et al: Circadian rhythms in depression and recovery: evidence for blunted amplitude as the main chronological abnormality. Psychiatry Res 28:263–278, 1989

Straub RE, Lehner T, Luo T, et al: A possible vulnerability locus for bipolar affective disorder on chromosome 21q22.3. Nat Genet 8:291–296, 1994

Thompson C, Franey C, Arendt J, et al: A comparison of melatonin secretion in depressed patients and normal subjects. Br J Psychiatry 152:260–265, 1988

Van Reeth O, Sturis J, Byrne MM, et al: Nocturnal exercise phase delays circadian rhythms of and thyrotropin secretion in normal men. Am J Physiol 266:E964–E974, 1994

Vitaterna MH, King DP, Chang A-M, et al: Mutagenesis and mapping of a mouse gene *clock* essential for circadian behavior. Science 264:719–725, 1994

Wehr TA, Goodwin FK: Desynchronization of circadian rhythms as a possible source of manic-depressive cycles. Psychopharmacol Bull 16:19–20, 1980

Wehr TA, Goodwin FK: Biological rhythms in psychiatry, in American Handbook of Psychiatry. Edited by Arieti S, Brodie HKH. New York, Basic Books, 1981, pp 46–67

Wehr TA, Wirz-Justice A, Goodwin FK, et al: Phase advance of the circadian sleep-wake cycle as an antidepressant. Science 206:710–713, 1979

Wehr TA, Muscettola G, Goodwin FK: Urinary 3-methoxy-4-hydroxyphenylglycol circadian rhythm. Arch Gen Psychiatry 37:257–263, 1980

Wehr TA, Goodwin FK, Wirz-Justice A, et al: 48-hour sleep-wake cycles in manic-depressive illness. Arch Gen Psychiatry 39:559–565, 1982

Wehr TA, Sack D, Rosenthal N, et al: Circadian rhythm disturbances in manic-depressive illness. Federal Proceedings 42:2809–2813, 1983

Wehr TA, Sack DA, Duncan WC, et al: Sleep and circadian rhythms in affective patients isolated from time cues. Psychiatry Res 15:327–339, 1985

Wetterberg L: The relationship between the pineal gland and the pituitary-adrenal axis in health, endocrine and psychiatric conditions. Psychoneuroendocrinology 8:75–80, 1983

Wetterberg L, Iselius L, Lindsten J: Genetic regulation of melatonin excretion in urine. Clin Genet 24:399–402, 1983

Wever RA: The Circadian System of Man: Results of Experiments Under Temporal Isolation. New York, Springer-Verlag, 1979

Whalley LJ, Perini T, Shering A, et al: Melatonin response to bright light in recovered, drug-free, bipolar patients. Psychiatry Res 38:13–19, 1991

Wirz-Justice A, Arendt J: Diurnal, menstrual cycle and seasonal indole rhythms in man and their modification in affective disorders, in Biological Psychiatry Today. Edited by Obiols J, Ballus C, Gonzalez Monclus E, et al. Amsterdam, Elsevier, 1979

Yocca FD, Lynch V, Friedman E: Effect of chronic lithium treatment on rat pineal rhythms: N-acetyltransferase, N-acetylserotonin and melatonin. J Pharmacol Exp Ther 226:733–737, 1983

Zimmermann RC, McDougle CJ, Schumacher M, et al: Effects of acute tryptophan depletion on nocturnal melatonin secretion in humans. J Clin Endocrinol Metab 76:1160–1164, 1993

Chapter 6

Melatonin in Eating and Panic Disorders

Gregory M. Brown, M.D., Ph.D., M.R.C.C.,
Richard P. Swinson, M.D., F.R.C.P.C., and
Sidney H. Kennedy, M.D., F.R.C.P.C.

Pineal function is of considerable interest in eating and panic disorders for several reasons: frequent comorbidity of eating disorders with panic disorder, pointing to a possible common etiology; increased output of melatonin in panic disorder, in acutely starving patients with anorexia nervosa and in acutely bingeing and purging patients with bulimia nervosa; and alterations of sympathetic nervous system regulation, along with a wide variety of other neuroendocrine abnormalities in these disorders. Pineal and neuroendocrine changes may be secondary to changes in neurotransmitter regulation, particularly regarding norepinephrine, serotonin, and opioids.

Epidemiological Aspects of Panic and Eating Disorders

Mood disorders, anxiety disorders, and substance use disorders are prevalent (Offord et al. 1994; Regier et al. 1990). A person who suffers from one mental disorder is at increased risk of suffering from at least one other mental disorder (Kessler et al. 1994). We will examine the relationships of eating disorders and panic disorder using data from population-based surveys, clinical sample comparisons, and symptom-structure investigations. Unfortunately, eating disorders have been omitted from examination in some recent large population-based studies, and subtypes of anxiety disorders have been omitted in others, although panic disorder has been reported in all.

Population-Based Surveys

Offord et al. (1994) reported the prevalence of mood disorders, eating disorders, alcohol and substance use disorders, and some of the anxiety disorders in the province of Ontario. Anxiety disorders without obsessive-compulsive disorder had the highest lifetime prevalence, followed by mood disorders. Details of the findings on eating disorders have been described by Garfinkel et al. (1995). Bulimia nervosa occurred almost exclusively in females, with a lifetime prevalence of 1.1% of the total female sample as compared with 2.6% for panic disorder. The purging subtype of bulimia nervosa was found to be associated with higher rates of comorbidity than the nonpurging subtype (Garfinkel et al. 1996).

Eating disorders and anxiety disorders both have their peak of onset in adolescence or early adulthood (Lewinsohn et al. 1993). Approximately 10% of subjects studied met diagnostic criteria for current mental disorder, and 33% had experienced a disorder at some time in their lives. Individuals found to have eating disorders had significantly increased rates of mood and anxiety disorders, but the specific relationship with panic disorder was not reported.

The lifetime prevalence for narrowly defined bulimia nervosa was 2.8% and 5.7% for possible bulimia nervosa in a population study of 2,163 female twins (Kendler et al. 1991). In individuals with bulimia nervosa, the occurrence of lifetime major depression is 51.2% and of panic disorder is 8.9%. The odds ratios for the co-occurrence of these disorders were statistically significant.

Further study in female twins using broad diagnostic definitions for bulimia nervosa and panic disorder revealed distinct effects of genetic, family environment, and individual-specific environmental factors for comorbidity (Kendler et al. 1995). Two genetic factors were found: the first loaded on phobia, panic disorder, and bulimia nervosa and the second on generalized anxiety disorder and alcoholism. A single familial-environmental factor identified loaded substantially only for bulimia nervosa. Three groups had varying degrees of genetic loading: bulimia nervosa, generalized anxiety disorder, and phobia had modest loading, major depression and panic disorder had moderate loading, and alcoholism had the highest loading. Bulimia nervosa and phobia received the genetic loading from the first factor and major depression mostly from the second factor. The data point to the possibility of a shared genetically mediated basis for phobia, panic disorder, and bulimia nervosa. Major depression was most strongly related to generalized anxiety disorder but not to panic disorder or bulimia nervosa. These data have to be interpreted cautiously, given the diagnostic criteria used for both panic disorder and bulimia nervosa.

Clinically Based Samples

Direct comparison of females with bulimia nervosa, panic disorder, and other eating and anxiety disorders revealed high levels of comorbidity between bulimia nervosa and anxiety disorders (Schwalberg et al. 1992) but not specifically panic disorder. A comorbid diagnosis of an anxiety disorder was found in 75% of bulimia nervosa subjects and in 63.6% of obese binge eaters. Panic disorder had a lifetime incidence of 10% and 13.6%, respectively, in the two eating disorders groups. In most cases, anxiety disorders had an onset before the eating disorder. No data from this study support a specific relationship between panic disorder and bulimia nervosa.

Within the eating disorders, various subtypes have different rates of comorbidity with other disorders (Laessle et al. 1989). Rates of lifetime comorbidity of bulimia nervosa were consistent across several subgroups and were higher than in restricting anorexia nervosa. Panic disorder occurred in 4%–11% of the subgroups. In 69 patients in New York (Fornari et al. 1992), 46% of anorexia nervosa patients had at least one lifetime anxiety disorder. In the other eating disorders groups, rates for mood and anxiety disorders were not significantly different. The rate of comorbidity for panic disorder was not reported separately.

Hudson et al. (1983a) reported a lifetime prevalence for panic disorder of 40% in an eating disorders population, whereas Piran et al. (1985) reported that 53% of bulimia nervosa patients had a lifetime history of panic disorder compared with 43% of anorexia nervosa subjects. In a study by S. Z. Yanovski et al. (1993), 34% of obese male and female subjects with binge-eating disorders had increased rates for lifetime major depression, panic disorder, and bulimia nervosa.

Follow-Up Studies

In a 10-year follow-up of 62 female anorexia nervosa patients, Halmi et al. (1991) reported that panic disorder was no more common than in the control population. In a 6-year follow-up study, Smith et al. (1993) reported that 43% of females with adolescent-onset anorexia nervosa continued to have eating disorders. Panic disorder was current in 17% of that group. There was considerable overlap for mood, eating, and anxiety disorders, with 17% of subjects meeting criteria for all three disorders. In another follow-up study of anorexia nervosa patients, 32% were still symptomatic (Toner et al. 1988). The lifetime prevalence of panic disorder was 40% among the symptomatic subjects, and 40% reported panic disorder in the past year. The majority with anxiety disorder developed panic disorder before onset of the eating disorder.

No cases of eating disorders were found by Kasvikis et al. (1986) in 83 female agoraphobic subjects. Caution must be taken in interpreting these data because no cases of bulimia nervosa were identified in the samples. Indirect evidence of a relationship between panic disorder and eating disorders has been investigated through the occurrence of mitral valve prolapse in the two diagnostic groups. The original finding of a close association between panic disorder and mitral valve prolapse was not strongly supported (Magraf et al. 1988). A direct comparison study of the frequency of mitral valve prolapse in patients with bulimia nervosa, anorexia nervosa, panic disorder, and control subjects showed that the patient groups had twice the rate of mitral valve prolapse of the control subjects and that the highest rates were in the anxious bulimia nervosa subjects (Kaplan et al. 1991).

Data from these clinical studies show that eating disorders and anxiety disorders are frequently comorbid. Genetic data point to a possible common etiological basis of panic disorder and eating disorders.

Pineal Function and Anorexia Nervosa

Although anorexia nervosa is believed to be multidetermined, involving psychological, social, and biological factors, there is conclusive evidence that the disorder is associated with a disturbance in hypothalamic function. Whether this disturbance is a consequence of starvation or a potential causative factor has been a source of ongoing debate (G. H. Anderson and Kennedy 1992). The relationship between melatonin and chronic low weight, mood disorder, reproductive function, and potential disruption of the sympathetic nervous system has been examined. A number of investigators have reported normal nocturnal melatonin profiles in anorexia nervosa (Baranowska et al. 1986; Bearn et al. 1988; Dalery et al. 1985; Kennedy et al. 1989). Fasting female volunteers with moderate weight loss also showed no alteration in the overnight profile (I. M. Anderson et al. 1990), nor did volunteers who fasted for 24 hours (Arendt et al. 1982). However, in some studies, melatonin levels were elevated in anorexia nervosa (Arendt et al. 1992; Brambilla et al. 1988; Ferrari et al. 1990; Tortosa et al. 1989). This finding is supported by animal studies in which food-restricted rats were found to have high levels of melatonin after 3 weeks (Chik et al. 1987).

A number of variables may explain seemingly contradictory findings. Patient status at the time of sampling; sampling procedures, in particular the frequency of determination of melatonin; and assay methods all must be considered.

Effect of Depression

The presence of concurrent depression appears to be particularly important. For example, in the study by Arendt et al. (1992), "none of the subjects met DSM-III-R criteria for a primary depressive illness" (p. 361). In contrast, Kennedy et al. (1989) examined the profiles of several groups of patients with anorexia nervosa of a restrictive and bulimic subtype, as well as bulimia nervosa patients, and compared them with control subjects. There were no differences in overnight levels of serum melatonin, but the eating disorders group with concurrent major depression had significantly lower elevations of nocturnal melatonin as compared with the depression-free group. This finding was confirmed using urinary 6-sulfatoxymelatonin (aMT6s) and is in agreement with other familial and biochemical studies in which differences between depressed and nondepressed eating disorders patients were studied (Biederman et al. 1984, 1985; Kassett et al. 1989).

Effect of Weight and Starvation

To examine the effect of weight change in anorexia nervosa patients, Kennedy et al. (1990) restudied nine anorexia nervosa patients who completed overnight melatonin sampling before and after weight restoration. There was no significant change in melatonin levels between the two sampling times, and at neither time did melatonin levels differ in the anorexia nervosa group from a female age-matched control group, suggesting that low weight alone does not alter melatonin release. Bearn et al. (1988) reported similar findings in anorexia nervosa patients before and after weight restoration.

However, the acute effects of starvation, possibly mediated through hypoglycemia, may be responsible for alterations in melatonin output. Arendt et al. (1992) suggested that hypoglycemia, which is known to be a potent stimulus to the noradrenergic neurons in the rat hypothalamus (Smythe et al. 1984), could be responsible for their findings. Kennedy et al. (1993) reported a disturbance in circadian rhythm of melatonin output in actively bingeing and purging anorexia nervosa patients. In this group, there was an elevation of daytime aMT6s during the first 24 hours of admission to the hospital. This abnormality had returned to normal 7 days later and was not present in acutely restricting anorexia nervosa patients. Hypoglycemia or the effect of altered protein intake on amino acid balance is a possible explanation.

Relationship to Amenorrhea

The relationship between melatonin and reproductive function has been of particular relevance among seasonal breeding animals. It is also known that melatonin levels peak in early childhood and then a significant decline occurs between prepubertal stage and early pubescence (see Shafii and Shafii, Chapter 7, in this volume). Mortola et al. (1993) compared melatonin levels in cycling and amenorrheic women with anorexia nervosa or bulimia nervosa with normal-cycling control women. There were no differences across groups, and the authors concluded that the frequent occurrence of amenorrhea in patients with eating disorders is not mediated through melatonin.

Melatonin and Panic Disorder

McIntyre et al. (1990) reported an increase in plasma melatonin between 4 A.M. and 7 A.M. in panic disorder patients who were previously unmedicated. We have recently examined a group of 10 unmedicated female patients with panic disorder in comparison with a group of 8 control subjects, measuring urinary output of aMT6s (G. M. Brown and R. P. Swinson, unpublished data, June 1997). Urine was collected during two time intervals: 11 P.M.–9 A.M. and 9 A.M.–11 P.M. There was a clear-cut increase in aMT6s in the patients with panic disorder during both the nocturnal and daytime collections. These increases, which support the findings of McIntyre et al. (1990), indicate continuing activation of melatonin synthesis in panic disorders both during the day and night. In anorexia nervosa, bulimia nervosa, and panic disorder, increases in pineal function may be found.

Neurochemical Mechanisms of Increased Pineal Function

Numerous neurotransmitters are involved in pineal regulation (J. Yanovski et al. 1987) (see also Reiter, Chapter 1, and Bhatnagar,

Chapter 2, in this volume). Alterations of these transmitter systems could occur in anorexia nervosa or bulimia nervosa because of hypoglycemia or altered amino acid balance, whereas in panic disorder, such alterations may be an integral part of the disorder.

Evidence suggests involvement of several neurotransmitters in the following disorders: in anorexia nervosa, opioids, dopamine, and muscarinic cholinergics; in bulimia nervosa, evidence is more limited but may point to opioids; and in panic disorder, serotonin, dopamine, and norepinephrine may be involved.

The increase in pineal function in patients with eating disorders and panic disorder could indicate that there is increased sympathetic activation. To determine whether there was a generalized increase in sympathetic activity in panic disorder, we measured urinary metanephrine. Metanephrine output in the panic disorder patients did not differ from that in control subjects during either the night or day. This finding indicates that if the increase in pineal activity in panic disorder is due to increased sympathetic input to the pineal gland, this increase is not generalized but is specific to that component of the sympathetic nervous system that innervates the pineal gland.

Neuroendocrine Abnormalities in Eating and Panic Disorder

Hypothalamic-Pituitary-Ovarian Axis

Disorders of the hypothalamic-pituitary-ovarian axis are one of the hallmarks of anorexia nervosa, with occurrence of amenorrhea accompanied by loss of libido and secondary sexual characteristics (Hurd et al. 1977). Up to 30% of bulimia nervosa patients who are at normal weight have amenorrhea or oligomenorrhea (Fairburn and Cooper 1984). Most underweight anorexia nervosa patients have low levels of plasma gonadotropins (Hurd et al. 1977; Jeuniewic et al. 1978). Regaining the adult pattern of plasma luteinizing hormone (LH) is correlated with weight restoration (Wakeling et al. 1977). In anorexia nervosa, the LH response to luteinizing hormone-releasing hormone (LHRH) is similar to that of the prepubertal state (Halmi et al. 1975; Palmer et al. 1975) and correlates highly with body weight (Palmer et al. 1975).

In contrast with anorexia nervosa and bulimia nervosa, in panic disorder, no abnormalities of the hypothalamic-pituitary-gonadal axis are reported.

Hypothalamic-Pituitary-Adrenal Axis

In anorexia nervosa, the normal circadian rhythm of cortisol is preserved at a higher level, with increased 24-hour urinary-free cortisol levels (Boyar et al. 1977). In bulimia nervosa, there is a similar elevation of the 24-hour rhythm of cortisol (Kennedy et al. 1989) and of adrenocorticotropic hormone (ACTH) (Mortola et al. 1989). In contrast, panic disorder patients have normal urinary-free cortisol (UFC) (Uhde et al. 1988), although increased UFC levels in some patients are accounted for by concomitant depression, agoraphobia, or both (Kathol et al. 1988). In most studies, anorexia nervosa patients fail to suppress cortisol output following dexamethasone (DEX) given at 11:00 P.M. (dexamethasone suppression test [DST]) (Walsh et al. 1978). Nonsuppression has been reported on the DST in 20%–60% of normal-weight bulimic patients (Hudson et al. 1983b; Kaplan et al. 1989; Musisi and Garfinkel 1985). Westberg et al. (1991) reported that post-DEX cortisol was normal in patients with panic disorder but significantly higher in patients with agoraphobic panic disorder, indicating an abnormality of DST suppression related to agoraphobic behavior rather than to panic attacks. Thus, there is no evidence for alteration of resting pituitary adrenal function or of responsiveness to DEX in panic disorder.

Anorexia nervosa (Cavagnini et al. 1986) and bulimia nervosa patients (Mortola et al. 1989) show blunted ACTH and cortisol responses to corticotropin-releasing hormone (CRH), suggesting that there is tonic hypersecretion of CRH, which leads to desensitization of pituitary corticotrophs in both conditions. Blunted responses also are reported in panic disorder (Roy-Byrne et al. 1986a).

Cortisol responses to the α_2-adrenergic agonist clonidine are unaltered in anorexia nervosa (Brambilla et al. 1987) and in panic disorder (Stein and Uhde 1988), although they differ between patients who have panic disorder with agoraphobia and control subjects (Brambilla et al. 1995b).

Cortisol responses to the serotonin agonists metachlorophenylpiperazine (m-CPP) and L-tryptophan are not altered in bulimia nervosa (Brewerton et al. 1992). Although in panic disorder patients, no alteration in hypothalamic-pituitary-adrenal (HPA) function is seen in the responses to the serotonin agonists L-5-hydroxytryptophan (Westenberg and den Boer 1989) and m-CPP (Charney et al. 1987; Klein et al. 1991), responses to oral fenfluramine (Targum and Marshall 1989) are increased in panic disorder patients who have an anxiogenic response. Moreover, a decreased corticotropin and cortisol release is seen following the 5-hydroxytryptamine$_{1A}$ (5-HT$_{1A}$) partial receptor agonist ipsapirone in patients with panic disorder (Lesch et al. 1992), supporting a role of 5-HT$_{1A}$ receptor–related serotonin dysfunction in the pathophysiology of panic disorder. Opioid regulation of the HPA axis is altered in anorexia nervosa patients; there is a decreased cortisol response to naloxone (Baranowska 1990) but an increased response in bulimia nervosa patients (Coiro et al. 1990b).

In summary, from HPA axis studies, there is evidence of altered opioid mechanisms in anorexia nervosa and bulimia nervosa patients and of changes in serotonin regulation in panic disorder patients.

Hypothalamic-Pituitary-Thyroid Axis

In anorexia nervosa patients, thyroxine levels are within the normal range (Miyai et al. 1975; Moshang et al. 1975) with normal levels of thyrotropin (thyroid-stimulating hormone [TSH]), although a few studies report decreased TSH (Hurd et al. 1977). Abnormally low levels of serum T_3 are found (Hurd et al. 1977; Moshang and Utiger 1977) with increased levels of inactive reverse T_3 (Leslie et al. 1978).

TSH responses to thyrotropin-releasing hormone (TRH) are normal or delayed in patients with anorexia nervosa (Aro et al. 1975; Vigersky and Loriaux 1977), with some reports of blunted responses (Maeda et al. 1976; Travaglini et al. 1976). Delayed and blunted responses occur with simple weight loss (Vigersky et al. 1977) and for the most part return to normal after weight gain (Leslie et al. 1978). Bulimic patients fail to demonstrate altered responses of TSH to TRH (Kaplan et al. 1989; Kiriike et al. 1987; Levy et al. 1988) when at normal weight. A decreased TSH response to TRH has been reported in patients with panic disorder (Roy-Byrne et al. 1986b). Among other factors, somatostatin and dopamine are major regulators of the hypothalamic-pituitary-thyroid (HPT) axis (Jackson 1984).

Growth Hormone

Growth hormone (GH) levels are elevated in many patients with anorexia nervosa. This elevation is related to caloric deficiency rather than reduced body weight because once caloric intake is increased, basal growth hormone levels return to normal (Brown et al. 1977; Garfinkel et al. 1975). Elevated GH levels also are seen in patients with bulimia nervosa (Coiro et al. 1990a). In patients with panic disorder, basal GH levels are normal (Brambilla et al. 1995b).

Administration of growth hormone-releasing hormone (GHRH) produces an exaggerated GH response in anorexia nervosa patients in most (Brambilla et al. 1989; Lomeo et al. 1989) but not all studies (De Marinis et al. 1991; Tamai et al. 1990). In contrast, a normal GH response is found in bulimia nervosa patients (Coiro et al. 1990a) and a decreased response in panic disorder patients (Rapaport et al. 1989; Uhde et al. 1992), although one study disagrees (Brambilla et al. 1995a).

The GH response to clonidine was normal in two studies of anorexia nervosa patients (Brambilla et al. 1987, 1989) but blunted in one study (Nussbaum et al. 1990), normal in bulimia nervosa patients (Coiro et al. 1990a), and blunted in the majority of studies of panic disorder patients (e.g., Charney and Heninger 1986a;

Schittecatte et al. 1988; Uhde et al. 1992). Because of these blunted GH responses in panic disorder patients, it has been postulated that there is a generalized hyporesponse of the hypothalamic GH system secondary to an abnormality of neurotransmitter regulation of the GH system or in somatomedin C regulation (Uhde et al. 1992). However, GH responses to apomorphine are increased in patients with panic disorder, suggesting a supersensitivity of dopaminergic mechanisms (Pitchot et al. 1992).

In patients with anorexia nervosa, muscarinic cholinergic blockade fails to decrease GHRH-stimulated GH responses as it does in control subjects (Rolla et al. 1990, 1991; Tamai et al. 1990). Studies with somatostatin inhibitors suggest that the basic defect may be a refractoriness to somatostatin-mediated cholinergic influence (Ghigo et al. 1994). Opioids may not be involved because naloxone inhibits the GH response to GHRH in anorexia nervosa and in healthy control subjects (De Marinis et al. 1991).

In summary, there is evidence of refractoriness to cholinergic influence in anorexia nervosa and of altered adrenergic and possibly dopaminergic regulation in panic disorder.

Prolactin

Resting morning levels of prolactin (PRL) are normal in anorexia nervosa patients (Beumont et al. 1974; Mecklenburg et al. 1974).

PRL response to administration of the dopamine antagonist metoclopramide is decreased in anorexia nervosa patients (Golden et al. 1992), whereas in bulimia nervosa patients there is a blunted response to m-CPP but not to L-tryptophan (Brewerton et al. 1992). Studies using tryptophan or m-CPP to stimulate PRL have shown no alteration in PRL responses in patients with panic disorder (Charney and Heninger 1986b; Charney et al. 1987), although one study (Kahn et al. 1991) indicated that there is an increased release in female patients. In contrast, there are increases in both anxiogenic and PRL responses to fenfluramine in patients with panic disorder (Apostolopoulos et al. 1993; Targum and Marshall 1989). Together with other evidence, these findings suggest that alterations in serotonin are one component of panic disorder (Coplan et al. 1992), whereas in patients with anorexia nervosa there may be an alteration of dopaminergic mechanisms.

Conclusions

There is now substantial evidence from clinical studies that eating disorders and anxiety disorders are frequently comorbid, and genetic studies suggest a common etiological basis of panic disorder and eating disorders. There is an increase in pineal function in patients with panic disorder, in acutely starving patients with anorexia nervosa, and in acutely bingeing and purging patients with bulimia nervosa. These changes in pineal function may be related to increased sympathetic activation of the pineal gland. This sympathetic activation is relatively specific to the pineal sympathetic input and not generalized to include other targets of the sympathetic system such as the adrenal medulla.

In considering the possibility of noradrenergic abnormalities related to anorexia nervosa and panic disorder, it is instructive to look at a neuroendocrine marker, the clonidine-GH challenge test. The GH response is normal in patients with anorexia nervosa and diminished in patients with panic disorder, providing no direct evidence of increased adrenergic activity in either group of patients. Alterations in serotonin regulation are another possible explanation for the increased pineal function in patients with panic disorder. The increased cortisol response to fenfluramine in patients with panic disorder is compatible with increased serotonergic activity in this disorder, and serotonin is known to modulate the amplitude of circadian rhythms (Gillette et al. 1993). However, there is no evidence of altered serotonin regulation in patients with eating disorders. Other neuroendocrine studies also fail to point to common features in these disorders.

Considering the foregoing studies, one may conclude that the increases in pineal function in panic disorder and in eating disorders are due to different factors and that they do not point to a common underlying mechanism.

References

Anderson GH, Kennedy SH: The Biology of Feast and Famine: Relevance to Eating Disorders. San Diego, CA, Academic Press, 1992

Anderson IM, Gartside SE, Cowen PJ: The effect of moderate weight loss on overnight melatonin secretion. Br J Psychiatry 156:875–877, 1990

Apostolopoulos M, Judd FK, Burrows GD, et al: Prolactin response to DL-fenfluramine in panic disorder. Psychoneuroendocrinology 18:337–342, 1993

Arendt J, Hampton S, English J, et al: 24-hr profiles of melatonin, cortisol, insulin, C-peptide and GIP following a meal and subsequent fasting. Clin Endocrinol (Oxf) 16:89–95, 1982

Arendt J, Bhanji S, Franey C, et al: Plasma melatonin levels in anorexia nervosa. Br J Psychiatry 161:361–364, 1992

Aro A, Lamberg BA, Pelkonen R: Dysfunction of the hypothalamic-pituitary axis in anorexia nervosa (letter). N Engl J Med 292:594–595, 1975

Baranowska B: Are disturbances in opioid and adrenergic systems involved in the hormonal dysfunction of anorexia nervosa? Psychoneuroendocrinology 15:371–379, 1990

Baranowska B, Soszynski P, Misiorowski W, et al: Circadian melatonin rhythm in women with hypothalamic amenorrhea. Neuroendocrinology Letters 8:295–300, 1986

Bearn J, Treasure J, Murphy M, et al: A study of sulphatoxy melatonin excretion and gonadotrophin status during weight gain in anorexia nervosa. Br J Psychiatry 152:372–376, 1988

Beumont PJV, Frieden HG, Gelder MG, et al: Plasma prolactin and luteinizing hormone levels in anorexia nervosa. Psychol Med 4:219–221, 1974

Biederman J, Herzog DB, Rivinus TM, et al: Urinary MHPG in anorexia nervosa patients with and without a concomitant major depressive disorder. J Psychiatr Res 18:149–160, 1984

Biederman J, Rivinus T, Kemper K, et al: Depressive disorders in relatives of anorexia nervosa patients with and without a current episode of nonbipolar major depression. Am J Psychiatry 142:1495–1496, 1985

Boyar RM, Hellman LD, Roffwarg H, et al: Cortisol secretion and metabolism in anorexia nervosa. N Engl J Med 296:190–193, 1977

Brambilla F, Lampertico M, Sali L, et al: Clonidine stimulation in anorexia nervosa: growth hormone, cortisol, and beta-endorphin responses. Psychiatry Res 20:19–31, 1987

Brambilla F, Fraschini F, Espasti G, et al: Melatonin circadian rhythm in anorexia nervosa and obesity. Psychiatry Res 23:267–276, 1988

Brambilla F, Ferrari E, Cavagnini F, et al: Alpha 2-adrenoceptor sensitivity in anorexia nervosa: GH response to clonidine or GHRH stimulation. Biol Psychiatry 25:256–264, 1989

Brambilla F, Perna G, Garberi A, et al: Alpha 2-adrenergic receptor sensitivity in panic disorder, I: GH response to GHRH and clonidine stimulation in panic disorder. Psychoneuroendocrinology 20:1–9, 1995a

Brambilla F, Bellodi L, Arancio C, et al: Alpha 2-adrenergic receptor sensitivity in panic disorder, II: cortisol response to clonidine stimulation in panic disorder. Psychoneuroendocrinology 20:11–19, 1995b

Brewerton TD, Mueller EA, Lesem MD, et al: Neuroendocrine responses to m-chlorophenylpiperazine and L-tryptophan in bulimia. Arch Gen Psychiatry 49:852–861, 1992

Brown GM, Garfinkel PE, Jeuniewic N, et al: Endocrine profiles in anorexia nervosa, in Anorexia Nervosa. Edited by Vigersky R. New York, Raven, 1977, pp 123–135

Cavagnini F, Invitti C, Passamonti M, et al: Impaired ACTH and cortisol response to CRH in patients with anorexia nervosa, in Advances in the Biosciences, Vol 60: Disorders of Eating Behaviour: A Psychoneuroendocrine Approach. Edited by Ferrari E, Brambilla F. Oxford, England, Pergamon, 1986, pp 229–233

Charney DS, Heninger GR: Abnormal regulation of noradrenergic function in panic disorders: effects of clonidine in healthy subjects and patients with agoraphobia and panic disorder. Arch Gen Psychiatry 43:1042–1054, 1986a

Charney DS, Heninger GR: Serotonin function in panic disorders: the effect of intravenous tryptophan in healthy subjects and patients with panic disorder before and during alprazolam treatment. Arch Gen Psychiatry 43:1059–1065, 1986b

Charney DS, Woods SW, Goodman WK, et al: Serotonin function in anxiety, II: effects of the serotonin agonist MCPP in panic disorder patients and healthy subjects. Psychopharmacology (Berl) 92:14–24, 1987

Chik CL, Ho AK, Brown GM: Effect of food restriction on 24-hr serum and pineal melatonin content in male rats. Acta Endocrinologica 115:507–513, 1987

Coiro V, Capretti L, Volpi R, et al: Growth hormone responses to growth hormone-releasing hormone, clonidine and insulin-induced hypoglycemia in normal weight bulimic women. Neuropsychobiology 23:8–14, 1990a

Coiro V, d'Amato L, Marchesi C, et al: Luteinizing hormone and cortisol responses to naloxone in normal weight women with bulimia. Psychoneuroendocrinology 15:463–470, 1990b

Coplan JD, Gorman JM, Klein DF: Serotonin related functions in panic-anxiety: a critical overview. Neuropsychopharmacology 6:189–200, 1992

Dalery J, Claustrat B, Brun J, et al: Plasma melatonin and cortisol levels in eight patients with anorexia nervosa. Neuroendocrinology Letters 7:159–164, 1985

De Marinis L, Mancini A, D'Amico C, et al: Influence of naloxone infusion on prolactin and growth hormone response to growth hormone-releasing hormone in anorexia nervosa. Psychoneuroendocrinology 16:499–504, 1991

Fairburn CG, Cooper PJ: The clinical features of bulimia nervosa. Br J Psychiatry 144:238–246, 1984

Ferrari E, Fraschini F, Brambilla F: Hormonal circadian rhythms in eating disorders. Biol Psychiatry 27:1007–1020, 1990

Fornari V, Kaplan M, Sandberg DE, et al: Depressive and anxiety disorders in anorexia nervosa and bulimia nervosa. Int J Eat Disord 12:21–29, 1992

Garfinkel PE, Brown GM, Stancer HC, et al: Hypothalamic-pituitary function in anorexia nervosa. Arch Gen Psychiatry 32:739–744, 1975

Garfinkel PE, Lin E, Goering P, et al: Bulimia nervosa in a Canadian community sample: prevalence and comparison of subgroups. Am J Psychiatry 152:1052–1058, 1995

Garfinkel PE, Lin E, Goering P, et al: Purging and non-purging forms of bulimia nervosa in a community sample. Int J Eat Disord 20:231–238, 1996

Ghigo E, Arvat E, Gianotti L, et al: Arginine but not pyridostigmine, a cholinesterase inhibitor, enhances the GHRH-induced GH rise in patients with anorexia nervosa. Biol Psychiatry 36:689–695, 1994

Gillette MU, DeMarco SJ, Ding JM, et al: The organization of the suprachiasmatic nucleus of the rat and its regulation by neurotransmitters and modulators. J Biol Rhythms 8 (suppl):S53–S58, 1993

Golden NH, Pepper GM, Sacker I, et al: The effects of a dopamine antagonist on luteinizing hormone and prolactin release in women with anorexia nervosa and in normal controls. J Adolesc Health 13:155–160, 1992

Halmi KA, Sherman BM, Zamudio R: LH and FSH response to gonadotropin-releasing hormone in anorexia nervosa: effect of nutritional rehabilitation. J Clin Endocrinol Metab 1:135–142, 1975

Halmi KA, Eckert E, Marchi P, et al: Comorbidity of psychiatric diagnoses in anorexia nervosa. Arch Gen Psychiatry 48:712–718, 1991

Hudson JI, Pope HG Jr, Jonas JM, et al: Hypothalamic-pituitary-adrenal axis hyperactivity in bulimia. Psychiatry Res 8:111–117, 1983a

Hudson JI, Pope HG Jr, Jonas JM, et al: Phenomenological relationship of eating disorders to major affective disorders. Psychiatry Res 9:345–354, 1983b

Hurd HP, Palumbo PJ, Gharib H: Hypothalamic-endocrine dysfunction in anorexia nervosa. Mayo Clin Proc 52:711–716, 1977

Jackson IMD: Hypothalamic releasing hormones: mechanisms underlying neuroendocrine dysfunction in affective disorders, in Neuroendocrinology and Psychiatric Disorder. Edited by Brown GM, Koslow SH, Reichlin S. New York, Raven, 1984, pp 255–266

Jeuniewic H, Brown G, Garfinkel P, et al: Hypothalamic function as related to body weight and body fat in anorexia nervosa. Psychosom Med 40:187–198, 1978

Kahn RS, Wetzler S, Asnis GM, et al: Pituitary hormone responses to meta-chlorophenylpiperazine in panic disorder and healthy control subjects. Psychiatry Res 37:25–34, 1991

Kaplan AS, Garfinkel PE, Brown GM: The DST and TRH test in bulimia nervosa. Br J Psychiatry 154:86–92, 1989

Kaplan AS, Goldbloom DS, Woodside DB, et al: Mitral valve prolapse in eating and panic disorder: a pilot study. Int J Eat Disord 10:531–537, 1991

Kassett JA, Gershon ES, Maxwell ME, et al: Psychiatric disorders in the first degree relatives of probands with bulimia nervosa. Am J Psychiatry 146:1468–1471, 1989

Kasvikis YG, Tsakiris F, Marks IM, et al: Past history of anorexia nervosa in women with obsessive-compulsive disorder. Int J Eat Disord 5:1069–1075, 1986

Kathol RG, Noyes R Jr, Lopez AL, et al: Relationship of urinary free cortisol levels in patients with panic disorder to symptoms of depression and agoraphobia. Psychiatry Res 24:211–221, 1988

Kendler KS, MacLean C, Neale M, et al: The genetic epidemiology of bulimia nervosa. Am J Psychiatry 148:1627–1637, 1991

Kendler KS, Walters EE, Neale MC, et al: The structure of the genetic and environmental risk factors for six major psychiatric disorders in women. Arch Gen Psychiatry 52:374–383, 1995

Kennedy SH, Garfinkel PE, Parienti V, et al: Changes in melatonin levels but not cortisol levels are associated with depression in patients with eating disorders. Arch Gen Psychiatry 46:73–78, 1989

Kennedy SH, Brown GM, McVey G, et al: Pineal and adrenal function before and after refeeding in anorexia nervosa. Biol Psychiatry 30:216–224, 1990

Kennedy SH, Brown GM, Ford C, et al: The acute effects of starvation on sulphatoxy-melatonin output in subgroups of patients with anorexia nervosa. Psychoneuroendocrinology 18:131–139, 1993

Kessler RC, McGonagle KA, Zhao S, et al: Lifetime and twelve month prevalence of DSM-III-R psychiatric disorders in the United States. Arch Gen Psychiatry 51:8–19, 1994

Kiriike N, Nishiwaki S, Izumiya Y, et al: Thyrotropin, prolactin, and growth hormone responses to thyrotropin-releasing hormone in anorexia nervosa and bulimia. Biol Psychiatry 22:167–176, 1987

Klein E, Zohar J, Geraci MF, et al: Anxiogenic effects of m-CPP in patients with panic disorder: comparison to caffeine's anxiogenic effects. Biol Psychiatry 30:973–984, 1991

Laessle RG, Wittchen HU, Fichter MM, et al: The significance of subgroups of bulimia and anorexia nervosa: lifetime frequency of psychiatric disorders. Int J Eat Disord 8:569–574, 1989

Lesch KP, Wiesmann M, Hoh A, et al: 5-HT$_{1A}$ receptor-effector system responsivity in panic disorder. Psychopharmacology (Berl) 106:111–117, 1992

Leslie RDG, Isaacs AJ, Gomez J, et al: Hypothalamo-pituitary-thyroid function in anorexia nervosa: influence of weight gain. BMJ 2:526–528, 1978

Levy AB, Dixon KN, Malarkey W: Pituitary response to TRH in bulimia. Biol Psychiatry 23:476–484, 1988

Lewinsohn PM, Hops H, Roberts RE, et al: Adolescent psychopathology, I: prevalence and incidence of depression and other DSM-III-R disorders in high school students. J Abnorm Psychol 102:133–144, 1993

Lomeo A, Mazzocchi G, Sessarego P, et al: Growth hormone and prolactin response to growth hormone-releasing in anorexia nervosa. Recenti Prog Med 80:569–573, 1989

Maeda K, Kato Y, Yamaguchi N, et al: Growth hormone release following thyrotropin-releasing hormone injection into patients with anorexia nervosa. Acta Endocrinologica 81:1–8, 1976

Magraf J, Ehlers A, Roth WT: Mitral valve prolapse and panic disorder: a review of the relationship. Psychosom Med 50:93–113, 1988

McIntyre IM, Judd FK, Burrows GD, et al: Plasma concentrations of melatonin in panic disorder. Am J Psychiatry 147:462–464, 1990

Mecklenburg RS, Loriaux DL, Thompson RH, et al: Hypothalamic dysfunction in patients with anorexia nervosa. Medicine 53:147–159, 1974

Miyai K, Yamamoto T, Azukizawa M, et al: Serum thyroid hormones and thyro-tropin in anorexia nervosa. J Clin Endocrinol Metab 40:334–338, 1975

Mortola JF, Rasmussen DD, Yen SS: Alterations of the adrenocorticotropin-cortisol axis in normal weight bulimic women: evidence for a central mechanism. J Clin Endocrinol Metab 68:517–522, 1989

Mortola JF, Laughlin GA, Yen SS: Melatonin rhythms in women with anorexia nervosa and bulimia nervosa. J Clin Endocrinol Metab 77:1540–1544, 1993

Moshang T Jr, Utiger RD: Low triiodothyronine euthyroidism in anorexia nervosa, in Anorexia Nervosa. Edited by Vigersky R. New York, Raven, 1977, pp 263–270

Moshang T Jr, Parks JS, Baker L: Low serum triiodothyronine in patients with anorexia nervosa. J Clin Endocrinol Metab 40:470–473, 1975

Musisi SM, Garfinkel PE: Comparative dexamethasone suppression test measures in bulimia, depression and normal controls. Can J Psychiatry 30:190–194, 1985

Nussbaum MP, Blethen SL, Chasalow FI, et al: Blunted growth hormone responses to clonidine in adolescent girls with early anorexia nervosa: evidence for an early hypothalamic defect. Journal of Adolescent Health Care 11:145–148, 1990

Offord DR, Boyle M, Campbell D, et al: One-year prevalence of psychiatric disorder in Ontarians 15 to 64 years of age. Can J Psychiatry 41:559–563, 1996

Palmer RL, Crisp AH, Mackinnon PCB, et al: Pituitary sensitivity to 50 μg LH/FSH-RH in subjects with anorexia nervosa in acute recovery stages. BMJ 1:179–182, 1975

Piran N, Kennedy S, Garfinkel PE, et al: Affective disturbance in eating disorders. J Nerv Ment Disease 173:395–400, 1985

Pitchot W, Ansseau M, Gonzalez Moreno A, et al: Dopaminergic function in panic disorder: comparison with major and minor depression. Biol Psychiatry 32:1004–1011, 1992

Rapaport MH, Risch SC, Gillin JC, et al: Blunted growth hormone response to peripheral infusion of human growth hormone-releasing factor in patients with panic disorder. Am J Psychiatry 146:92–95, 1989

Regier DA, Burke JD, Christie KA: Comorbidity of affective and anxiety disorders in population-based studies: the National Institute of Mental Health Epidemiological Catchment Area (ECA) program, in Comorbidity of Anxiety and Depressive Disorders. Edited by Maser JD, Cloninger CR. Washington, DC, American Psychiatric Press, 1990

Rolla M, Andreoni A, Belliti D, et al: Effects of cholinergic muscarinic antagonist pirenzepine on GH response to GHRH 1-40 in patients with anorexia nervosa. Endocrinologia Experimentalis 24:195–204, 1990

Rolla M, Andreoni A, Belliti D, et al: Blockade of cholinergic muscarinic receptors by pirenzepine and GHRH-induced GH secretion in the acute and recovery phase of anorexia nervosa and atypical eating disorders. Biol Psychiatry 29:1079–1091, 1991

Roy-Byrne PP, Uhde TW, Post RM, et al: The corticotropin-releasing hormone stimulation test in patients with panic disorder. Am J Psychiatry 143:896–899, 1986a

Roy-Byrne PP, Uhde TW, Rubinow DR, et al: Reduced TSH and prolactin responses to TRH in patients with panic disorder. Am J Psychiatry 143:503–507, 1986b

Schittecatte M, Charles G, Depauw Y, et al: Growth hormone response to clonidine in panic disorder patients. Psychiatry Res 23:147–151, 1988

Schwalberg MD, Barlow DH, Alger SA, et al: Comparison of bulimics, obese binge eaters, social phobics, and individuals with panic disorder on comorbidity across DSM-III-R anxiety disorders. J Abnorm Psychol 101:675–681, 1992

Smith C, Feldman SS, Naserbakht A, et al: Psychological characteristics and DSM-III-R diagnoses at 6-year follow-up of adolescent anorexia nervosa. J Am Acad Child Adolesc Psychiatry 32:1237–1245, 1993

Smythe GA, Grunstein HS, Bradshaw JE, et al: Relationship between brain noradrenergic activity and blood glucose. Nature 308:65–67, 1984

Stein MB, Uhde T: Cortisol response to clonidine in panic disorder: comparison with depressed patients and normal controls. Biol Psychiatry 24:322–330, 1988

Tamai H, Komaki G, Matsubayashi S, et al: Effect of cholinergic muscarinic receptor blockade on human growth hormone (GH)-releasing hormone-(1-44)-induced GH secretion in anorexia nervosa. J Clin Endocrinol Metab 70:738–741, 1990

Targum SD, Marshall LE: Fenfluramine provocation of anxiety in patients with panic disorder. Psychiatry Res 28:295–306, 1989

Toner B, Garfinkel PE, Garner DM: Affective and anxiety disorders in the long-term follow-up of anorexia nervosa. Int J Psychiatry Med 18:357–364, 1988

Tortosa F, Puig-Domingo M, Peinado M-A, et al: Enhanced circadian rhythm of melatonin in anorexia nervosa. Acta Endocrinologica 120:574–578, 1989

Travaglini P, Beck-Peccoz P, Ferrari C, et al: Some aspects of hypothalamic-pituitary function in patients with anorexia nervosa. Acta Endocrinologica 81:252–262, 1976

Uhde TW, Joffe RT, Jimerson DC, et al: Normal urinary free cortisol and plasma MHPG in panic disorder: clinical and theoretical implications. Biol Psychiatry 23:575–585, 1988

Uhde TW, Tancer ME, Rubinow DR, et al: Evidence for hypothalamo-growth hormone dysfunction in panic disorder: profile of growth hormone (GH) responses to clonidine, yohimbine, caffeine, glucose, GRF and TRH in panic disorder patients versus healthy volunteers. Neuropsychopharmacology 6:101–118, 1992

Vigersky RA, Loriaux DL: Anorexia nervosa as a model of hypothalamic dysfunction, in Anorexia Nervosa. Edited by Vigersky R. New York, Raven, 1977, pp 109–122

Vigersky RA, Andersen AE, Thompson RH, et al: Hypothalamic dysfunction in secondary amenorrhea associated with simple weight loss. N Engl J Med 297:1141–1145, 1977

Wakeling A, DeSouza VA, Beardwood CJ: Assessment of the negative and positive feedback effects of administered oestrogen and gonadotropin release in patients with anorexia nervosa. Psychol Med 7:397–405, 1977

Walsh BT, Katz JL, Levin J, et al: Adrenal activity in anorexia nervosa. Psychosom Med 40:499–506, 1978

Westberg P, Modigh K, Lisjo P, et al: Higher postdexamethasone serum cortisol levels in agoraphobic than in nonagoraphobic panic disorder patients. Biol Psychiatry 30:247–256, 1991

Westenberg HG, den Boer JA: Serotonin function in panic disorder: effect of L-5-hydroxytryptophan in patients and controls. Psychopharmacology (Berl) 98:283–285, 1989

Yanovski J, Witcher J, Adler N, et al: Stimulation of the paraventricular nucleus area of the hypothalamus elevates urinary 6-hydroxymelatonin during daytime. Brain Res Bull 19:129–133, 1987

Yanovski SZ, Nelson JE, Dubbert BK, et al: Association of binge eating disorder and psychiatric comorbidity in obese subjects. Am J Psychiatry 150:1472–1479, 1993

Part III

Melatonin in Children and Adolescents

Chapter 7

Melatonin in Healthy and Depressed Children and Adolescents

Mohammad Shafii, M.D., and
Sharon Lee Shafii, R.N., B.S.N.

In Copenhagen, Krabbe (1923) published the first article noting the relationship between the pineal gland and sexual development. With the advancement of surgical procedures during the twentieth century, neurosurgeons associated pineal gland tumors with signs of precocious puberty. Kitay (1954) further noticed that precocious puberty was associated with destructive tumors of the pineal gland, whereas delayed pubescence was associated with hyperactive tumors.

The Pineal Gland and Melatonin

Lerner et al. (1958) isolated from the pineal gland and peripheral nerves of humans, cows, and monkeys a new hormone, *N*-acetyl-5-methoxytryptamine, which they called melatonin. A year later, McIssac and Page (1959) observed the in vivo conversion of serotonin (5-hydroxytryptamine [HT]) to *N*-acetylserotonin using the enzyme *N*-acetyltransferase (NAT). A few months later, Axelrod and Weissbach (1960), in a less-than-one-page article, reported the isolation of the enzyme hydroxyindole-*O*-methyltransferase (HIOMT) from the pineal gland of cows and thus made the discovery that melatonin was synthesized from *N*-acetylserotonin in the pineal gland. Wurtman et al. (1964) observed that darkness mediated by the sympathetic nervous system stimulates the synthesis of melatonin from serotonin and tryptophan in the pinealocytes of the pineal gland and that light inhibits this synthesis.

From that time on, the search began in earnest to find effective and accurate methods of measuring melatonin in various body fluids and tissues and to understand the function of melatonin and the pineal gland (see Reiter, Chapter 1, and Wetterberg, Chapter 3, in this volume).

Developing sensitive methods of measuring melatonin such as radioimmunoassay (RIA) (Arendt et al. 1975, 1977; Wetterberg et al. 1978) and gas chromatography mass spectrometry (Lewy and Markey 1978) took a few years. Careful studies with these new methods revealed that most melatonin is synthesized during darkness in the pineal gland of mammals, including humans, and immediately secreted into the blood and distributed throughout the cells and other body fluids such as spinal fluid, saliva, and urine. We now know that most melatonin is secreted in darkness when the lights are turned off from 11 P.M. to 3 A.M., peaking around 2 A.M. (Wetterberg et al. 1978). Darkness stimulates noradrenergic neurons of the retina, which in turn, through a circuitous route, stimulate the β- and to a lesser extent α-adrenergic receptors of the pinealocyte membranes of the pineal gland, resulting in the synthesis of N-acetylserotonin and melatonin from serotonin and tryptophan. Although close to 90% of melatonin is synthesized in the pineal gland, a small amount in humans is also synthesized in the cells of the retina and gastrointestinal tract among others (see Reiter, Chapter 1, and Bhatnagar, Chapter 2, in this volume).

Recently, receptor sites of melatonin have been discovered in the suprachiasmatic nuclei (SCN) of the hypothalamus (Rivkees et al. 1990; Stankov et al. 1991, 1993; Vanecek 1988; Viswanathan et al. 1990). SCN are pacesetters of circadian rhythm, having a slightly more than 24-hour cycle. Melatonin has a regulating effect through its receptor sites on the SCN, resulting in the entrainment of the circadian rhythm to a 24-hour cycle. Reiter (1994) further observed, "Once in the blood melatonin has access to every cell in the body. . . . The same feature of the molecule which allowed it to escape readily from the pinealocytes, i.e., its high lipophilicity, permits it to pass quickly through cell membranes and into every subcellular compartment. Melatonin seems to have receptors on the membranes of a few cells and in the nucleus of all cells" (p. 173).

Melatonin in Infancy, Childhood, and Adolescence

In some hibernating mammals, such as the Syrian hamster, seasonal light changes in the fall stimulate the enlargement of the pineal gland and increase melatonin production. This increased melatonin production influences biological rhythms and results in increased eating, weight gain, shrinkage of gonads, decreased body temperature, and eventually hibernation. When daylight lengthens in late winter and early spring, the size of the pineal gland and the amount of melatonin decrease, resulting in the enlargement of the gonads and increases in sexual hormones, body temperature, and body activity, leading to mating behavior. These observations in animals have made some investigators wonder whether there is a direct relationship in humans between emerging pubescence and decreased pineal gland function.

Arendt (1978) measured serum melatonin in nine children and adolescents—six prepubertal and three pubertal. Two blood samples were drawn—noon and midnight. No difference was found in the serum melatonin level between these two groups. Silman et al. (1979) carried out a much more extensive study on 51 males and females, ages 11½–14 years. In females, blood samples were taken at 11 A.M. and in males at 1 P.M. They found "the concentration of melatonin in schoolgirls ranged from < 5 to 280 pg mL–1 and did not change with development. In contrast, the concentration of melatonin in boys, which ranged from < 10 to 2,300 pg mL–1, showed a marked change during adolescent development" (Silman et al. 1979, p. 301). Particularly, they noticed a significant decline of serum melatonin from Tanner stage I (no sign of pubescence) to Tanner stage II (early sign of pubescence). But there was no difference in the serum melatonin level in Tanner stages II, III, and IV. Silman et al. (1979) also noticed more variability in the serum melatonin levels in females as opposed to males. They postulated that this variability could be related to the morning blood sampling in the females as opposed to the early afternoon sampling in males. They concluded, "Our findings show that in young boys there is an abrupt fall in the concentration of melatonin with advancing development suggesting that it may play an important physiological role in the control of human puberty" (Silman et al. 1979, p. 301).

Lemaitre et al. (1981) in Paris assayed urine melatonin (not the metabolite, a6-hydroxymelatonin sulfate [aMT6s]) in 58 healthy males from ages 1 day to 30 years. They calculated urine melatonin in nmol•24h–1•kg–1 body weight, and their findings are shown in Table 7–1.

Lemaitre et al. (1981) concluded that urine melatonin is high in newborns but decreases during the first year of life. Interestingly, the serum melatonin level in the newborn umbilical artery and/or vein is significantly higher than the mother's melatonin level (Mitchell et al. 1979). Lemaitre et al. (1981) found that from age 1 year, an individual's urine melatonin gradually increases until age 13 years or pubescence. During pubescence and adulthood, urine melatonin declines.

Fevre et al. (1978) were the first investigators to do frequent blood sampling at 20-minute intervals for 24 hours to measure the secretion of melatonin and luteinizing hormone (LH) in four adolescents, ages 12–17 years. They found that there was a nocturnal increase in melatonin and LH, with a positive correlation between them. Lenko et al. (1982), in Geneva, studied daytime serum melatonin levels in 83 males and 79 females, ages 7–17 years—representing prepubescence (Tanner stage I)—to full development or Tanner stage V. The authors found no difference in serum melatonin levels between males and females or in various stages of prepubescence and pubescence. They recognized that because the serum melatonin level during the day is very low, daytime sampling does not reflect the differences between the groups.

Gupta et al. (1983), in Tübingen, Germany, reported on the serum melatonin levels of 87 children. A blood sample was taken at noon and at midnight. They noticed a significant serum melatonin decline between prepubertal stage I and early pubescence, stage II. In another study, they divided prepubertal stage I chil-

Table 7–1. Urine melatonin in males

Developmental level	Newborns	Babies	Young children	Older children	Adults
Age	1–15 days	21 days–6 months	1–4 years	4–13 years	22–30 years
N	18	7	11	10	12
Melatonin nmol • 24h^{-1} • kg^{-1}	.044	.018	.035	.044	.028
Standard Deviation (SD)	±.029	±.010	±.013	±.012	±.008

Source. Adapted from Lemaitre et al. 1981, p. 80.

dren into two groups. One group included the less skeletally mature preschool children and the second group the more skeletally mature, school-age prepubescent children, which they referred to as "PI." Gupta (1986) found a significant decline of nocturnal serum melatonin level "from the less skeletally mature children to the more [skeletally] mature" prepubescents (p. 222). The author concluded, "It appears that the decline in melatonin peak from infancy to maturity has two different characteristics. The first decline from infancy to skeletally more mature PI children is rather steep, while later with increasing skeletal development the decline is slow but steady" (Gupta 1986, p. 222).

Attanasio et al. (1985) reported on the circadian rhythm of serum melatonin in 38 children and adolescents, ages 1–18 years. A blood sample was collected at noon, 9 P.M., midnight, 3 A.M., and 6 A.M. They found that serum melatonin was significantly higher at midnight and at 3 A.M. in children ages 1–5 years as compared with children ages 6–10 years (PI—skeletal development but no pubescence). Also, they noticed that serum melatonin of children ages 6–10 years was significantly higher than that of children ages 9–12 years (PII—early stage of pubescence). They found a small decline from PII to PIV and PV, the later stages of pubescence. They concluded, " . . . the decline in the nocturnal melatonin surge is not exclusively related to pubertal development, but begins in infancy" (Attanasio et al. 1985, p. 388).

Waldhauser et al. (1984, 1988), from Vienna, measured the serum melatonin levels of 367 subjects, ages 3 days to 90 years. A daytime blood sample was collected between 7 A.M. and 10 A.M. and a nighttime sample between 11 P.M. and 1 A.M. They found that mean serum melatonin was low in the first 6 months of life (27.3 ± 5.4 pg/mL or .12 ± .02 nmol/L). The highest level occurred between ages 1 and 3 years (329.5z ± 42.0 pg/mL or 1.43 ± .18 nmol/L). Gradually, as the individual grew older, the mean serum melatonin declined. In individuals ages 15–20 years old, mean serum melatonin was significantly lower (62.5 ± 9.0 pg/mL or .27 ± .04 nmol/L). The lowest mean serum melatonin was between ages 70 and 90 years (29.2 ± 6.1 pg/mL or .13 ± .03 nmol/L).

Based on all of these studies, we now think that the decline of serum melatonin during physical growth from childhood to young adulthood is related to an increase in body mass, weight, and musculoskeletal development. The role of pubescence in the decline of serum melatonin is still being debated by some authors. Cavallo (1991, 1992a, 1992b, 1993) and Cavallo et al. (1992) studied 30 males and 32 females, ages 5–17 years. Cavallo et al. (1992) did multiple blood sampling by constant withdrawal at hourly intervals from 6 P.M. to 8 A.M. and found a significant decline in the melatonin peak and mean serum melatonin with age. The highest melatonin levels occurred between ages 1 and 5 years. Cavallo (1992b) also found " . . . a significant trend for decreasing melatonin concentrations with pubertal development" (p. 376). Cavallo (1992b) added that this trend was not associated with ". . . a significant time shift or change in the duration of the nocturnal surge. The quantitative changes, however, could not be linked exclusively to puberty, as age was a significant covariate. Therefore, in normal development, the effect of age on melatonin concentrations may mask the interactions between melatonin and puberty" (p. 378).

Melatonin in Adult Depression

Wetterberg and his colleagues at St. Göran's Hospital, Karolinska Institute, Stockholm, Sweden, are pioneers in studying the relationship between melatonin and depressive disorders in adults (see Wetterberg, Chapter 3, in this volume). They found that in patients with major depression along with a positive dexamethasone suppression test (DST), the nocturnal serum melatonin was significantly lower than that in patients with major depression who did not have early cortisol escape from the DST (Beck-Friis et al. 1983, 1984, 1985a, 1985b, 1985c; Wetterberg et al. 1979, 1981, 1990; Wirz-Justice and Arendt 1979). Wetterberg et al. (1990) succinctly summarized these works in a chapter titled "Melatonin as a Marker for a Subgroup of Depression in Adults," published in our earlier book, *Biological Rhythms, Mood Disorders, Light Therapy, and the Pineal Gland* (Shafii and Shafii 1990).

There have been a number of studies in the United States, Canada, and Europe that have confirmed Wetterberg et al.'s (1979) findings in adult depression (Brown et al. 1985; Kennedy et al. 1989; Nair et al. 1984, 1985). There also have been a few studies that have not confirmed Wetterberg et al.'s (1979) findings. Jimerson et al. (1977), in a bioassay of urine melatonin in six adult patients with primary depression as compared with six control subjects, did not see any difference between the two groups. Also, Thompson et al. (1988), in RIA of serum melatonin in nine patients with a diagnosis of "endogenous depression" and paired control subjects, found no difference between the two groups.

Two studies in adult depression showed an increase of melatonin. Stewart and Halbreich (1989), in a study of 113 patients with Research Diagnostic Criteria for major depression and minor intermittent depression, found that daytime serum melatonin levels were increased in these patients. There was no control group. Rubin et al. (1992) found a significant increase in the nocturnal melatonin level in premenopausal women, ages 22 years and older, with major depression as compared with a control group. Also, they found no difference in the nocturnal melatonin levels in postmenopausal women with major depression or in males with major depression as compared with control subjects. In addition, Rubin et al. (1992) found a higher diurnal serum melatonin level in both male and female depressed patients.

Kennedy et al. (1989) studied 33 females, ages 18–30 years, with anorexia. RIA serum melatonin was performed. There was no control group. The authors divided the anorexic patients into two groups: anorexic patients without depression and anorexic patients with depression. They found that the serum melatonin level in anorexic patients without depression was significantly higher than in those with depression (see Brown et al., Chapter 6, in this volume).

Stanley and Brown (1988) assayed melatonin in the pineal gland of 19 individuals who committed suicide (gunshot wounds, hanging, carbon monoxide poisoning, and drug overdose) versus 19 control subjects who died of sudden death (gunshot wounds, myocardial infarctions, and car accidents). Both groups had 17 males and two females. The results of the measurement of pineal melatonin were divided according to the time of death into three periods: 6 A.M.–2 P.M., 2 P.M.–10 P.M., and 10 P.M.–6 A.M. The authors found that "... melatonin levels in the pineal glands of suicide victims are significantly lower than those of nonsuicide controls ... the greatest group difference during the 2200–0600-hour interval...." (Stanley and Brown 1988, p. 485). They did not report whether or not a psychological autopsy was performed in order to establish a postmortem psychiatric diagnosis.

Melatonin in Child and Adolescent Depression

Compared with studies in adults, neuroendocrinological studies of depression in children and adolescents are limited. This is particularly true with studies of serum or urine melatonin and its metabolite, (aMT6s).

In the United States, there is no accurate estimate of the prevalence of depressive disorders in children and adolescents younger than age 19 years. However, the prevalence of depression in preschool- and school-age children younger than age 12 years is estimated to be close to 2% and in adolescents ages 13–18 years close to 5% (Kashani and Schmid 1992). Conservatively, 1–3 million children and adolescents younger than age 19 years suffer from depressive disorders. Longitudinal studies in recent years have shown that these disorders are mostly cyclic, intermittent, and chronic. They are usually associated with other comorbid psychiatric disorders such as anxiety, phobia, oppositional defiant, attention-deficit/hyperactivity, and conduct disorders. Depressive disorders often continue into adulthood in the form of various mood disorders with comorbidity of antisocial disorders and drug and alcohol abuse (Harrington et al. 1990; Kovacs et al. 1984, 1994; Poznanski 1980; Rohde et al. 1994; Shafii and Shafii 1992). In the psychological autopsies of children and adolescents who committed suicide, between 50% and 75% had a postmortem diagnosis of mood disorder, particularly major depression and/or bipolar disorder (Brent et al. 1988, 1992; Shafii and Shafii 1992; Shafii et al. 1985, 1988).

Symptoms of major depression, such as disturbances in appetite, sleep, concentration, mood changes, and the rest and activity cycle suggest disturbances in the circadian rhythm. As discussed by Reiter, Chapter 1, and Wetterberg, Chapter 3, in this volume, the SCN of the hypothalamus set the pace of circadian rhythms, which is slightly more than 24 hours. Melatonin is immediately distributed through the blood throughout the body's cells and organs. Melatonin has a regulating effect through its receptor sites on the SCN, resulting in the entrainment of the circadian rhythm to a 24-hour cycle.

In healthy individuals, whether children or adults, melatonin is low during daylight. In darkness, melatonin secretion surges. The highest secretion occurs between 11 P.M. and 3 A.M., with a peak at 1 A.M.–2 A.M. (Wetterberg 1978; Wetterberg et al. 1979). It is estimated that between 1% and 5% of melatonin is secreted in the urine, but most of the melatonin is conjugated in the liver and secreted in the urine in the form of inactive aMT6s. Melatonin also can be measured in saliva and in cerebrospinal fluid. The secretion of melatonin is fairly resistant to daily stress. Measurement of serum or urine melatonin reflects the function of the pineal gland. An increase or decrease of melatonin reflects a dysregulation of the pineal gland, which may result in symptoms of biological rhythm disturbances, such as in mood disorders, in children, adolescents, and adults.

Regarding measurement of melatonin in children and adolescents with depressive disorders, Cavallo et al. (1987) reported the first RIA study of serum melatonin. They studied nine males, ages 7–13 years, with a diagnosis of major depression, "atypical depression," or dysthymic disorder. The authors compared these patients with 10 males, ages 9–15 years, of short or normal stature or delayed pubescence. Blood was drawn through continuous sampling over a 24-hour period, and data were reported for every hour. Cavallo et al. (1987) found that mean nocturnal serum melatonin was lower in the depressed group as opposed to the control group. In an earlier report, we have discussed the methodological problems with this study (Shafii et al. 1990). The number of subjects was small, and close to half of the patients had atypical depression. The diagnosis of atypical depression does not have the specificity and accuracy of other types of depressive disorders and has different meanings to different investigators. Comorbid diagnosis, which is often present in child and adolescent depressive disorders, was not discussed. Most of the control subjects were not healthy because they had been referred due to short stature or delayed pubescence. Also, the use of an integrated blood sampling method blurs the specificity of the time sample, whereas intermittent sampling is time specific.

Shafii et al. (1988, 1990) measured bedtime and overnight urine melatonin in 96 children and adolescents, ages 6–16 years (33%, 6–11 years; 67%, 12–16 years). In regard to developmental stages of puberty, "39% were in Tanner stages I and II and 61% were in Tanner stages III–V" (Shafii et al. 1990, p. 108). The male-to-female ratio was 56%:44%. These 96 patients were divided into three groups: group I, primary depression ($N = 21$), consisted of major depression, major depression plus dysthymia, or dysthymia; group II, secondary depression ($N = 36$), consisted of major depression and/or dysthymia along with anxiety, conduct, adjustment, psychosis, and identity disorders; group III, control group ($N = 39$), consisted of conduct, oppositional defiant, and attention-deficit/hyperactivity disorders. In RIA of bedtime and overnight urine in these groups, we found that there was no significant difference in mean bedtime urine melatonin. To our surprise, mean melatonin in the overnight urine in group I, primary depression, was significantly higher than in the other two groups: $\bar{x}_I = .438$ nmol/L $\pm .147$ (SE .031); $\bar{x}_{II} = .275$ nmol/L $\pm .121$ (SE .024); $\bar{x}_{III} = .273$ nmol/L $\pm .156$ (SE .023), $P < .001$. When simultaneous adjustments for age, sex, race, height, and weight were made, mean melatonin in the overnight urine of group I, primary depression, continued to be significantly higher than that of the other two groups ($P < .01$). Adjustment for seasons and Tanner stages did not affect the results.

This study had some methodological problems. The control group was a nondepressed psychiatric group instead of a healthy control group. Although we used various depressive rating scales and child behavior checklists, in addition to reviewing the patients' psychiatric and medical records during hospitalization, we did not use structured diagnostic interviews.

Waterman et al. (1992) measured aMT6s in 31 children and adolescents, ages 6–14 years, with major depression and 15 healthy control subjects. They found that there was no significant difference between the two groups. These investigators also had some methodological problems with their study. They measured aMT6s after giving their subjects insulin 12 hours earlier as a challenge test for growth hormone studies. The use of insulin may have affected the synthesis of melatonin in the pineal gland, the metabolism of melatonin in the liver, and the excretion of its metabolite, aMT6s, in the urine. Waterman et al. (1992) did not measure aMT6s in the bedtime urine to establish a baseline. Also, they did not measure melatonin in the urine to compare it with its metabolite.

In a recent study, Shafii et al. (1995, 1996) measured nocturnal serum melatonin from 6 P.M. to 7 A.M. using RIA. Intermittent blood sampling was drawn through an indwelling catheter every half hour to establish a specific time for the sample. The subjects ranged in age from 8–17 years. There were 41 subjects divided into two groups: a depressed group ($N = 22$), consisting of patients with major depression ($n = 18$), dysthymia ($n = 1$), and depressive-phase bipolar disorder ($n = 3$) and a healthy control group ($N = 19$). There were no significant differences in the two groups regarding the number of males and females. We used Tanner stages I and II to delineate prepubescence and Tanner stages III–V for pubescence. The ratio of prepubescence to pubescence was slightly less than 1:2.

Based on our earlier study of melatonin in overnight urine, we hypothesized that mean nocturnal serum melatonin in depressed children and adolescents would be higher than in the control subjects (Shafii et al. 1988, 1990). Analysis of overall nocturnal serum melatonin data in our latest study supported this hypothesis.

Lights were turned off at 10 P.M. and subjects were awakened at 7 A.M. We calculated mean serum melatonin during darkness from 10:30 P.M. to 7 A.M. We found that mean serum melatonin during darkness in the depressed group continued to be significantly higher than that in the control group.

In post hoc analysis, the depressed group was divided into two subgroups: depression with psychosis ($n = 7$) and depression without psychosis ($n = 15$). In the depressed group with psychosis, nocturnal serum melatonin was lower than that in the control group, and in the depressed group without psychosis, the nocturnal melatonin continued to be high.

Discussion

Based on our studies, and using diabetes mellitus as a model, we speculate that depressive disorders in children and adolescents may be of two types. Type I would be high melatonin major depression (HMMD). In our studies, 68% of children and adolescents had a significant increase in their nocturnal serum melatonin profile. HMMD usually occurs in childhood but also may occur throughout life. The increase of serum melatonin might be related to a higher synthesis of melatonin from serotonin in the pineal gland or to a decrease in the metabolic degradation of melatonin in the liver. If there were degradation of melatonin in the liver, there should be a significant decrease of aMT6s in the urine of the HMMD group as compared with the control group, which was not the case. Our findings suggest dysregulation of the pineal gland in the form of hyperfunction, resulting in hypermelatoninemia.

Type II would be low melatonin major depression (LMMD) or normal melatonin major depression (NMMD). Type II usually occurs in adults but also may occur in children and adolescents. Wetterberg and other investigators found decreased melatonin in a subset of patients who have major depression; these patients may have a type II depressive disorder. In our study, 32% of depressed children and adolescents were type II. Type II depression in youths may be associated with psychotic features. Low nocturnal serum melatonin may be related to the hypofunctioning of the pineal gland in the form of a decrease in synthesis of melatonin from serotonin, or it could be related to a higher degradation of melatonin in the liver. Again, if there were a higher metabolism of melatonin in the liver, there also should have been a significant increase of aMT6s in the urine. This was not the case.

Based on the nocturnal serum melatonin profile, we speculate that in children and adolescents there may be two types of major depression—either hypermelatoninemia (HMMD) or hypomelatoninemia (LMMD). These types of major depression also might occur in adults. If future clinical investigators confirm these findings, it may have a significant impact in making a more accurate diagnosis and providing specific treatment for various types of depressive disorders, whether in youths or adults.

References

Arendt J: Melatonin assay in body fluids. J Neural Transm Suppl 13:265–278, 1978

Arendt J, Paunier L, Sizonenko PC: Melatonin radioimmunoassay. J Clin Endocrinol Metab 40:347–350, 1975

Arendt J, Wirz-Justice A, Bradtke J: Annual rhythm of serum melatonin in man. Neurosci Lett 7:327–330, 1977

Attanasio A, Borrelli P, Gupta D: Circadian rhythms in serum melatonin from infancy to adolescence. J Clin Endocrinol Metab 61:388–390, 1985

Axelrod J, Weissbach H: Enzymatic O-methylation of N-acetylserotonin to melatonin. Science 131:1312, 1960

Beck-Friis J, Hanssen T, Kjellman BF, et al: Serum melatonin and cortisol in human subjects after the administration of dexamethasone and propranolol. Psychopharmacol Bull 19:646–648, 1983

Beck-Friis J, vonRosen D, Kjellman FJ, et al: Melatonin in relation to body measures, sex, age, season and the use of drugs in patients with major affective disorders and healthy subjects. Psychoneuroendocrinology 9:261–277, 1984

Beck-Friis J, Ljunggren J-G, Thoren M, et al: Melatonin, cortisol and ACTH in patients with major depressive disorder and healthy humans with special reference to the outcome of the dexamethasone suppression test. Psychoneuroendocrinology 10:173–186, 1985a

Beck-Friis J, Borg G, Wetterberg L: Rebound increase of nocturnal melatonin levels following evening suppression by bright light exposure
  in healthy men: relationship to cortisol levels and morning exposure.
  Ann N Y Acad Sci 453:371–375, 1985b

Beck-Friis J, Kjellman BF, Aperia B, et al: Serum melatonin in relation to
  clinical variables in patients with major depressive disorders and a
  hypothesis of a low melatonin syndrome. Acta Psychiatr Scand
  71:319–330, 1985c

Brent DA, Perper JA, Goldstein CE, et al: Risk factors for adolescent
  suicide. Arch Gen Psychiatry 45:581–588, 1988

Brent DA, Perper JA, Moritz G, et al: Psychiatric effects of exposure to
  suicide among the friends and acquaintances of adolescent suicide
  victims. J Am Acad Child Adolesc Psychiatry 31:629–640, 1992

Brown RP, Kocsis JH, Caroff S, et al: Differences in nocturnal melatonin
  secretion between melancholic depressed patients and control subjects. Am J Psychiatry 142:811–816, 1985

Cavallo A: Plasma melatonin rhythm in disorders of puberty: interactions of age and pubertal stages. Horm Res 35:16–21, 1991

Cavallo A: Melatonin secretion during adrenarche in normal human
  puberty and in pubertal disorders. J Pineal Res 12:71–78, 1992a

Cavallo A: Plasma melatonin rhythm in normal puberty: interactions of
  age and pubertal stages. Neuroendocrinology 55:372–379, 1992b

Cavallo A: Melatonin and human puberty: current perspectives. J Pineal
  Res 15:115–121, 1993

Cavallo A, Holt KG, Hejazi MS, et al: Melatonin circadian rhythm in
  childhood depression. J Am Acad Child Adolesc Psychiatry 26:395–
  399, 1987

Cavallo A, Richards GE, Smith ER: Relation between nocturnal melatonin profile and hormonal markers of puberty. Horm Res 37:185–
  189, 1992

Fevre M, Segel T, Marks JF, et al: LH and melatonin secretion patterns in
  pubertal boys. J Clin Endocrinol Metab 47:1383–1386, 1978

Gupta D: The pineal gland in relation to growth and development in
  children. J Neural Transm Suppl 21:217–232, 1986

Gupta D, Riedel L, Frick HJ, et al: Circulating melatonin in children: in
  relation to puberty, endocrine disorders, functional tests and racial
  origin. Neuroendocrinology Letters 5:63–78, 1983

Harrington R, Fudge H, Rutter M, et al: Adult outcomes of childhood and adolescent depression, I: psychiatric status. Arch Gen Psychiatry 47:465–473, 1990

Jimerson DC, Lynch HJ, Post RM, et al: Urinary melatonin rhythms during sleep deprivation in depressed patients and normals. Life Sci 20:1501–1508, 1977

Kashani JH, Schmid LS: Epidemiology and etiology of depressive disorders, in Clinical Guide to Depression and Children and Adolescents. Edited by Shafii M, Shafii SL. Washington, DC, American Psychiatric Press, 1992, pp 43–64

Kennedy SH, Garfinkel PE, Parienti V, et al: Changes in melatonin levels but not cortisol levels are associated with depression in patients with eating disorders. Arch Gen Psychiatry 46:73–78, 1989

Kitay JJ: Pineal lesions and precocious puberty: a review. J Clin Endocrinol Metab 15:622–625, 1954

Kovacs M, Feinberg TL, Crouse-Novak MA, et al: Depressive disorders in childhood, I. Arch Gen Psychiatry 41:229–237, 1984

Kovacs M, Akiskal HS, Gatsonis C, et al: Childhood-onset dysthymic disorder. Arch Gen Psychiatry 51:365–374, 1994

Krabbe KH: The pineal gland especially in relation to the problem of its supposed significance in sexual development. Endocrinology 7:379–414, 1923

Lemaitre BJ, Bouillie J, Hartmann L: Variations of urinary melatonin excretion in humans during the first 30 years of life. Clin Chim Acta 110:77–82, 1981

Lenko H, Lang C, Aubert ML, et al: Hormonal changes in puberty, VII: lack of variation of daytime plasma melatonin. J Clin Endocrinol Metab 54:1056–1058, 1982

Lerner AB, Case JD, Takahashi Y, et al: Isolation of melatonin: the pineal gland factor that lightens melanocytes. Journal of the American Chemical Society 80:2587, 1958

Lewy AJ, Markey SP: Analysis of melatonin in human plasma by gas chromatography: negative chemical ionization mass spectrometry. Science 201:741–743, 1978

McIssac M, Page IH: The metabolism of serotonin (5-hydroxytryptamine). J Biol Chem 234:858, 1959

Mitchell MD, Bibby JG, Sayers L, et al: Melatonin in the maternal and umbilical circulations during human parturition. Br J Obstet Gynaecol 86:29–31, 1979

Nair NPV, Hariharasubramanian N, Pilapil C: Circadian rhythm of plasma melatonin in endogenous depression. Prog Neuropsychopharmacol Biol Psychiatry 8:715–718, 1984

Nair NPV, Hariharasubramanian N, Pilapil C: Circadian rhythm of plasma melatonin in endogenous depression, in Advances in the Biosciences, Vol 53: The Pineal Gland: Endocrine Aspects. Edited by Brown GM, Wainwright SD. Oxford, England, Pergamon, 1985, pp 339–345

Poznanski E: Childhood depression: the outcome. Acta Paedopsychiatrica 46:297–304, 1980

Reiter RJ: Melatonin suppression by static and extremely low frequency electromagnetic fields: relationship to the reported increased incidence of cancer. Rev Environ Health 10(3–4):171–186, 1994

Rivkees SA, Carlson LL, Reppert SM: Guanine nucleotide-binding protein regulation of melatonin receptors in lizard brain. Proc Natl Acad Sci U S A 86:3882–3891, 1990

Rohde P, Lewinsohn PM, Seeley JR: Are adolescents changed by an episode of major depression? J Am Acad Child Adolesc Psychiatry 33:1289–1298, 1994

Rubin RT, Heist EK, McGeoy SS, et al: Neuroendocrine aspects of primary endogenous depression. Arch Gen Psychiatry 49:558–567, 1992

Shafii M, Shafii SL (eds): Biological Rhythms, Mood Disorders, Light Therapy, and the Pineal Gland. Washington, DC, American Psychiatric Press, 1990

Shafii M, Shafii SL: Clinical manifestations and developmental psychopathology of depression, in Clinical Guide to Depression in Children and Adolescents. Edited by Shafii M, Shafii SL. Washington, DC, American Psychiatric Press, 1992, pp 3–42

Shafii M, Carrigan S, Whittinghill JR, et al: Psychological autopsy of completed suicide in children and adolescents: a comparative study. Am J Psychiatry 142:1061–1064, 1985

Shafii M, Foster MB, Greenberg RA, et al: Urinary melatonin in depressed children and adolescents, in 1988 Syllabus and Proceedings Summary, 141st Annual Meeting of the American Psychiatric Association. Washington, DC, American Psychiatric Association, 1988, p 188

Shafii M, Foster MB, Greenberg RA, et al: The pineal gland and depressive disorders in children and adolescents, in Biological Rhythms, Mood Disorders, Light Therapy, and the Pineal Gland. Edited by Shafii M, Shafii SL. Washington, DC, American Psychiatric Press, 1990, pp 97–116

Shafii M, MacMillan DR, Key MP, et al: Serum melatonin in early onset depression, in Syllabus and Proceedings Summary, 148th Annual Meeting of the American Psychiatric Association. Washington, DC, American Psychiatric Association, 1995, pp 131–132

Shafii M, MacMillan DR, Key MP, et al: Nocturnal serum melatonin profile in major depression in children and adolescents. Arch Gen Psychiatry 53:1009–1013, 1996

Silman LE, Leone RM, Hooper RJL, et al: Melatonin, the pineal gland and human puberty. Nature 282:301–303, 1979

Stankov B, Fraschini F, Reiter RJ: Melatonin binding sites in the central nervous system. Brain Res Brain Res Rev 16:245–256, 1991

Stankov B, Fraschini F, Reiter RJ: The melatonin receptor: distribution, biochemistry and pharmacology, in Melatonin: Biosynthesis, Physiological Effects, and Clinical Applications. Edited by Yu H-S, Reiter RJ. Boca Raton, FL, CRC Press, 1993, pp 155–186

Stanley M, Brown GM: Melatonin levels are reduced in the pineal glands of suicide victims. Psychopharmacol Bull 24:484–488, 1988

Stewart JW, Halbreich U: Plasma melatonin levels in depressed patients before and after treatment with antidepressant medication. Biol Psychiatry 25:33–38, 1989

Thompson C, Franey C, Arendt J, et al: A comparison of melatonin secretion in normal subjects and depressed patients. Br J Psychiatry 152:260–266, 1988

Vanecek J: Melatonin binding sites. J Neurochem 51:1436–1440, 1988

Viswanathan M, Laitinen JT, Saavdra JM: Expression of melatonin receptors in arteries involved in thermoregulation. Proc Natl Acad Sci U S A 87:6200–6204, 1990

Waldhauser F, Weiszenbacher G, Frisch H, et al: Fall in nocturnal serum melatonin during prepuberty and pubescence. Lancet 1:362–365, 1984

Waldhauser F, Weiszenbacher G, Tatzer E, et al: Alterations in nocturnal serum melatonin levels in humans with growth and aging. J Clin Endocrinol Metab 66:648–652, 1988

Waterman GS, Ryan ND, Perel JM, et al: Nocturnal urinary excretion of 6-hydroxymelatonin sulfate in prepubertal major depressive disorder. Biol Psychiatry 31:581–590, 1992

Wetterberg L: Melatonin in humans: physiological and clinical studies. J Neural Transm Suppl 13:289–310, 1978

Wetterberg L, Eriksson O, Friberg Y, et al: A simplified radioimmunoassay for melatonin and its application to biological fluids: preliminary observations on the half-life of plasma melatonin in man. Clin Chim Acta 86:169–177, 1978

Wetterberg L, Beck-Friis J, Aperia B, et al: Melatonin/cortisol ratio in depression. Lancet 2:1361, 1979

Wetterberg L, Aperia B, Beck-Friis J, et al: Pineal-hypothalamic-pituitary function in patients with depressive illness, in Steroid Hormone Regulation of the Brain. Edited by Fuxe K, Gustafsson JA, Wetterberg L. Oxford, England, Pergamon, 1981, pp 397–403

Wetterberg L, Beck-Friis J, Kjellman BF: Melatonin as a marker for a subgroup of depression in adults, in Biological Rhythms, Mood Disorders, Light Therapy, and the Pineal Gland. Edited by Shafii M, Shafii SL. Washington, DC, American Psychiatric Press, 1990, pp 69–95

Wirz-Justice A, Arendt J: Diurnal, menstrual cycle and seasonal indole rhythms in man and their modification in affective disorders, in Biological Psychiatry Today. Edited by Obiols J, Ballús C, Gonzàles Monclús E, et al. Amsterdam, Elsevier North-Holland, 1979, pp 294–302

Wurtman RJ, Axelrod J, Fischer JE: Melatonin synthesis in the pineal gland: effect of light mediated by the sympathetic nervous system. Science 143:1328–1330, 1964

Chapter 8

Melatonin in Sleep Disorders in Children With Neurodevelopmental Disabilities

James E. Jan, M.D., F.R.C.P.C., Hilary Espezel, R.N., B.S.N., and Keith J. Goulden, M.D., F.R.C.P.C.

Sleep disturbances in children and adolescents are a common concern of pediatricians (McGarr and Hovell 1980; Mindell et al. 1994). There are numerous surveys on sleep problems in children without neurodevelopmental disabilities (Dahl et al. 1991; Fisher et al. 1989; Johnson 1991; Kahn et al. 1989; Kaplan et al. 1987; Kataria et al. 1987; Klackenberg 1982; Lozoff et al. 1985; Scott and Richard 1990; and Zuckerman et al. 1987). It would be difficult to compare these studies even with each other because of various methodologies and definitions. Difficulties in going to sleep and night awakenings are the most common sleep disturbances, affecting about 20% of the population. Sleep disturbances tend to be age related and transient, and, in most instances, children who have sleep disturbances respond well to the treatment advice given to parents.

Sleep disturbances are present in up to 80% of children with neurodevelopmental disabilities. This statistic is not surprising because sleep requires neurological control. Prevalence studies have focused on individuals with mental retardation (Bartlett et al. 1985; Quine 1991; Stores 1992), Down's syndrome (Cunningham et al. 1986), Rett's syndrome (Piazza et al. 1990, 1991), tuberous sclerosis (Hunt and Stores 1994), Tourette's syndrome (Allen et al. 1992), brain damage (Okawa et al. 1986), and blindness (Espezel et al. 1996; Jan et al. 1994; Sasaki et al. 1992). The sleep disorders associated with disabilities are often chronic and resistant to strict bedtime scheduling, various psychological measures, and sedatives. Some of these children have difficulty falling asleep, and some sleep in a fragmented fashion throughout the day, whereas others have varying sleep-onset problems or sleep during the daytime rather than during the night. When the children are awake, they tend to fuss, cry, play, and demand attention from their exhausted parents. Such chronic sleep disturbances can seriously affect the caregivers and siblings. The parents, who already experience significant stress from the amount of care they have to provide for their disabled child, also may have their own health problems along with other psychological and economic strains. In addition, the parents may have chronic sleep difficulties themselves because of their child's chronic sleep disturbances, which may become a major factor in their inability to cope and to provide care for their child (Espezel et al. 1996).

A few years ago, a blind child with multiple neurological disabilities had severe chronic fragmented sleep disorder and did not respond to the conventional treatments. His parents were sleep deprived and in crisis. On compassionate grounds, we decided to prescribe melatonin as a possible treatment (Palm et al. 1991). The treatment was successful, far beyond expectations, so we began to use it for other children.

Methodology

This research was carried out as two independent studies. One research team was located in Vancouver, British Columbia, and the second in Edmonton, Alberta. The Vancouver study was done by British Columbia Children's Hospital Visually Impaired Program, which is a provincial facility where children with visual loss are referred for interdisciplinary medical, developmental, and educational assessments and habilitative services. As part of their evaluation, caregivers were interviewed, with specific inquiry concerning the children's sleep disturbances. If the children had sleep disturbances, they were assessed further and treated with melatonin. Although the medical community has become more aware of this project, and some children with normal sight also have been accepted for melatonin treatment, our study is biased toward the visually impaired.

Polysomnographic studies are exceedingly difficult and expensive to perform in children with multiple disabilities because of their lack of cooperation. Many such patients cannot tolerate attached electrodes because of their tactile defensiveness. Changes in environment, especially hospital admissions, tend to cause deterioration in their sleep pattern. Blood samples are difficult to obtain because the children are often terrified of needles. The success of maintaining an intravenous access site is unlikely for similar reasons. Urine collections frequently require indwelling catheters, and the subjects need to be restrained during that period. We have been criticized for the lack of polysomnographic testing in our study, but these criticisms do not take into account the extreme difficulty of getting disabled children to cooperate with the requirements of polysomnographic recording and the burdens on their parents.

In our studies, we had to rely heavily on the parents or caregivers for sleep charting. In the Vancouver study, sleep charting was done for 7–10 days before and 7–10 days after the melatonin treatment was initiated. Although such measurements appear to be inexact, we and the parents felt that they were accurate because their multidisabled children, when awake during the night, tended to rouse them by their crying and demands. Therefore, the sleep charts also represented the sleep disturbances of one or both parents (Figure 8–1). Adults can record their own sleep patterns with acceptable accuracy; such measurements correlate rather well with polysomnographic testing (Haynes et al. 1981). It also has been documented that, with sleep charting, the parents can accurately record the aberrant sleep patterns of their multidisabled children (Piazza et al. 1990). A member of the Vancouver team also has begun a study to compare the accuracy of sleep recording in children with multiple disabilities done by parental

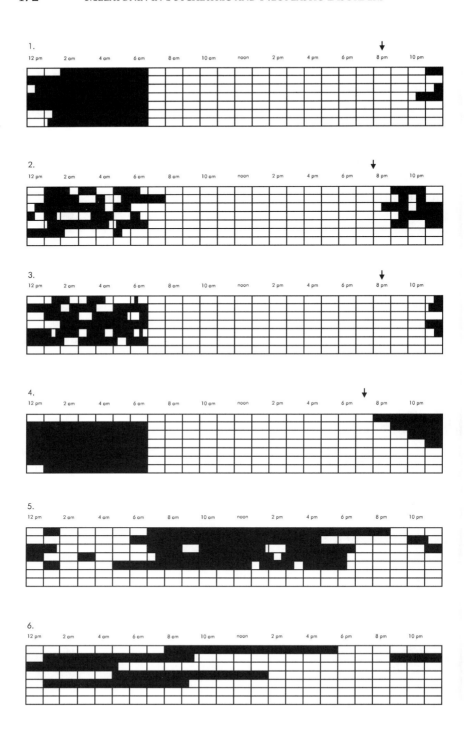

somnologs and by computerized actigraphs. So far, no conclusions can be drawn.

During the early days of the Vancouver study, oral fast-release melatonin or a placebo was administered in a double-blind, randomized fashion for 7–10 days, with a washout period of 5 days. However, with melatonin treatment, in most instances the effects were so obvious and immediate that everyone knew when placebo or melatonin was given. Therefore, the use of placebo became superfluous. Subsequently, the majority of the patients had 7–10 days of sleep charting done by the caregivers before and during treatment, and then the results were compared. This method of sleep charting appeared to be a practical and reasonably accurate measurement of changes in the sleep pattern. Some might say that 7–10 days of sleep charting in both phases is too short, but in clinical practice it is difficult to request more from the exhausted caregivers.

Initially, only a 3-week supply of oral synthetic melatonin was prescribed, and the families were contacted by telephone every 2–3 days. After this phase, if the response was successful, prescriptions were given at 3-month intervals to ensure follow-up. Melatonin is an investigational drug, although it is widely available in many health food stores. For these studies, it is supplied by Sigma Company, St. Louis, Missouri, in a powder form, which is then prepared as 5-mg capsules. More recently, tablets have been made available.

The Edmonton study developed after the Vancouver experi-

Figure 8–1. Samples of sleep-wake cycle disturbances. *(From top)* 1. Delayed sleep onset, 2. fragmented sleep pattern, 3. combination of delayed sleep onset and fragmentation, 4. free-running sleep-wake rhythm cycle, 5. day-night reversal, and 6. variable sleep onset. The sleep charts are recorded by the caregivers. The horizontal squares indicate hours from midnight to midnight, and the vertical divisions represent days. Black spaces show when the child is asleep, and the arrows indicate when the child is put to bed. The first four children are regularly woken up in the morning at the same time.

ence but involved placebo control and blinded outcome analysis. All children needing assistance with refractory sleep disorders were included and, because the investigators are located at a rehabilitation hospital, most had significant developmental disabilities. Consenting families were offered (blindly) either melatonin/lactose capsules or lactose placebo for 6 weeks and then crossed over to the other. Baseline 4-week sleep charting was compared with sleep diaries and clinical response during both treatment and placebo phases and afterward. If the long-term need for therapy had not been demonstrated already, children were withdrawn from treatment until the sleep disorder returned, usually within a day or two, and then without breaking the blind, families were offered the "effective" treatment long term. Our minimum of 6 months' follow-up, so far, has shown continued response in all long-term "responders." Clinical examination and wrist radiographs for bone age were completed on all prepubertal children at baseline and after 6 months of therapy.

Results

Since the fall of 1991, the Vancouver team has treated 90 children with melatonin for their chronic sleep-wake disorders—52 males and 38 females. Their ages ranged from 3 months to 21 years, with an average age of 10.3 years. Approximately 20 additional families requested help for their children, but they were not enrolled in the study because the parents or caregivers failed to complete the sleep charting, the sleep difficulties were minor or subsided, or the sleep disturbances could be treated with conventional methods. Visual loss was documented in 47 of the 90 subjects (15 ocular, 25 cortical, and 7 combined cases). There were 79 subjects with multiple neurodevelopmental disabilities such as mental retardation, cerebral palsy, deaf-blindness, and epilepsy. The causes were chromosomal abnormalities, hypoxic-ischemic and other types of diffuse brain damage, head injury, autism, various forms of epilepsy, or degenerative central nervous system disorders, such as Rett's syndrome and infantile Refsum's disease. There were only

11 subjects who were not multidisabled, and their diagnoses were attention-deficit/hyperactivity disorder (4), anxiety disorder (1), ulcerative colitis (1), brain tumor (2), severe sleep myoclonus (1), head injury (1), and total ocular blindness (1).

The duration of the sleep disorders ranged from a few weeks to 20 years. The treatment was successful in 87% (78 of 90) of the children. The sleep-wake cycle disturbances are shown in Table 8–1. The following factors might have been responsible for the failure of treatment in nonresponders: recurrent pain (2), destroyed suprachiasmatic nucleus (3), noisy sleep environment (1), psychological reasons for delayed sleep onset (1), multiple bedtime medications (1), extreme organically driven behavior (1), and unclear (2). Several responders initially failed until their multiple sedatives were discontinued or until their pain, due to esophageal reflux, was corrected.

The Edmonton study has included treatment of 16 children and 1 parent (8 males and 9 females). The childrens' ages ranged from 3½ to 15 years, with a mean age of 6.7 years. Eight of these children had visual impairment and the remaining eight had multiple disabilities: cerebral palsy (2), learning disability (2), mental retardation (2), autism (1), and optic nerve hypoplasia with autism (1). The mother of one child with multiple disabilities had a chronic delayed sleep-onset disorder. This disorder severely limited her ability to assess the outcome for her child because she was

Table 8–1. Sleep-wake cycle disturbances ($N = 107$)

	Vancouver study	Edmonton study
Fragmented	44	6
Delayed sleep onset	18	8
Combined fragmented and delayed	20	2
Free running	5	1
Variable sleep onset	1	0
Night-day reversal	1	0
Markedly reduced sleep time	1	0

awake already and her activity awakened him. Both she and her son have benefited from treatment.

Two subjects were withdrawn from the study during treatment, one because of medical problems requiring admission to the hospital and surgery and the other because of psychiatric admission of a parent, leaving $N = 14$. One child's response could not be determined because of his caregiver's own sleep disorder as mentioned previously. Nine of the 14 subjects were long-term responders, with 8 on melatonin and 1 on placebo (57% versus 7%, $P < .05$). Three children (21%) did not respond or had only transient response to treatment: one with autism had unusual "cycles" of sleep disturbance, and two with mental retardation had fragmented sleep patterns. Two cases (14%) were undetermined: one because the mother herself had sleep difficulties, and one showed short-term improvement but not impressive enough for the parents to maintain the child on long-term treatment. Of the 17 parents, 13 (76%) could differentiate whether or not the child was on the "active" drug, 2 (12%) identified the placebo as the "active" drug ($P < .01$), and 2 other parents (12%) were unable to give an opinion.

Caregivers Before Treatment

The status of the caregivers before melatonin treatment is described to show the adverse effect that childrens' chronic sleep-wake disorders can exert on their families. In 24 of 86 families in the Vancouver study, the children were placed in alternate care. Many birth parents cited the chronic sleep disturbances of their children as the reason for this placement. Several of these subjects were subsequently transferred to group homes because even the foster parents were unable to look after them. It was often impossible for families to leave their children with baby-sitters, and they consequently rarely had a break. Some families were fortunate enough to be able to hire government-subsidized caregivers who stayed with the children two to three nights per week while their parents rested. Although such an arrangement affected the privacy of the family, it allowed them to carry on. Many caregivers looked exhausted, with dark circles around their eyes, and drank coffee continuously to fight their sleep deprivation. In several families, one of the partners left the family unit. One mother angrily stated during her initial interview that her family was abused for years by her child's sleep disorder. Another mother admitted that for 12 years she and her husband had not slept together because their child, with multiple disabilities and a chronic sleep disorder, required constant supervision. The majority of caregivers felt that physicians, other professionals, and advice books on sleep offered little or no help. Usually, although not always, the mother carried the brunt of the caregiving. Some children were given five to six nighttime sedatives and lived in a drugged state. Relatives often implied that since sleep was natural, something had to be wrong with the parents' care. Two mothers were contemplating suicide. Some caregivers constructed intricate yet safe beds for their children so that they would not be able to crawl out when awake during the night.

Dosage

The dose of oral fast-release melatonin in the Vancouver study ranged from 2.5 mg to 20 mg, with the majority of children given 5 mg. None of these subjects were treated with slow-release melatonin. Calculating the dose according to body weight was not necessary. Infants and toddlers were generally started on 2.5 mg, whereas older children were started on 5 mg. During the initial stages of the treatment, higher quantities of melatonin were sometimes used until a satisfactory sleep pattern was developed, then it was reduced to an optimum level. Because adverse side effects have not been observed, the caregivers were allowed some freedom in increasing or reducing the amount of melatonin. For example, many parents noticed that larger doses were required when their children had an upper respiratory tract infection or during a change in the daily routine, such as traveling, visitors to the home, vacations, and moving.

In the Edmonton study, the dosage was titrated during treatment, starting at 2.5 mg for smaller children and 5 mg for children above 25 kg. If a child responded to the initial dose, it was decreased. A lack of response was titrated upward by doubling the starting dose. Long-term responders took 2.5–10 mg (two took 2.5 mg, four took 5 mg, two took 10 mg), which was a mean of 0.25 mg/kg (range 0.1–0.4 mg/kg). Predictably, the subjects went to sleep a short time after administration of melatonin, usually within 10–20 minutes.

Administration of Melatonin

The "desired" bedtime for each child was worked out together with the parents, taking the age of the child into consideration and realizing that if the child went to sleep too early, he or she would wake up too early. Melatonin usually was administered orally at the desired bedtime. At times, it was also given by gastrostomy tube, as was the case for several children. None of the patients objected to the taste of the medication. Some caregivers administered melatonin when the subject was already in bed, whereas others did so 15–30 minutes before bedtime. When the children resisted going to bed, the medication was given earlier and, as they became sleepy, the resistance often quickly diminished. Several parents observed that melatonin taken on an empty stomach usually produced sleep within 15–20 minutes; when melatonin was taken with a meal, the sleep onset could be delayed by a half hour. When melatonin was administered with other medications, such as anticonvulsants or various feeding formulas, the absorption of the melatonin often appeared to be delayed and at times had no effect. Therefore, the caregivers were carefully instructed to give other drugs 1 or 2 hours earlier than melatonin, with melatonin given either 30 minutes before or 1½ hours after a tube feeding. Melatonin treatment appeared to be more effective when given regularly and always at the same time, combined with a strict sleep schedule and strong clues indicating bedtime and awakening.

Normalization of Sleep

Most children's sleep improved as the treatment began, but their sleep pattern often did not normalize until 1–4 weeks later; occasionally, the process took several months. Surprisingly, chronic sleep-wake cycle disorders in some cases responded immediately to the first dose of melatonin. The majority of caregivers described the response to treatment as "great." It is noteworthy that the parents continued to sleep poorly at times for several weeks after the normalization of their children's sleep patterns, even though they were no longer awakened during the night. Early morning awakening was frequently seen and was difficult to treat by increasing the bedtime dosage of "fast-release" melatonin.

As expected, because the Edmonton drug trial was a blinded study, the success rate was lower than that of the Vancouver study, which was an open trial. Also, the Edmonton study group was smaller and came from a more varied background.

Adverse Side Effects of Melatonin

Adverse side effects of melatonin, including drowsiness in the morning, were not seen in the Vancouver study. However, on two occasions, during the first few days of treatment, the parents reported restlessness and irritability shortly after the administration of melatonin. We felt that this restlessness and irritability might be due to increased drowsiness in these sleep-deprived children, who were struggling to fall asleep.

In the Edmonton drug trial, as well, there were no adverse side effects of melatonin. It is of note that four of the children (25%) had baseline abnormalities of bone age: two with advanced bone age, having already gone through a precocious puberty, and two with significantly delayed bone age—one of whom had pituitary growth hormone deficiency. Another subject had recognized abnormalities of the pituitary and was taking hormonal replacement. These findings suggest that the children who are "at risk" for refractory sleep disorders because of their multiple disabilities are also at risk for hormonal abnormalities.

Drug Interactions With Melatonin

Our studies were not designed for the analysis of complex drug interactions, but it appeared that many medications could interact with the effectiveness of melatonin. When children were taking several sedatives because of their chronic sleep disorders, melatonin was often ineffective, or less effective, until some of these drugs were discontinued. Drugs such as vigabatrin appeared to promote sleeplessness. Drug interaction must be carefully studied in the future.

Mood and Cognitive Changes

As our subjects began to sleep normally, their parents saw them as less irritable, calmer, happier, more playful, content, and affectionate, with fewer temper tantrums. They were able to socialize better and were more gentle with their siblings and pets. They also became more attentive, while their cognitive abilities and mobility improved. On rare occasions, lethargy changed to hyperactivity and, as a result, more care was required to look after them. In the majority of children, there was a close relationship between better sleep and better mood. However, in a couple of children, as the melatonin treatment began, the improved behavior was evident even without a significant change in their sleep pattern. A common comment from parents was that it was now easier to get a baby-sitter. Self-injurious and self-stimulating behaviors, which had often been seen in our multidisabled patient population, tended to diminish with melatonin treatment.

Health Benefits

Parents consistently commented that their children seemed to have fewer infections while taking melatonin than before treatment and were generally healthier. Increased appetite and growth rate were also commonly noted. Unexpected improvements were seen in esophageal reflux (2), gastrointestinal symptoms of ulcerative colitis (1), cystic fibrosis (1), and nonspecific chronic diarrhea (3). Thus, it appears that melatonin may have some as yet unclear function on the gastrointestinal tract. Children who had uncontrolled epilepsy appeared to have, at times, significantly fewer seizures.

Impact of Successful Treatment on Family and Other Caregivers

The normalization of sleep in our subjects meant major benefits for the families and for other caregivers. The following statements seem to represent their feelings:

- "There is improved quality of life for all of us."
- "We can't see life without melatonin."
- "The family bonds are closer."
- "It saved our sanity."
- "Melatonin treatment saved our family from falling apart."
- "There is less stress on the marriage."
- "We are more patient with the other children."
- "We spend more time together."
- "I am not as tired."
- "I didn't realize how tired I was."
- "I am more efficient in my job, and I can now work in the evening."

There were some sad comments as well, such as "Unfortunately, it is too late for my marriage." Therapists, teachers, and other caregivers also confirmed an improvement in the functioning of these children.

Duration of Treatment With Melatonin

The aim of melatonin treatment, together with careful restructuring of sleep routines, was to establish a normal sleep pattern. Once this developed in the Vancouver study, melatonin was gradually withdrawn without any apparent side effects. However, the majority of children with severe disabilities could not maintain their normalized sleep without continuous treatment with melatonin, even with strong environmental enforcement. There were exceptions. A few patients only needed melatonin for a few days and some only for several months. As melatonin was introduced and the subjects' sleep normalized, other sedatives were successfully discontinued. In a few patients, the dose of melatonin needed to be increased over time, but the development of tolerance was not seen.

Discussion

Chronic sleep disorders, commonly seen in children with multiple neurodevelopmental disabilities, can have a devastating effect on the family unit. Children with multiple disabilities are predisposed to sleep-wake rhythm disturbances because they may not be able to perceive or interpret a multitude of cues for synchronizing their sleep with the environment (Arendt 1993). Observing the subjects' rapid response to melatonin treatment, we could hypothesize that they have abnormal melatonin secretion, although we have not measured their melatonin levels. Further studies should also include melatonin measurements, even though it is very difficult to do in the disabled.

Desynchronization of sleep patterns with the environment can occur at any age from infancy to old age. It is not isolated to individuals with vision loss or with specific neurological diseases (Sahelian 1995). Therefore, melatonin treatment offers hope to individuals with chronic disabilities, head injuries, autism, psychiatric disorders (Brown 1995), and degenerative neurological conditions (Jan and Espezel 1995; Jan et al. 1994) and also to those whose sleep is desynchronized because of shift work (Folkard et al. 1993), traveling (Arendt et al. 1987; Petrie et al. 1993), or unstructured sleep habits (Dahlitz et al. 1991; Weitzman et al. 1981).

Melatonin treatment does not correct all sleep disorders, but it is simple, effective, quick, and safe in some sleep-wake rhythm disturbances. The benefits from normalizing sleep in children with disabilities are significant, and there appear to be additional independent gains (Sahelian 1995).

In any clinical drug trial, it is useful to study both the responders and nonresponders. Recurring pain, the cause of which is often hidden in the disabled, can produce fragmentation of sleep. The most common example of this appears to be esophageal reflux (Heine et al. 1995), which causes discomfort, especially when the child lies down to sleep. Melatonin does not appear to help these patients.

Noise, psychological factors, and multiple medications also may result in treatment failure. Children with multiple disabilities frequently have treatment-resistant seizure disorders, which often result in momentary arousals. At the beginning of our studies, we speculated that melatonin is unlikely to help these patients. However, more than half of the responders had epilepsy and their seizures significantly diminished.

It is noteworthy that three subjects, after surgery for their optic nerve gliomas, had a damaged suprachiasmatic nucleus and developed severe sleep fragmentation. All forms of treatment, including melatonin, failed to help these children. In rats, entrainment of circadian rhythm by melatonin does not occur after lesion of the suprachiasmatic nucleus (Cassone et al. 1986). From the previous discussions, it is clear that the key to successful treatment is proper selection of patients.

We are not aware of any published studies of melatonin levels in children with disabilities, but in healthy volunteers, after oral administration, the peak plasma concentration of melatonin occurs within 1 hour (Waldhauser et al. 1990). Most of our patients were indeed asleep within 30 minutes. Melatonin has a short half-life of 30–53 minutes (Aldhous et al. 1985); therefore, the dosages of fast-release melatonin initially must result in supraphysiological levels. It is reasonable to assume that by early morning melatonin would be metabolized, but most of our subjects still eventually slept through the night. Slow-release oral melatonin may have the advantage that smaller doses would be required without early morning awakening, although this has not been studied.

We have been struck with the plight of families caring for children with chronic sleep disorders. So many sleep-deprived parents desperately and most often unsuccessfully try to obtain help. Many novice professionals are ready to criticize them because of their own lack of experience in sleep management. Our research shows that, in the majority of instances, oral fast-release melatonin (2.5 mg–10 mg) given at the desired bedtime can quickly improve the sleep pattern of these children if it is combined with structured sleep routines. The point needs to be emphasized that melatonin is *not* a sedative. Also, melatonin does not always need to be given indefinitely. Once a satisfactory sleep pattern is established, with a well-structured sleep environment the treatment may be withdrawn without side effects and sometimes without recurrence of sleep problems. It is critical for parents to actively promote structured sleep habits for children with multiple disabilities to synchronize their sleep-wake rhythms with the environment.

Interest in melatonin is exploding; close to 1,000 articles a year are being published (Sahelian 1995). Yet, there is need for far more research. In our view, melatonin is now what penicillin was years ago. Melatonin will revolutionize the management of sleep disorders. Despite the fact that there have been no adverse side effects observed, the number of subjects involved in our studies is not yet sufficient to prove the safety of this treatment. Long-term side effects still may be discovered; therefore, melatonin should be used with the scientific discipline that major drugs deserve. It is ironic that although melatonin treatment can literally rescue from despair families who have children with sleep disturbances, physicians cannot prescribe this hormone, and at the same time the sale of melatonin is being withdrawn from health food stores.

Summary

Children with neurodevelopmental disabilities frequently have refractory chronic sleep disorders, which can seriously affect their own health, as well as that of their caregivers and siblings. The sleep-wake cycle disorders of 107 patients with disabilities were treated with oral melatonin and with different methodologies by two independent research teams, one in Vancouver, British Columbia, and the other in Edmonton, Alberta. Eighty-seven subjects responded to doses of 2.5 mg–20 mg given at the desired bedtime, resulting in major health, psychological, and economic benefits for the whole family. Adverse side effects were not observed. In a few cases, melatonin did not need to be given indefinitely once a satisfactory sleep pattern was established within a well-structured sleep environment. The treatment was most effective when combined with strict environmental sleep structuring.

Chronic sleep disorders of children with disabilities must not be ignored because they can have a devastating effect on the child and the entire family. Oral administration of synthetic melatonin appears to be a safe, effective, cost-efficient treatment. Melatonin treatment can rescue families from despair.

References

Aldhous M, Franey C, Wright J, et al: Plasma concentrations of melatonin in man following oral absorption of different preparations. Br J Clin Pharmacol 4:517–521, 1985

Allen RP, Singer HS, Brown JE, et al: Sleep disorders in Tourette syndrome: a primary or unrelated problem? Pediatr Neurol 8:275–280, 1992

Arendt J: Some effects of light and melatonin on human rhythms, in Light and Biological Rhythms in Man. Edited by Wetterberg L. Oxford, England, Pergamon, 1993, pp 203–214

Arendt J, Aldhous M, English J, et al: Some effects of jet-lag and their alleviation by melatonin. Ergonomics 30:1379–1393, 1987

Bartlett LB, Rooney V, Spedding S: Nocturnal difficulties in a population of mentally handicapped children. British Journal of Mental Subnormality 31:53–59, 1985

Brown GM: Melatonin in psychiatric and sleep disorders: therapeutic implications. Central Nervous System Drugs 3:209–226, 1995

Cassone VM, Chesworth MJ, Armstrong SM: Entrainment of rat circadian rhythms by daily injection of melatonin depends upon the hypothalamus suprachiasmatic nuclei. Physiol Behav 36:1111–1121, 1986

Cunningham C, Slope T, Rangecroft A, et al: The effects of early intervention on the occurrence and nature of behavior problems in children with Down's syndrome: final report to DHSS. Manchester, England, Hester Adrian Research Centre, University of Manchester, 1986

Dahl RE, Pelham WE, Wierson M: The role of sleep disturbances in attention deficit disorder symptoms: a case study. J Pediatr Psychol 16:229–239, 1991

Dahlitz M, Alvarez B, Vignau J: Delayed sleep phase syndrome response to melatonin. Lancet 333:1121–1124, 1991

Espezel H, Jan JE, O'Donnell ME, et al: Sleep-wake rhythm disorders of visually impaired children and their treatment with melatonin. Journal of Visual Impairment and Blindness 90:43–50, 1996

Fisher BE, Pauley C, McGuire K: Children's sleep behaviour scale: normative data on 870 children in grades 1 to 6. Percept Mot Skills 68:227–236, 1989

Folkard S, Arendt J, Clark M: Can melatonin improve shift workers' tolerance of night shift? preliminary findings. Chronobiol Int 10:315–320, 1993

Haynes SN, Adam AE, West S, et al: The stimulus control paradigm in sleep-onset insomnia: a multimethod assessment. J Psychosom Res 26:601–606, 1981

Heine RG, Reddihough DS, Catto-Smith AG: Gastro-oesophageal reflux and feeding problems in children with severe neurological impairment. Dev Med Child Neurol 37:320–329, 1995

Hunt A, Stores G: Sleep disorder and epilepsy in children with tuberous sclerosis: a questionnaire-based study. Dev Med Child Neurol 36:108–115, 1994

Jan JE, Espezel H: Melatonin treatment of chronic sleep disorders. Dev Med Child Neurol 37:279–280, 1995

Jan JE, Espezel H, Appleton RE: The treatment of sleep disorders with melatonin. Dev Med Child Neurol 36:97–107, 1994

Johnson CM: Infant and toddler sleep: a telephone survey of parents in one community. J Dev Behav Pediatr 12:108–114, 1991

Kahn A, Van de Merckt C, Rebuffat E, et al: Sleep problems in healthy preadolescents. Pediatrics 84:542–546, 1989

Kaplan BJ, McNichol J, Conte RA, et al: Sleep disturbance in preschool-aged hyperactive and nonhyperactive children. Pediatrics 80:839–844, 1987

Kataria S, Swanson MS, Trevathan GE: Persistence of sleep disturbance in preschool children. J Pediatr 110:642–646, 1987

Klackenberg G: Sleep behaviour studied longitudinally. Acta Paediatrica Scandinavica 71:501–506, 1982

Lozoff B, Wolf AW, Davis NS: Sleep problems seen in pediatric practice. Pediatrics 75:477–483, 1985

McGarr RJ, Hovell MF: In search of the sandman: shaping an infant to sleep. Education and Treatment of Children 3:173–182, 1980

Mindell JS, Moline ML, Zendell SM, et al: Pediatricians and sleep disorders: training and practice. Pediatrics 94:194–200, 1994

Okawa M, Takahashi K, Sasaki H: Disturbance of circadian rhythms in severely brain-damaged patients correlated with CT findings. J Neurol 233:274–282, 1986

Palm L, Blennow G, Wetterberg L: Correction of non-24-hour sleep wake cycle by melatonin in a blind retarded boy. Ann Neurol 29:336–339, 1991

Petrie K, Dawson A, Thompson L, et al: A double-blind trial of melatonin as a treatment for jet lag in international cabin crew. Biol Psychiatry 33:526–530, 1993

Piazza CC, Fisher W, Kiesewetter K, et al: Aberrant sleep pattern in children with Rett Syndrome. Brain Dev 12:488–493, 1990

Piazza CC, Fisher W, Moser H: Behavioral treatment of sleep dysfunction in patients with Rett Syndrome. Brain Dev 13:232–237, 1991

Quine L: Sleep problems in children with mental handicaps. Journal of Mental Deficiency Research 35:269–290, 1991

Sahelian R: Melatonin: Nature's Sleeping Pill. Marina Del Rey, CA, Be Happier Press, 1995

Sasaki H, Nakata H, Murakami S, et al: Circadian sleep-waking rhythm disturbance in blind adolescents (abstract). Jpn J Psychiatry Neurol 46:209, 1992

Scott G, Richard MPM: Night waking in 1-year-old children in England. Child Care Health Dev 16:283–302, 1990

Stores G: Sleep studies in children with a mental handicap. J Child Psychol Psychiatry 33:1303–1317, 1992

Waldhauser F, Saletu B, Trinchard-Lugan I: Sleep laboratory investigations on hypnotic properties of melatonin. Psychopharmacology (Berl) 200:333–336, 1990

Weitzman ED, Czeisler CA, Coleman RA, et al: Delayed sleep phase syndrome, a chronobiological disorder with sleep-onset insomnia. Arch Gen Psychiatry 38:737–746, 1981

Zuckerman B, Stevenson J, Bailey V: Sleep problems in early childhood: continuities, predictive factors and behavioural correlates. Pediatrics 80:664–671, 1987

Part IV

Melatonin and Neoplastic Disorders

Chapter 9

Melatonin at the Neoplastic Cellular Level

Steven M. Hill, Ph.D., Prahlad T. Ram, Ph.D., Tina M. Molis, Ph.D., and Louaine L. Spriggs, Ph.D.

Melatonin (*N*-acetyl-5-methoxytryptamine) is a ubiquitously acting indolamine that exhibits daily rhythms in the pineal gland and serum of almost all vertebrates examined (Reiter 1991a). The pineal gland, an end organ of the visual system, translates the photoperiodic message into a neuroendocrine hormone, melatonin, which serves as a signal to other organs and tissues (Reiter 1980). The ability of the pineal gland to emit a nighttime melatonin signal has been well documented in a variety of mammalian species, including humans. This indolamine is an important neuroendocrine transducer, which, under certain experimental conditions, produces an inhibitory effect on gonadal function. Current evidence supports the concept that under appropriate photoperiodic conditions, melatonin signals the neuroendocrine system to modulate physiological events critical to the regulation of endocrine functions, most notably those related to the control of seasonal reproduction (Reiter 1980, 1987) (see Reiter, Chapter 1, and Bhatnagar, Chapter 2, in this volume).

In the pineal gland, melatonin synthesis is determined primarily by the nighttime release of norepinephrine from nerve endings whose cell bodies are located in the superior cervical ganglia. The mechanisms involved in melatonin release are poorly understood. Because of its high lipophilicity, melatonin most likely diffuses out of the pinealocytes into the circulation, where plasma melatonin levels parallel the pineal melatonin concentration (Reiter 1991b). Thus, blood melatonin is elevated during the dark phase of the

191

light-dark cycle and, because the light-dark ratio changes on a daily basis, the endocrine message that the pineal gland sends to the organism also varies both daily and seasonally (Reiter 1980). The high lipophilicity of melatonin is a critical component in the rapid dissemination of melatonin.

The role of melatonin in coordinating information about day length with the timing of reproduction in photoperiodic animals (Reiter 1987) and with thermoregulatory and locomotor rhythms in reptiles and birds (Ralph 1984) is now firmly established. Melatonin appears to participate as a mediator of circadian variations in mood and sleep in humans (Wurtman and Lieberman 1985). As the major secretory product of the pineal gland, melatonin is unique because not only is it a central regulator of chronobiology, but also, as has been shown in numerous systems, it possesses potent antineoplastic activity. The antitumorigenic actions of melatonin have been observed both in vitro and in vivo in a broad spectrum of tumor types, such as melanoma, ovarian, prostate, pituitary, uterine, and breast. The concept of the pineal gland as an oncostatic endocrine organ is further supported by the fact that in addition to melatonin, which possesses antitumorigenic activity, many other products are secreted from the pineal gland (H. Bartsch et al. 1987). However, the mechanisms through which melatonin acts to mediate these effects have not been clearly elucidated (see Blask, Chapter 10, in this volume).

Currently, we are just beginning to understand some of the molecular and signal transduction pathways that may mediate the actions of melatonin at the cellular level. For example, in the pituitary gland, particularly in cells of the pars tuberalis, evidence suggests that melatonin's signal is transmitted by the interaction of melatonin with a membrane-bound receptor coupled to an inhibitory guanine nucleotide G-binding protein (P. J. Morgan et al. 1989). However, unlike melatonin's actions on the neuroendocrine substrates controlling reproductive physiology, virtually nothing is known regarding the signaling and downstream gene modulatory events initiated or controlled by melatonin that produce its oncostatic effects. A few laboratories have reported the presence of low-affinity melatonin-binding sites in melanoma and breast cancer cells (Burns et al. 1990; Pickering and Niles 1992; Stankov et al. 1991); however, these sites are apparently not linked to adenylate cyclase. In breast cancer, melatonin's antitumorigenic action has been linked to the modulation of both humoral and growth factor response pathways (Blask et al. 1994; Cos and Blask 1994; Molis et al. 1995). Several recent reports have provided evidence that the retinoic acid receptor response pathway may be involved in mediating some of melatonin's actions; however, no definitive signal transduction pathways have been clearly elucidated to account for the antiproliferative effect of melatonin in neoplastic tissues. The aim of this chapter is to describe and outline known aspects of melatonin's actions on the molecular and cellular biology of various neoplastic cells and, based on our current understanding, to define pathways through which these actions are mediated. Because breast cancer has been a key area of focus for melatonin's oncostatic effects, much of the discussion will be drawn from our understanding of melatonin's influence on breast cancer cell biology.

General Effects of Melatonin on Neoplastic Cells

A number of in vitro studies have strongly indicated the presence of active compounds within the pineal gland that are capable of suppressing cellular replication in a number of tissues and tumor types. The tissue types inhibited by various pineal extracts range from renal epithelium to breast areolar epithelium and adipose tissue (Bindoni et al. 1976). From these studies, Bindoni and colleagues suggested that the pineal gland contains an antimitotic factor that is able to restrict cell proliferation in vivo. Early reports (Tapp 1982) postulated a colchicine-like action for melatonin because both colchicine and melatonin appeared to inhibit the formation of mitotic spindles. Follow-up studies by other laboratories have clearly shown that although melatonin's actions are almost always associated with growth arrest or suppression, its effects in the different tissues are not always identical to those of colchicine (Poffenbarger and Fuller 1976). Numerous studies have shown that the surgical removal of the pineal gland from animal models results in the accelerated growth of a variety of experimental tumors. In rats, surgical removal of the pineal gland is associated with the accelerated growth of Ehrlich ascites tumors (Bindoni et al. 1976), Walter 256 transplantable tumors, and 7,12-dimethylbenzanthracene (DMBA) and N-nitrosomethylurea (NMU)-induced mammary tumors (Blask et al. 1991; Kothari 1987). When Syrian hamsters were inoculated subcutaneously with melanoma, the tumor cells proliferated at a significantly elevated rate in pinealectomized hamsters as compared to intact animals (Das Gupta and Terz 1967).

Although most studies regarding melatonin and oncogenesis have focused on either breast cancer or melanoma, numerous studies in recent years have demonstrated an influence of melatonin on tumor growth in various experimental model systems, including bladder carcinoma, colon carcinoma, Ehrlich's tumor, epidermoid carcinoma, fibrosarcomas, pituitary tumors, leukemias, lung carcinoma, neuroblastoma, prostatic carcinoma, and uterine tumors (see Table 9–1). Depending on the tumor and the conditions, effects ranging from growth stimulation to growth inhibition have been observed with melatonin treatment.

Prostatic Carcinoma

The first demonstration that melatonin could inhibit the proliferation of androgen-sensitive prostate tumors was provided by Buzzell and colleagues (Buzzell et al. 1988; Toma et al. 1987). Using the transplantable Dunning (R3327) prostatic tumor in Copenhagen-Fisher male rats sensitized to the antireproductive effects of melatonin by olfactoribulbectomy as a tumor model, this group demonstrated that daily late afternoon injections of melatonin significantly inhibited the growth of these androgen-sensitive tumors. These effects were not associated with changes in nuclear or cytosolic androgen-binding activity or levels of testosterone, prolactin, or serum gonadotropins. A follow-up study by Philo and Berkowitz (1988) showed that melatonin was more effective in inhibiting tumor growth when administered at an elevated dosage to animals maintained under long-day conditions (14L:10D). In this particular study, serum testosterone levels were signifi-

Table 9–1. Neoplasms affected by melatonin

Tumor type	Model	Dose	Results
Bladder carcinoma cells	RT112 cells	525 µg/mL	Decreased growth
Breast cancer	MCF-7 cells	10^{-9}–10^{-11} M	Decreased growth
	Carcinogen-induced rat mammary tumors	500 µg/day	Decreased incidence and growth
Fibrosarcomas	DBF1 mouse	3.5 µg/kg/day	Decreased growth
Leukemia	LSTRA cells Balb/c mice	100 µg/day	Decreased growth
Ovarian carcinoma cells	SKOV-3 and JA-1 cells	600–370 µg/mL	Decreased growth
Pituitary tumors tumor	DES-induced	10^{-7}–10^{-11} M	Decreased growth

Note. DES = diethylstilbestrol.

cantly decreased. Analysis of melatonin's effects on androgen-insensitive tumors reveals a more convoluted picture. Melatonin's effects on these tumors range from inhibitory to stimulatory depending on numerous factors, including whether or not the animals were castrated (Blask and Nodelman 1979; Buzzell et al. 1988; Philo and Berkowitz 1988). Although more detailed analysis of melatonin's effects on models of prostate cancer has been provided by others, the previously mentioned studies clearly demonstrate that melatonin can inhibit the proliferation of hormone-sensitive prostate tumors (see Blask, Chapter 10, in this volume).

Melanoma

The Syrian hamster is a photoperiodically sensitive species that serves as a good animal model for melanoma. Employing this model, Das Gupta and Terz (1967) and Stanberry et al. (1983) found that surgical removal of the pineal gland (pinealectomy) in hamsters inoculated with transplantable hormone-responsive melanoma cells (MM1) promoted tumor growth as well as the metastases of these tumors. Daily injections of melatonin into pinealectomized animals for 2–3 weeks resulted in differential effects, depending on the photoperiodic environment of the animals. Melatonin administration was associated with inhibition of tumor growth and metastasis in animals housed under short-day conditions (6L:18D), whereas melatonin stimulated tumor growth in animals maintained under long-day conditions (14L:10D). A growth-inhibitory effect of melatonin was observed when melatonin was fed to athymic nude mice transplanted with B16 mouse melanoma cells.

In vitro studies by Mayskens and Salmon (1981) found that increasing concentrations of melatonin, ranging from 10-15 M to 10-5 M, inhibited anchorage-independent growth of human melanoma cells in a linear and dose-dependent manner in 6 of 11 tumors, as measured in a soft-agar clonogenic assay. Of the five tumors not growth-inhibited by melatonin, two were stimulated to grow in response to melatonin, whereas three tumors showed no growth. This differential response was supported by the studies of H. Barstch et al. (1986, 1987), who found that human melanoma cells grown in vitro exhibited differential responses to melatonin depending on the length of time in culture (passage number). Cells from early passages were growth inhibited by physiological levels of melatonin but could be stimulated by pharmacological doses. Cells from later passages were growth inhibited only by concentrations of melatonin in the millimolar range. Although the results obtained with melatonin treatment depend on the photoperiodic environment of the animal, route and timing of melatonin administration, and even presence of endogenous melatonin, these studies highlight the fact that the pineal gland via its hormone, melatonin, can inhibit or suppress the development, growth, and metastasis of melanoma (see Table 9–1).

Breast Cancer

A number of studies have examined the role of the pineal gland in mammary tumorigenesis and have found that via its hormone, melatonin, the pineal exerts an inhibitory influence on the development and growth of carcinogen-induced rat mammary tumors (Chang et al. 1985; Tamarkin et al. 1982). The majority of these studies have employed the 7,12-DMBA-induced rat mammary tumor model, which produces hormone-responsive mammary tumors (Welsch and Nagasawa 1977). In general, maximum stimulation of pineal melatonin secretion by binding and removal of the olfactory bulbs significantly decreases both the incidence and volume of DMBA-induced rat mammary tumors and, in some cases, induces the regression of established mammary tumors, as compared with intact DMBA-treated control subjects. Surgical removal of the pineal prevents this oncostatic effect so that tumor incidence and volume are essentially equivalent to intact DMBA-treated control subjects. It should be noted that blinding and anosmia also markedly reduce the levels of estradiol and prolactin, both of which are critical regulators of tumor growth and are most likely modulated by melatonin (Blask 1984; Chang et al. 1985). Additional evidence for a role of the pineal and melatonin in mammary cancer is found in a variety of studies showing that chronic daily late-afternoon injections of melatonin (250 µg/mg/day) suppress both the development and growth of NMU-induced and transplanted R3230 AC rat mammary tumors (Blask et al. 1991; Tamarkin et al. 1981).

In contrast to animal studies, only a marginal amount of work has been conducted with respect to the role of the pineal and melatonin in human breast cancer. A few clinical studies have assessed pineal function in patients with breast cancer. C. Bartsch et al. (1981) found that postmenopausal Indian women with advanced breast cancer have diminished urinary levels of melatonin as compared with those levels in healthy control subjects. Tamarkin et al. (1982) also have shown that the normal nocturnal rise in plasma melatonin is significantly reduced in women with estrogen-receptor (ER)-positive breast tumors as compared with patients who have ER-negative breast tumors or with age-matched control subjects. Furthermore, this group showed an inverse correlation between ER levels and peak nighttime melatonin values. Subsequent studies by Hill and Blask (1988) have shown that physiological concentrations of melatonin, corresponding to peak nighttime plasma levels seen in humans, are able to inhibit the growth and alter the morphology of estrogen-responsive MCF-7 human breast cancer cells in vitro. The direct growth-inhibitory effect of melatonin on breast cancer cell lines has been confirmed by other groups (Cos et al. 1991) who have found, using flow cytometric analyses, that the antiproliferative effect of melatonin, like that of the antiestrogen tamoxifen (Sutherland et al. 1983), is cell cycle–specific, inducing a G/GI-S transition delay in MCF-7 human breast cancer cells. Furthermore, melatonin is able to block the estrogen release of cells inhibited by tamoxifen (Cos et al. 1991). This information, along with our recent evidence (Hill et al. 1991) and that of others, that only ER-positive human breast tumor cell lines are responsive to the antiproliferative effects of melatonin, suggests that melatonin's actions may be linked to the cell's estrogen-response pathway (see Blask, Chapter 10, in this volume).

Melatonin Receptors: Tissue and Subcellular Localization

Binding sites for melatonin have been identified in numerous tissues, including the brain, dermal melanophores, and even breast tissue. The identification and characterization, both structurally and functionally, of these binding sites proceeded at a slow rate until the last decade. Before that time, a clear picture of tissues to which melatonin bound was not available. Vakkuri et al. (1984) demonstrated that melatonin can be iodinated to a high specific activity with iodine-125 (^{125}I), leading to the formation of 2-[^{125}I]-iodomelatonin (I-MEL). This radioligand, I-MEL, has been used extensively to determine both tissue and subcellular localization of melatonin binding. I-MEL has two main advantages over earlier radiolabeled melatonin ligands. First, its high specific activity ensures its ability to detect receptors, which exhibit a high affinity for melatonin but may be present in low abundance, and second, this iodinated ligand retains its biological activity (Weaver et al. 1988).

These properties of I-MEL have now been used by numerous laboratories in identifying and characterizing melatonin receptors. For this purpose, two principal techniques have been employed: ligand-binding assays using homogenized cellular and membrane preparations and in vitro autoradiography. Employing these approaches, high-affinity binding sites were first identified in the hypothalamus of the rat brain (Vanecek et al. 1987). Subsequent studies have demonstrated melatonin-binding sites in other regions of the mammalian brain, with the most intense labeling being found in the pars tuberalis of the hypothalamus (P. J. Morgan et al. 1994). Binding sites for melatonin also have been identified in various peripheral tissues, including the liver, skin, and breast, and in certain neoplasms, including breast tumors (see review by P. J. Morgan et al. 1994). Throughout the literature, two different binding sites with significantly different binding affinities have been reported: a high-affinity binding site with a K_d in the picomolar range and a low-affinity binding site with a K_d in the nanomolar range. The high-affinity binding site has been shown to be sensitive to guanosine 5'-triphosphate (GTP) indicating that these receptors are coupled to G-proteins (Carlson et al. 1989; Dubocovich 1991; Laitinen and Saavedra 1990; P. J. Morgan et al. 1989; Rivkees et al. 1989). Although these studies have identified binding sites, the identity, molecular structure, and mechanism of action of the melatonin receptors remained unknown until only recently.

Melatonin is highly lipophilic (Lerner et al. 1959) and, as such, is capable of diffusing through both the cell and nuclear membranes and entering intracellular compartments, including the nucleus, much like the steroid hormones (Menendez-Pelaez and Reiter 1993). Although most melatonin binding has been localized to the cell membrane, the lipophilic nature of melatonin suggests that receptors for this indolamine could be located in intracellular compartments as well. Within the last couple of years, two distinct classes of melatonin receptors have been identified. The first to be characterized were the G-protein-linked receptors, which are expressed at the cell membrane (Reppert et al. 1994), and the second were the nuclear orphan receptors belonging to the retinoic acid receptor class of the steroid/thyroid hormone receptor superfamily (Becker-André et al. 1994). Both receptors specifically bind melatonin, although with different affinities, and transduce their signals within the cell by significantly different mechanisms. The membrane-bound receptor binds melatonin and transmits its signal through second messengers to affect protein and enzyme activity and possibly even the transcription of specific genes. The intracellular receptors, on the other hand, are localized to the nucleus and, like other members of the steroid receptor superfamily, act as ligand-inducible trans-acting transcription factors.

Membrane-Associated, G-Protein-Linked Melatonin Receptors

Using an expression cloning strategy, melatonin receptor complementary DNAs (cDNAs) have been isolated from *Xenopus laevis* dermal melanophores (Ebisawa et al. 1994)(see Figure 9–1). These receptors exhibit high affinity for I-MEL, with a K_d of approximately 0.06 nM, and have subsequently been identified in Syrian golden hamsters, sheep, and humans (Reppert et al. 1994). Structural analysis of these receptors suggests that they belong to the G-protein-linked superfamily, although they possess unique sequences that do not allow them to be grouped into any known subfamily. This class of surface receptor utilizes heteromeric G-proteins to transmit signals between the receptor and its effector enzymes (Birnbaumer 1990) and includes a number of receptors that share some common features, including an extracellular ligand-binding domain located at the *N*-terminal, seven hydrophobic segments representing the transmembrane domain, and a C-terminal, G-protein-coupled intracellular domain (Pearson 1990). The cDNA for the Mel$_a$ receptor, cloned from *X. laevis* dermal melanophores, encodes a protein of 426 amino acids in *Xenopus,* a protein of 366 amino acids in sheep, and, in humans, a protein of approximately 350 amino acids, with a predicted molecular mass of approximately 39 kilodaltons for the human receptor. The human melatonin Mel_{1a} membrane receptor shows 65% sequence identity to the *Xenopus* melatonin membrane receptor and 85% identity to the sheep receptor. This finding suggests that human and sheep receptor clones are species homologues of the same receptor (Reppert et al. 1994). Recently, Reppert et al. (1995) have cloned and isolated a second melatonin membrane receptor, the Mel_{1b}, that has approximately 40% identity to the Mel_{1a} receptor. These receptor proteins maintain a consensus site for N-linked glycosylation, a common feature of G-protein-associated receptors. Although the melatonin membrane receptor shares general features with other G-protein-linked receptors, it does not belong to any known receptor family. The highest degree of homology is shared with the mu opioid and somatostatin type 2 receptors, which show 25% identity to the human melatonin membrane receptor (Ebisawa et al. 1994). In addition, the carboxyl end of the membrane melatonin receptor also contains consensus sites for protein kinase C phosphorylation, which may play a critical role in receptor regulation. Transfection and expression of the Mel_{1a} membrane receptor into COS-7 cells shows I-MEL binding affinities of 24 pM and a Bmax of about 210 fmol/mg of protein for the human receptor (Reppert et al. 1994). Both the cloned Mel_{1a} and Mel_{1b} receptors inhibit adenylate cyclase through a pertussis toxin–sensitive mechanism (Reppert et al. 1994) and thus appear to be synonymous with the high-affinity binding sites observed in earlier ligand-binding studies (Carlson et al. 1989; P. J. Morgan et al. 1990; Stankov et al. 1991, 1992; White et al. 1987). Recent studies have found a limited distribution of these melatonin membrane receptors. In situ hybridization studies using the cloned Mel_{1a} melatonin membrane receptor cDNA show the highest levels of expression of this receptor in the pars tuberalis of the hypothalamus (Reppert et al. 1994). Expression also is seen in the suprachiasmatic nucleus and the paraventricular nucleus of the thalamus, confirming earlier melatonin-binding studies by other researchers (Bittman and Weaver 1990; P. J. Morgan et al. 1989; Vanecek et al. 1987; Williams et al. 1989). Northern blot analysis of RNA isolated from the pars tuberalis defined a major transcript of > 9.5 kb and a minor messenger RNA (mRNA) of 4 bn (Reppert et al. 1994).

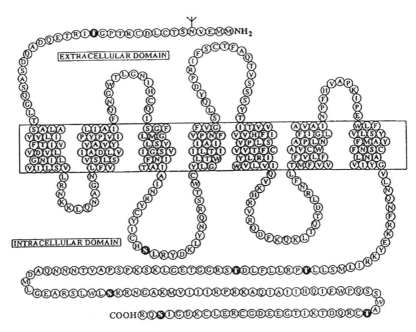

Figure 9–1. Proposed membrane structure of the *Xenopus* melatonin receptor. Deduced amino acid sequence is shown. Ψ = potential *N*-linked glycosylation site; solid circles = consensus sites for protein kinase C phosphorylation.

Source. Reprinted from Ebisawa T, Karne S, Lerner MR, et al.: "Expression Cloning of a High-Affinity Melatonin Receptor From *Xenopus* Dermal Melanophores. *Proceedings of the National Academy of Sciences of the Unites States of America* 91:6133–6137, 1994.

Nuclear Melatonin Receptors

In addition to the melatonin membrane receptor identified by Reppert et al. (1994), recent studies on different tissues have shown nuclear localization of melatonin binding (Burns et al. 1990; Stankov et al. 1991). For example, Acuña-Castroviejo et al. (1993, 1994) have observed melatonin-binding sites in rat liver nuclei. Recently, Becker-André et al. (1994) found that I-MEL was able to specifically bind to a class of nuclear orphan receptors, the retinoid Z receptors α and β (RZRα and RZR β) and the retinoic orphan receptor α (RORα), for which no ligand had previously been identified (Wiesenberg et al. 1995). Unlike the melatonin membrane receptor, these receptors appear to have a lower binding affinity for I-MEL, with a K_d of approximately 50–70 nM. RZRα and RORα belong to the steroid/thyroid hormone receptor superfamily and show considerable sequence conservation with the retinoic acid receptor (RAR) and retinoid X receptor (RXR) (Becker-André et al. 1993; Giguere et al. 1994). Considerable commonality is shared in both structure and function among all members of this receptor superfamily. As with the other steroid hormone receptors, the RZR/RORαs exhibit four domains, three of which are key functional domains (shown in bold in the following diagram): 1) an activation function domain (AF-1) located at their N-terminal, 2) an internal DNA-binding domain (DBD), 3) a hinge domain, and 4) a C-terminal hormone-binding domain (HBD).

Similar to other steroid hormone receptors, there are subdomains located within the DBD and HBD that are critical to the functioning of the receptor. Located in the DBD is a basic region containing a constitutively active, hormone-independent, nuclear localization subdomain A; a second nuclear localization signal that is ligand dependent is contained with the HBD. Also located in the HBD are a dimerization domain, a heat shock protein-binding region, and a hormone-dependent region of activation function termed AF-2. As with all steroid receptors, the hinge domain, located between the DBD and HBD, is the least conserved of all the regions and is involved in receptor folding. The aporeceptor or unliganded receptor exhibits a conformation such that the HBD is in close proximity to the DBD, sterically interfering with the ability of the receptor to bind ligand. In this conformation, the receptor is not competent for transcriptional activation and the subdomains, such as the dimerization domain, are inactive. Upon binding of ligand, the receptor unfolds and the conformation of the HBD is such that specific sites are available for phosphorylation, leading to activation of the AF-2 domain, dimerization, and DNA binding. The activated receptor recognizes and binds cis-acting domains in the upstream region of responsive genes called hormone response elements (HREs). Most members of the steroid hormone receptor superfamily recognize and bind HREs as dimers, either as hetero- or homodimers. However, most data to date suggest that unlike most steroid receptors, the RZR/RORαs bind DNA as monomers (Becker-André et al. 1994; Giguere et al. 1994) to regulate the transcription of specific sets of genes. Initial studies by Giguere et al. (1994) have suggested that RZR/RORαs do not form heterodimers with RXR, RAR, thyroid receptor (TR), or vitamin D receptor (VDR). Because this is not an exhaustive list, there may be other members of the steroid receptor superfamily that could dimerize with RZR/RORα.

Two species of RZR receptors have been identified, the RZRα and RZRβ receptors (Becker-André et al. 1993). In addition, there are four isoforms of the RORα receptors: RORα1, RORα2, RORα3 (Giguere et al. 1994), and RORα4. RZRα is, in fact, a splice variant of the ROR family and as such can be considered as RORα4 and a member of the RORα family. The tissue distribution of RZRβ is considerably different from that of RZRαs and the RORαs. RZRβ expression has only been localized to tissues of the central nervous system and does not appear to be expressed elsewhere in the body (Becker-André et al. 1994). RZRαs and RORαs, on the other hand, are expressed in a number of tissues, including the brain, ovary, testes, kidney, spleen, prostate, thymus, liver, lung, heart, and, most abundantly, in peripheral blood leukocytes (Becker-André et al. 1993; Forman et al. 1994; Steinhilber et al. 1995). In addition, Wiesenberg et al. (1995), as well as our laboratory (Ram and Hill 1995), have identified RORα transcripts in the MCF-7 human breast cancer cell line. Transcriptional activation of RZR/RORα by melatonin has been reported to occur at the midnanomolar range (Becker-André et al. 1994; Wiesenberg et al. 1995). All the isoforms of RZR and RORαs, with the exception of RORα1, bind melatonin and are transcriptionally activated by this indolamine (Becker-André et al. 1994; Wiesenberg et al. 1995). The RORα1 isoform exhibits a significantly different activation function than the other RORα isoforms, exhibiting constitutive transcriptional activity, whereas the other isoforms appear to be modulated in response to melatonin binding. Functionally, RZRα/RORs have been shown to be biologically responsive to melatonin treatment in human B lymphocytes, modulating the transcription of the 5-lipoxygenase gene (Steinhilber et al. 1995). At present, no selective gene activation has been noted for the different receptor forms; however, differential recognition of DNA-binding sites retinoid orphan response elements (ROREs) has been described for the various receptor isoforms (Giguere et al. 1994). This strongly suggests that each receptor isoform may recognize specific versions of the RORE and thus may activate somewhat different sets of genes. A major caveat in this story of RZR and RORα as melatonin receptors is the recent report by Tini et al. (1995) that melatonin binding to the RORα receptors cannot be repeated. Only further studies will prove if RORαs and RZRs are in fact functional melatonin receptors.

Effects of Melatonin on the Estrogen-Response Pathway of Breast Tumor Cells

Studies with animal models of mammary cancer, breast tumors maintained in organ culture, and established breast tumor cell lines have shown that the growth of many breast tumors is clearly estrogen responsive (Daniel and Prichard 1963; Lippman et al. 1976). For example, the MCF-7 human breast cancer cell line is responsive to estrogen but is not totally dependent on estrogen for growth in culture. Yet, when implanted into ovariectomized nude mice, MCF-7 cell growth and solid tumor formation are dependent on concomitant estrogen administration (Bates et al. 1986). The presence or absence of specific ER proteins can be used to identify human breast tumors that are hormone responsive or autonomous (Edwards et al. 1979; McGuire et al. 1975) and thus predict which tumors will successfully respond to endocrine therapy. Approximately 60%–70% of all primary breast tumors are ER positive; of these, approximately 60% respond to endocrine therapy directed toward blockage of estrogenic stimulation (Edwards et al. 1979).

Estrogen receptors represent a class of trans-acting regulatory proteins that bind to the genome and activate specific sets of responsive genes, thereby inducing changes in expression of specific mRNAs and proteins involved in regulating cell proliferation, differentiation, and physiological function (Dickson and Lippman 1987; Dickson et al. 1987). The mechanisms by which estrogen promotes the growth of breast cancer are not completely understood; however, several lines of evidence suggest that polypeptide growth factors and even oncogenes mediate estrogen's mitogenic effect (Dickson et al. 1987). Human breast cancer cells in culture synthesize and secrete a variety of growth factors, such as transforming growth factors α (TGFα) and β (TGFβ), insulin-like growth factors (IGFs), and cathepsin D (a lysosomal protease), among others. The expression, and sometimes secretion, of these growth factors has been found to be modulated by estrogen. In addition to specific growth factors, estrogen also induces the expression of the immediate early genes c-myc (Dubik and Shiu 1988) and c-fos (Weisz and Bresciani 1988), as well as progesterone receptor (PgR) (Horwitz and McGuire 1978) and the protein product of pancreatic spasmolytic polypeptide (pS2) mRNA (Brown et al. 1984).

The expression of ER has been shown to be regulated both in vivo and in vitro by a number of factors, including the cell cycle, cell density, and even growth factors and hormones (retinoic acid). Both insulin and progesterone can alter ER expression to various degrees (Horwitz and McGuire 1978) and, in turn, can affect the growth of breast cancer cells. Because the influence of estrogen on breast cancer cell proliferation is modulated via the ER, it is therefore of interest to identify the mechanisms through which ER expression can be regulated and thus a tumor cell response to estrogen. With the advent of cDNA and antibody probes for ER, PgR (Greene et al. 1986; Misriahi et al. 1987), and other estrogen-induced transcripts and proteins, it is now possible to study the functional significance of alterations in ER expression and the usefulness of these estrogen-regulated products as functional markers of ER activation or deactivation.

Melatonin Modulation of Estrogen Receptor Expression

Past studies have suggested that there is a correlation, although not always consistent, between melatonin and ER expression. For example, studies by Danforth et al. (1983a) found that melatonin is able to suppress the estrogen-induced growth of MCF-7 human breast cancer cells in vitro and that this effect is apparently associated with a rapid but transient increase in estrogen-binding activity. Conversely, Sanchez-Barcelo et al. (1988) observed that in the rat, pineal activation by blinding and olfactory bulbectomy results in a significant decrease in estrogen-binding activity in DMBA-induced mammary tumors as compared with that in non-stimulated and pinealectomized control subjects. This inhibitory effect is supported by studies in other tissues, such as hamster brain, in which melatonin-induced suppression of estrogen-binding activity has been described (Danforth et al. 1983b; Lawson et al. 1992). These data suggest that the pineal gland via its hormone, melatonin, can modulate ER expression in various tissues, including human breast cancer cells; however, the nature and significance of this modulation have not been clearly defined. To test the hypothesis that melatonin inhibits the growth of estrogen-responsive breast cancer via modulation of the cells' estrogen-response pathway, Molis et al. (1993) examined ER expression in MCF-7 breast cancer cells. In these studies, nanomolar concentrations of melatonin, previously found to be effective in inhibiting the proliferation of the ER-positive MCF-7 human breast cancer cell line, were able to significantly suppress both ER protein (Molis et al. 1995) and ER mRNA (Molis et al. 1994) in a time-dependent manner, beginning as early as 6 hours after treatment. The inability of melatonin to compete with labeled estrogen for binding to the ER and its inability to activate the ER in a yeast transcriptional assay (Molis et al. 1993) suggests that the down-regulation of ER by melatonin is not mediated through its binding to the HBD of the receptor and its subsequent activation. More recent studies have shown that the down-regulation of ER mRNA levels is a result of decreased transcription of the ER gene (Molis et al. 1994).

The mechanism by which melatonin suppresses ER gene transcription, however, remains to be elucidated. To fully understand the role of the pineal gland and melatonin in regulating the growth of breast cancer and possibly other endocrine-responsive tissues, it will be necessary to examine and clarify their role in controlling ER expression, as well as the functional significance of this modulation. One possible mechanism by which melatonin may regulate ER gene transcription is via interaction with the 5'-regulatory region of the ER gene. Recent analysis of the 5'-flanking region of the ER gene by Sullivan et al. (1995) has identified a response element for the RORα receptors, an RORE. This finding, combined with the observations of Ram and Hill (1995) and Carlberg et al. (1994) that transcripts for these receptors are expressed in the MCF-7 breast cancer cell line and the observation by Becker-André et al. (1994) that these receptors are activated in response to melatonin, suggests that melatonin-activated RORαs may bind to this RORE to regulate the transcription of the ER gene. A potential caveat in the RORα story is that we and others have not been able to demonstrate melatonin binding to or transactivation of the RORαs.

Modulation of Estrogen-Regulated Genes by Melatonin

It has become increasingly apparent that an important component of breast tumor cell growth involves locally synthesized growth factors and their autocrine or paracrine actions. In the human breast cancer cell line, MCF-7, 17-β estradiol stimulates cell proliferation and synthesis and, in some cases, secretion of specific proteins. The estrogen-induced proliferation of breast tumor cells has been hypothesized to be mediated by the induction of autocrine polypeptide growth factors (Dickson and Lippman 1987). For example, estrogen stimulation of MCF-7 cell growth is accompanied by changes in the expression of several genes, including an elevation of PgR (Eckert and Katzenellenbogen 1982); enhanced transcription and secretion of the mitogenic growth factor, TGFα (Bates et al. 1986, 1988); and secretion of the lysosomal protease, cathepsin D (Cavailles et al. 1988), which also has been shown to be mitogenic. In addition to the induction of various mitogenic factors, estrogens also decrease the synthesis and expression of the potent growth-inhibitory factor, TGFβ. Estrogen also has been shown to be autoregulatory, down-regulating the expression of its own receptor in MCF-7 breast tumor cells (Saceda et al. 1986). Thus, it is clear that the mitogenic activity of estrogen in human breast tumor cells is mediated by the induction of a number of growth-stimulatory factors, as well as the inhibition of specific growth-inhibitory factors.

Based on the hypothesis that melatonin may inhibit the proliferation of breast cancer cells via the suppression of the tumor cells' estrogen-response pathway, it follows that if melatonin down-regulates ER expression, it will likely modulate the downstream expression of estrogen-regulated gene products, including critical growth-modulatory factors such as TGFa and TGFb, oncogenes c-myc and c-fos, and other estrogen-regulated cellular products (PgR and pS2). Initial studies by Molis et al. (1995) have found that melatonin treatment of MCF-7 breast cancer cells results in a biphasic modulation of TGFa, with a transient increase after 3 and 6 hours, followed by a transient but significant decrease in the steady-state mRNA levels of TGFa at 12 hours and a return to control values by 24 hours. Thus, there does not appear to be a significant long-term effect of melatonin on TGFa mRNA expression in this breast cancer model. Conversely, melatonin treatment was found to induce a significant and long-term increase in the steady-state mRNA levels of the proto-oncogene, c-myc, beginning as early as 1 hour and continuing through 48 hours, while significantly decreasing the long-term expression (6–48 hours) of c-fos steady-state mRNA levels. Considering that both c-myc and c-fos have been implicated as regulators of cellular proliferation and are induced by estrogen, the induction of c-myc by melatonin, which is growth inhibitory, is somewhat confusing. However, a report by Armstrong et al. (1992) has shown that c-myc expression is significantly stimulated in response to the growth-inhibitory effects of epidermal growth factor (EGF) in the ER-negative MDA-MB-468 breast tumor cell line. Thus, an induction of c-myc may correlate with growth inhibition. It is also interesting to note that in the Armstrong et al. (1992) study, PgR mRNA levels, which are enhanced in response to estrogen, were significantly suppressed by melatonin treatment at the same time and with the same amplitude as reported earlier for the ER (Molis et al. 1994). This finding is in contrast to the expression pattern of the pS2 transcript, another estrogen-induced mRNA, which showed significant stimulation after 3 hours of melatonin treatment. Thus, the effects of melatonin on the expression of some of these transcripts (*c-myc* and pS2) do not completely support the hypothesis that all of melatonin's growth-inhibitory effects are mediated via the estrogen-response pathway. In fact, the rapid modulation of most of these transcripts (3–6 six hours) prior to melatonin's down-regulation of ER indicates that in addition to the ER gene, melatonin may directly modulate the expression of these gene products.

TGFβ is a potent growth inhibitor of breast tumor cells whose expression is suppressed by estrogen. Molis et al. (1995) found that melatonin treatment of MCF-7 cells resulted in a rapid and protracted induction of TGFβ mRNA expression. Although induction of mRNA expression does not always correlate with increased protein expression, these data clearly suggest that a key mechanism by which melatonin inhibits MCF-7 breast cancer growth is via the induction of this growth-inhibitory factor. The early modulation of TGFβ expression and the expression of other gene products by melatonin is clearly too rapid to be mediated through melatonin's down-regulation of ER expression. It is possible that melatonin directly regulates the transcription of specific sets of genes, given its effects on ER gene transcription. This possibility is further supported by the recent identification of melatonin's binding to members of the steroid receptor superfamily of transcription factors. It is probable that later effects, beginning as early as 12 hours and 24 hours, are mediated by melatonin's regulation of ER levels and subsequent downstream effects on the cell's estrogen-response pathway. Studies by Cos and Blask (1994) support this concept, showing that the growth-inhibitory effects of melatonin on MCF-7 cells in cultured media supplemented with EGF are reversed by estrogen but not by EGF. This finding suggests that melatonin's effects, mediated via the cell's estrogen-response pathway, are to inhibit the action or release of growth-stimulatory factors, as well as stimulate the release of growth-inhibitory factors.

Antioxidant Effects of Melatonin

Neoplastic Cell Metabolism, Glutathione, and Melatonin

Numerous studies have pointed to the oncostatic effects of melatonin in several in vivo and in vitro tumor models. However, no definitive mechanism has yet been identified through which melatonin exerts its anticarcinogenic activity. There is increasing evidence that elevated intracellular concentrations of bioreactive oxygen, organic peroxidases, and radicals initiate and promote the growth of tumors. In specific tumor types, such as melanomas (H. Bartsch et al. 1986), melatonin's inhibition of tumor cell growth occurs in the micro- and millimolar range, suggesting, but not proving, that these antiproliferative actions are not mediated by a melatonin receptor pathway. As described earlier in this chapter, binding sites (receptors) for melatonin, both membrane-associated and nuclear, have been identified in numerous tissues, including melanoma cells and rodent and human breast cancer cells (Burns et al. 1990; Stankov et al. 1991). Given that melatonin is highly lipophilic and that its effects in some tumor types (melanoma) are observed only at concentrations significantly higher than the receptors binding, it is possible that these effects occur independent of melatonin's receptor-mediated pathways. A small but growing body of evidence suggests that some of melatonin's anticancer actions may result from the antioxidant effects of this indolamine.

DNA damage induced by oxidative stress and free radicals is believed to be a major contributor to the development of a malignant phenotype. Thus, considerable interest has been generated in compounds that function as antioxidants and factors that regulate the expression of endogenous antioxidants. One such antioxidant, critical in regulating the cells' oxidation-reduction (redox) state, is γ-glutamylcysteineglycine or glutathione (GSH), a ubiquitous nonprotein thiol produced at high levels in mammalian cells. The antioxidant actions of GSH protect cells from damage by oxidation and free radicals, in addition to other oxidants. GSH also has been shown to be an essential component of DNA synthesis, as well as protein and enzyme structure and function. In addition, the metabolism of both hormones and drugs has been shown to be affected by GSH via its conjugation of these compounds.

GSH is synthesized from γ-glutamyl amino acids in the glutamyl cycle. The rate-limiting step of GSH production is catalyzed by γ-glutamylcysteine synthase (case) to produce γ-glutamylcysteine, which is subsequently converted to GSH by γ-glutamylcysteineglycine synthetase (GSHase) (Meister 1991). The reduced state of GSH is the predominant intracellular form, accounting for greater than 99.5% of the total, whereas glutathione disulfide (GSSG) accounts for the remainder of the intracellular GSH. Buthionine sulfoximine (BSO) is a specific transition state inactivator of Gcase and as such is able to inhibit GSH synthesis. BSO is thus able to induce intracellular depletion of GSH by blocking GSH synthesis despite continued GSH secretion. Blask et al. (1994) have reported that in vitro growth-inhibitory effects of physiological concentrations of melatonin (10–9 M) are abrogated by the addition of BSO (10–6 M) to the culture medium. The observation that the depletion of intracellular GSH by BSO treatment negates the oncostatic effects of melatonin suggests that these effects occur through a GSH-mediated pathway. This hypothesis is supported by the restoration of melatonin's antiproliferative effects on MCF-7 breast cancer cells in BSO-containing media by the addition of GSH (10–6 mol/L). Further confirmation is found in that approximately a fivefold induction of GSH was observed after melatonin-induced growth inhibition in these MCF-7 cells. A similar induction of GSH has been observed by D. E. Blask and co-workers (D. Blask, personal communication) in MCF-7 cells in response to the antiestrogen tamoxifen. Blask et al. (1994) suggest that melatonin enhances the reductive milieu of these breast tumor cells, thereby providing the proper redox environment for melatonin to inhibit cell proliferation (see Blask, Chapter 10, in this volume).

Neoplastic Cell Metabolism, Nitric Oxide, and Melatonin

Another pathway through which melatonin's antioncogenic effects might be mediated is via its modulation of intracellular nitric oxide (NO) levels. This modulation is possibly enhanced by the observed genotoxic effects of NO on the in vitro proliferation of tumor cells. NO is synthesized from L-arginine by a family of enzymes that are homologous to cytochrome P450 reductase and are collectively known as NO synthase (NOS) (Rettori et al. 1992). L-arginine is converted to NO and citrulline by the oxidation of five electrons of a terminal quanidine nitrogen and the insertion of a pair of oxygen atoms into the arginine substrate. Thus, NO is a free radical, having only one unpaired electron, and readily reacts with other molecules (Lowenstein and Snyder 1992; Stamler et al. 1992). For example, NO can react with superoxide anion radicals, leading to the formation of peroxynitrite anion (ONOO–) (Lipton et al. 1993), which can induce DNA damage (Beckman 1994). Furthermore, OCOO– oxidizes sulfhydryl groups, releasing the highly reactive •OH (Beckman et al. 1990; Radi et al. 1991). In addition, NO can independently induce genomic alterations (Victorin 1994; Wink et al. 1991) through multiple mechanisms, including deamination of deoxynucleosides, deoxynucleotides, and intact DNA (Wink et al. 1991), or possibly through the activation of poly(adenosine 5'-diphosphate [ADP]-ribose) synthetase (Zhang et al. 1994). The functions of NO appear to be diverse and include acting as a biological messenger or neurotransmitter involved in signal transduction mechanisms (Lowenstein and Snyder 1992), a vasodilator, an activator of macrophage cytotoxicity, an enzyme regulator, and an immune regulator (Lowenstein and Snyder 1992; Maragos et al. 1993; Stamler et al. 1992). The antitumorigenic action of NO is thought to be mediated via its ability to inhibit the activity of the rate-limiting enzyme ribonucleotide reductase in DNA synthesis (Stamler et al. 1992).

The protective effects of melatonin against oxidative damage have been examined both in vivo and in vitro in a number of models (Reiter 1995; Reiter et al. 1995). To test if NO is involved in the mechanisms of melatonin's antiproliferative effects on MCF-7 breast cancer cells, Blask et al. (1994) incubated MCF-7 cells with melatonin (10–9 M) in the presence or absence of the NOS inhibitor *N*-monomethyl-L-arginine (NMMA) (300 Tmol/L). After 5 days of treatment, melatonin's growth-inhibitory activity was completely blocked in the presence of NMMA, whereas NMMA alone had no effects on the proliferation of these cells. This inhibition of melatonin-induced growth inhibition by NMMA could be reversed in a dose-dependent fashion by the addition of sodium nitroprusside (200 Tmol/L, 500 Tmol/L, and 1 mmol/L), which delivers NO to the cells. A similar abrogation of melatonin's growth-inhibitory effects was seen when cells were treated concomitantly with hemoglobin (2 Tg/mL), an activator shown to inactivate endogenous NO (Rettori et al. 1992).

Other recent reports (Barlow-Walden et al. 1995; Pablos et al. 1995; Sewerynek et al. 1995a, 1995b) show that melatonin protects against lipopolysaccharide (LPS)-induced lipid peroxidation in vivo by reducing resultant lipid degradation products and by lowering GSSG levels (Sewerynek et al. 1995b) and that melatonin stimulates the activity of the antioxidant enzyme GSH peroxidase. In addition, Tan et al. (1993) reported that melatonin can inhibit safrole-induced DNA adduct production in the rat liver. The lipophilicity of melatonin and its associated entry into subcellular compartments, as well as the noted elevated accumulation of both endogenous and exogenous melatonin in the nucleus as compared with cytosol of mammalian tissues (Menendez-Pelaez and Reiter 1993), potentially support the hypothesis that melatonin can rapidly diffuse into the nucleus where it can protect the cell from oxidative damage. Taken together, these data tentatively support the hypothesis that NO and GSH are important components of human breast cancer cells.

The Role of the Pineal Gland in Immunity

In the past, the nervous, endocrine, and immune systems were believed to function independently. However, over the last several years, evidence has emerged of a possible functional interrelationship among these three systems (Cardarelli 1990; Dunn 1989; Maestroni 1993). Recently, the possible physiological interaction between the immune system and the pineal gland via its hormone, melatonin, has received great interest.

Much of the early evidence pointing to an interaction between the pineal gland and the immune system came from in vivo studies examining the effects of pinealectomy, or other experimental methods that inhibit melatonin synthesis and secretion, on cells and organs of the immune system. Inhibition of melatonin synthesis and secretion was shown to result in a state of immunodepression, which could be reversed by exogenous administration of melatonin.

Several parameters of the immune system are apparently affected by melatonin. In addition to the disruption of circadian rhythmicity, pinealectomized mice exhibit an inhibition of interleukin-2 (IL-2) production (del Gobbo et al. 1989) and the inability to form a humoral response against sheep red blood cells (SRBCs) (Becker et al. 1988). Vermeulen et al. (1993) showed that antibody-dependent cellular cytotoxicity (ADCC) levels are significantly reduced in adult mice pinealectomized in the first week of life, which can be restored by subsequent exogenous melatonin administration. Interestingly, this impairment of the immune system first appears in the mature adult around 60 years of age, suggesting that reproductive hormones may be involved in the pineal effect.

In addition to pinealectomy, inhibition of melatonin synthesis also can be produced by environmental (permanent lighting) or pharmacological (late-day administration of β-blockers) manipulations because the synthesis and secretion of melatonin by the pineal gland occur via nocturnal postsynaptic activation of β-adrenergic receptors (Deguchi and Axelrod 1973).

Maestroni and colleagues (Maestroni and Pierpaoli 1981; Maestroni et al. 1986, 1987a, 1987b) found that mice kept under constant light, or given evening injections of the β-adrenergic blocker propranolol to inhibit melatonin synthesis, exhibited an inability to mount a primary antibody response to SRBCs, a depressed autologous mixed lymphocyte reaction, and a decreased cellularity in the thymus and spleen, all of which could be reversed by late-afternoon administration of exogenous melatonin.

The pineal's involvement in immunoregulation in mice has been confirmed by many investigators, and similar effects on immune function have been reported in rats (Paciotti et al. 1987;

Radosevic-Stasic et al. 1993) and other rodent species. The Syrian hamster, a highly photoperiodic-responsive species, has also been used as a model to study the role of the pineal gland on immune function (Brainard et al. 1988; Peters et al. 1989; Vaughan et al. 1987). These studies found that in hamsters exposed to short photoperiods, spleen weight, total number of splenic lymphocytes, and total number of splenic macrophages were increased. In another study, hamsters injected with propranolol to inhibit endogenous melatonin synthesis and secretion showed a reduction in spleen weight and decreased concanavalin A–induced T-cell blastogenesis, both of which could be reversed by administration of melatonin (Champney and McMurray 1991).

Melatonin administration also has been reported to produce an immunopotentiating effect in animals with normal endogenous melatonin production. Late-afternoon injections of melatonin increase both the primary and secondary antibody response to SRBCs and potentiate the secondary cytotoxic T-cell response to *vaccinia* virus. However, the immunoenhancing effects are seen only when melatonin is administered in the late afternoon or in the presence of T-dependent antigen stimulation (Maestroni et al. 1987a, 1988).

The mechanisms by which the pineal and its hormone, melatonin, affect the immune system are not yet clearly defined. It has been hypothesized that melatonin may act both directly at the immune cellular level and indirectly through modulation of hormonal systems that can subsequently impact on immune function.

For example, melatonin has been shown to directly affect specific immune cells, inhibiting blastogenesis and natural killer (NK) cell activity (Arzt et al. 1988; Lewinski et al. 1989). Lopez-Gonzalez et al. (1992) reported that melatonin can bind to melatonin receptors present on lymphocytes in culture, activating cyclic guanosine monophosphate (cGMP) and potentiating cyclic adenosine monophosphate (cAMP) levels. And Steinhilber et al. (1995) showed that 5-lipoxygenase, which is involved in the inflammatory immune response, is down-regulated by melatonin in B lymphocytes, which express an isoform of the RZR/RORα nuclear receptor that binds to the 5-lipoxygenase response element. These data suggest that there may be at least two possible mechanisms by which melatonin can directly affect immune cell function, one mediated via a membrane-associated receptor and the other by a nuclear receptor.

There have been two hypotheses proposed to explain how melatonin could indirectly modulate immune function. First, melatonin could affect the immune system by modulating other endocrine systems. For example, melatonin could modify steroid hormone levels, which are known to alter immune function (Grossman 1984; Paciotti et al. 1987; Reiter 1991a). Second, melatonin's effects on the immune system may be mediated via the endogenous opiate system, as has been demonstrated in the mouse (Maestroni 1993; Maestroni and Conti 1990).

Effect of Melatonin on Acquired Immunity

Even though melatonin's immunomodulatory effects appear to be mediated by several parameters, such as lymphokines, hormones, and, possibly, opiates, the thymus gland seems to be a primary target of melatonin's action. Early studies found that pinealecto-mized mice underwent accelerated involution of the thymus (Csaba and Barath 1975). Conversely, thymic hormones are capable of modulating melatonin synthesis by the pineal gland. In addition, melatonin's effects on the thymus are not species specific. In chickens, thymic weight is considerably reduced, and the primary and secondary immune responses are significantly lowered by subcutaneous injections of melatonin. Direct administration of melatonin into the bursa of Fabricius of chickens causes a decrease in bursal weight and reduction in antibody production involving the primary immune response (Giannessi et al. 1992). Liu and Pang (1992) have reported the presence of melatonin-binding sites in membrane preparations of duck thymus that are stable, saturable, reversible, and of high affinity.

Melatonin also can exert direct effects on specific cells of the immune system. Administration of melatonin significantly inhib-its proliferation of normal mouse and human lymphocytes and T-lymphoblastoid cell lines in culture (Persengiev and Kyurkchiev 1993). In addition, blastogenesis, human NK cell activity, and γ-interferon (γ-IFN) synthesis are all inhibited by melatonin in vitro (Arzt et al. 1988; Lewinski et al. 1989). These findings, however, are not consistent with the stimulation of immune function by melatonin observed in rodent models in vivo (Maestroni 1993).

Melatonin's effects on human monocytes also have been studied. Melatonin alone and synergistically with LPS activates monocytes—apparently via the protein kinase C pathway—leading to stimulation of human monocyte cytotoxicity, induction of both interleukin-1α (IL-1α) and interleukin-1β (IL-1β) activity, and production of reactive oxygen intermediates (Morrey et al. 1994).

Although the mechanisms responsible for immunodepression following pinealectomy are not yet defined, inhibition of IL-2 production appears to be one of the primary factors. IL-2, a lymphokine released by activated T-helper cells, plays an important role in the development and modulation of the immune response (D. A. Morgan et al. 1976; Watson and Mochizuki 1980) and in the differentiation and proliferation of various immune effector cells. Antigen injection or mitogen administration activates the immune system by stimulating the production of IL-2 from T-helper lymphocytes, type 1. After its release, IL-2 stimulates almost all immune cells, including T-cytotoxic lymphocytes, NK cells, B lymphocytes, monocytes and macrophages, and T-helper lymphocytes, type 2, which are the main source of other lymphokines (Lissoni et al. 1993c). Pinealectomized mice exhibit a significant inhibition of IL-2 production by T cells and reduced NK cell activity (del Gobbo et al. 1989). These inhibitory effects of pinealectomy can be reversed by a single subcutaneous injection of melatonin. Chronic injection of melatonin into young or immunodepressed mice also has been shown to increase induction of T-helper cell activity and IL-2 production and to enhance the antibody response to a T-dependent antigen (Caroleo et al. 1994).

Other lymphokines have been implicated in melatonin's modulation of immune function. Preliminary data suggest that interleukin-3 (IL-3) alone or in association with melatonin may decrease IL-2-induced macrophage activation and alter macrophage function during cancer immunotherapy with IL-2 (Lissoni et al. 1993a).

Melatonin also stimulates T-helper cells, type 2, to release inter-leukin-4 (IL-4). IL-4 is a T-cell cytokine that may exert a selective inhibitory effect on primitive progenitor cells by affecting the pro-liferation of pluripotent stem cells in the bone marrow and induc-ing activated macrophages and stromal cells to produce colony-stimulating factors (Banchereau 1991; Maestroni et al. 1994; Wieser et al. 1989).

Melatonin has been shown to influence the secretion of γ-IFN, a lymphokine secreted by antigen-stimulated T-helper lympho-cytes. Interferons are known to heighten natural immunity by stimulating NK cell activity and cytotoxic T cells and could inhibit tumor growth, either directly or by modifying other parameters of the host's immune system (Angeli et al. 1992; Caroleo et al. 1992; del Gobbo et al. 1989).

Effect of Melatonin on Natural Immunity

Studies show that melatonin can modulate several aspects of natu-ral immunity. For example, melatonin treatment has been re-ported to stimulate ADCC (Giordano and Palermo 1991), lymphocyte blastogenesis (Champney and McMurray 1991; Fraschini et al. 1990), and IL-2 production (Caroleo et al. 1992; del Gobbo et al. 1989) and to enhance the T-helper to T-suppressor ratio in vivo (Lissoni et al. 1987).

One of the important functions influenced by melatonin's ef-fects on lymphokine production is that of NK cell activity. NK cells are immune effectors that can recognize and kill a variety of cellu-lar targets, including neoplastic and virus-infected cells. Thus, NK cells play an important role in the immunosurveillance against tumors and their metastases, as well as resistance to viral infec-tions (Heberman and Ortaldo 1981; Trinchieri and Perussia 1984). However, the data on the effects of melatonin on NK cell activity are often conflicting. Lewinski et al. (1989) reported that in vitro exposure of peripheral blood lymphocytes from healthy subjects to melatonin resulted in an inhibition of NK activity, as estimated by measurement of radioactive chromium (^{51}Cr) release from K562 human leukemia target cells. Others have shown that the alteration in NK cell activity correlates with IL-2 production. NK cells are under direct T-cell control through IL-2 production, which influences their proliferation and activity. Pinealectomy, which results in a significant reduction in IL-2 production, also significantly inhibits NK cell activity in vivo (Angeli et al. 1992; del Gobbo et al. 1989; Hanney et al. 1981). However, Maestroni and Conti (1991) reported that melatonin has no effect on NK cytotoxic activity on virally infested target cells.

Despite these conflicting data, it seems clear that melatonin possesses unique immunoregulatory actions on the body's natural immunity, although the mechanisms are difficult to explain. Melatonin has been shown to inhibit IL-2-induced macrophage activation, as suggested by the lower increase in the specific macrophage marker neopterin following treatment with IL-2 and melatonin as compared with IL-2 alone. Because activated macrophages have been shown to inhibit NK cells and IL-2-dependent immune functions and are responsible for platelet destruction, inhibition of macrophage activation may explain the increase in NK cells and activated lymphocytes, as well as the prevention of thrombocytopenia, observed with melatonin administration (Lissoni et al. 1993c).

It also has been suggested that melatonin may stimulate the body's natural immune cytolytic effectors indirectly by modulating the production of hormones such as growth hormone (GH) and prolactin (PRL), both of which have been shown to increase NK cell activity (del Gobbo et al. 1989).

Melatonin as an Immunotherapeutic Agent in Cancer

Recently, activation of the body's own natural immune mechanisms has been investigated for use in cancer immunotherapy. NK cells and T-cytotoxic cells attack malignant or virus-infected cells (Heberman and Ortaldo 1981), and IL-2 has been shown to activate NK and T-cytotoxic cells (Rosenberg and Terry 1987). To date, IL-2 represents the principal cytokine responsible for the generation of the antitumor cytotoxic immune reaction, and its use constitutes the basis of modern immunotherapies for cancer.

However, the use of IL-2 in clinical trials has been limited by the potential toxicity of the high concentrations at which its antineoplastic effects are observed. The finding that the pineal gland can have powerful oncostatic effects (Barni et al. 1992; Blask 1984, 1993; Blask and Hill 1988; Regelson and Pierpaoli 1987; Ying et al. 1993) and that melatonin can stimulate IL-2 production and amplify its antitumor activity led to speculation that melatonin might act synergistically with IL-2 in the treatment of cancer. This hypothesis was first tested in animal experiments designed to evaluate the effect of melatonin alone and in combination with IL-2 on the development and growth of established pulmonary metastases. Melatonin alone exerted a significant antitumor effect, and, combined with IL-2, melatonin appeared to potentiate the IL-2 oncostatic effects in an additive manner (Maestroni and Conti 1993). This regimen would thus allow treatment with less toxic, low-dose IL-2.

Based on the promising data from the animal studies, clinical trials have been conducted examining the influence of melatonin on IL-2-induced immune effects in patients with various cancers, including advanced human malignant melanoma (Gonzalez et al. 1991), metastatic colorectal carcinoma (Barni et al. 1992), locally advanced or metastatic hepatocellular carcinoma (Aldeghi et al. 1988), and metastatic gastric carcinoma (Lissoni et al. 1993d). The data were consistent with the hypothesis that melatonin can restore T-cell responses and increase NK cell activity, both of which are frequently depressed in cancer patients, by triggering endogenous cytokine production, especially IL-2 (Wanebo et al. 1985). Subsequently, the influence of melatonin on IL-2-induced immune effects was examined in patients with metastatic solid neoplasms who did not respond to previous chemotherapy. Tumor histotypes included nonsmall-cell lung cancer, renal cell carcinoma, colon adenocarcinoma, and mammary carcinoma. The patients were divided into three treatment groups: one group (14 patients) was treated with IL-2 alone, a second group received melatonin alone, and the third was treated with IL-2 plus melatonin. The patients receiving IL-2 plus melatonin exhibited a significantly higher increase in mean number of lymphocytes,

T lymphocytes, NK cells, CD25-positive cells, and eosinophils than those given IL-2 alone. Conversely, mean serum levels of neopterin, a macrophage marker, were significantly higher in patients treated with IL-2 alone. There was no significant effect on either immune cell number or on neopterin secretion in those patients receiving melatonin alone, suggesting that melatonin acts by enhancing IL-2-mediated immune effects rather than by inducing immune responses directly (Lissoni et al. 1991, 1993a, 1993b, 1993c, 1993d).

Recently, a phase II pilot study was performed with low-dose IL-2 plus melatonin in 14 patients with untreatable endocrine tumors, including carcinoid tumor, thyroid and pancreatic islet cell carcinomas, and adrenal and neuroendocrine lung tumors. The results of this preliminary study suggest that low-dose IL-2 immunotherapy in association with melatonin may constitute a new well-tolerated and potentially active therapy for untreatable advanced endocrine tumors (Lissoni et al. 1995).

In a preliminary clinical study by Tommasi et al. (1993) on 16 patients with advanced solid tumors treated with melatonin as a single agent, marked increases in circulating levels of α-tumor necrosis factor, γ-IFN, and IL-2 were found. In a follow-up study, the antitumor efficacy and toxicity of a combination of human lymphoblastoid IFN with melatonin in patients with renal cell carcinoma was undertaken. The overall response rate for the group was 33%, with a median response duration of 16 months, median time to tumor progression of 11 months, and median survival time of 18 months. Moreover, the IFN-melatonin combination was characterized by low toxicity, enabling therapy to be prolonged over a 12-month period (Neri et al. 1994).

Clinical trials also have been conducted to determine the efficacy of melatonin treatment versus supportive care alone in patients with brain metastases due to solid neoplasms. Results showed that mean survival time is significantly higher, and complications lower, with melatonin treatment than with supportive care alone (Lissoni et al. 1994).

All the evidence to date supports the hypothesis that the pineal gland and its hormone, melatonin, possess immunoenhancing and antineoplastic functions, although the mechanisms by which these functions occur are not yet clear (see Figure 9–2). Studies further defining the mechanisms involved are essential, particularly given the nontoxic and positive responses observed in the wide range of clinical trials that have been conducted thus far, and could conceivably lead to new strategies in the prevention and treatment of diseases that involve immunosuppression (e.g., HIV) or a high risk of developing cancer (e.g., breast cancer) (see Blask, Chapter 10, in this volume).

Conclusions

A considerable number of studies strongly implicate the pineal gland and its key hormone, melatonin, in the etiology of various neoplasms, particularly those known to be responsive to other hormones, such as breast, uterine, ovarian, and prostate cancer. In addition, other types of tumors not typically associated with endocrine responsiveness, such as colon cancer and melanoma, have been reported to be affected by melatonin. Although a handful of studies has suggested a stimulatory effect of melatonin in tumor development and growth, most have supported the general hypothesis that the effects of the pineal and melatonin on cancer, in general, are inhibitory. Although over the last decade considerable efforts have been extended toward understanding melatonin's role as an oncostatic agent, little is truly known regarding the mechanisms by which this indolamine inhibits tumor growth.

The most frequently studied tumor model that is responsive to the oncostatic effects of melatonin is breast cancer. Both carcinogen-induced animal tumor models and human breast cancer cell line models have been extensively used to examine the potential pathways by which melatonin inhibits the development and growth of these tumors. Given the general effects of melatonin on the reproductive system, three possible pathways for melatonin's action can be envisioned. One such pathway involves an indirect neuroendocrine mechanism by which melatonin affects higher endocrine centers, the hypothalamus and pituitary, and the

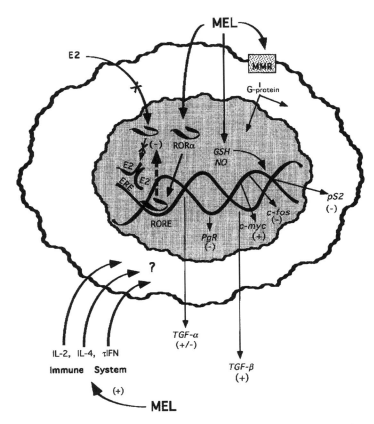

Figure 9–2.   Schematic of possible cellular-molecular pathways involved in melatonin's effects on neoplastic cells. Five major input pathways have been suggested, including melatonin's interaction with its membrane-bound receptor (MMR), its nuclear receptor (RORα receptors), the immune system, the glutathione system (GSH), or the nitric oxide (NO) pathway to protect the cell from oxidative damage. MEL = melatonin; E_2 = 17 β-estradiol; ER = estrogen receptor; ERE = estrogen-response element; RORα = retinoic acid orphan receptor-α; RORE = RORα-response element; *c-myc* and *c-fos* = proto-oncogenes (estrogen regulated); PgR = progesterone receptor; pS2 = pancreatic spasmolytic polypeptide (estrogen-regulated gene); IL-2 = interleukin-2; IL-4 = interleukin-4; τIFN = interferon; TGFα = transforming growth factor-α (estrogen-stimulated growth factor); TGFβ = transforming growth factor-β (a growth-inhibitory factor of epithelial cells, whose expression is suppressed by estrogen).

subsequent downstream development and growth of various reproductive tissues, including the breast, via the hypothalamic-pituitary-gonadal axis. For example, melatonin may suppress the circulating levels of estrogen and PRL, two hormones critical for the development and proliferation of carcinogen-induced mammary cancers. This suppression of estrogen and PRL would significantly impair the development and slow the growth of these tumors (see Blask, Chapter 10, in this volume).

The second major pathway is a direct one, by which melatonin affects reproductive tissues at the cellular and molecular level. Because melatonin's actions have most frequently been reported in endocrine-responsive neoplasms and because these effects are most often associated with growth inhibition, it seems likely that the direct effects of melatonin on these tumor cells might be mediated via disruption of stimulatory endocrine signals. This scenario has been indirectly demonstrated in MCF-7 human breast tumor cells, wherein melatonin is able to block estrogen-induced proliferation, much like the antiestrogen tamoxifen (Cos et al. 1991). However, unlike tamoxifen, melatonin does not bind to the ER; rather, melatonin appears to inhibit the transcription of the ER gene (Molis et al. 1994), thereby down-regulating ER levels and suppressing the estrogen-responsive pathway of the tumor cell. Because 60%–70% of all human breast tumors express quantifiable levels of ER and these tumors are typically responsive to the mitogenic effects of estrogen via estrogen's induction of various growth-regulatory factors, the disruption of the tumor cell's estrogen-response pathway could prove an effective mechanism for suppressing breast tumor development.

With the recent cloning of the melatonin membrane receptor (Ebisawa et al. 1994; Reppert et al. 1994) and the identification of the nuclear orphan receptors RZRα, RZRβ, and RORα as nuclear transcription factors activated by melatonin (Becker-André et al. 1994; Wiesenberg et al. 1995), cellular and molecular pathways by which melatonin can directly affect the estrogen-response pathway and breast tumor growth can now be envisioned. For example, by activating the G-protein-linked membrane receptor on breast cancer cells, melatonin could initiate signal transduction pathways resulting in the activation/deactivation of transcription factors that regulate the expression of key genes. In the case of breast cancer, the membrane receptor pathway does appear to be an important one for melatonin's oncostatic effect, as we have characterized the expression of the Mel_{1a} receptor at both the MRNA and protein levels in MCF-7 breast cancer cells. In addition, using melatonin membrane receptor-specific agonists and antagonists, we have reconstituted and antagonized, respectively, the growth-inhibitory effects of melatonin. In addition, mRNA transcripts for the RORα receptors have been identified in MCF-7 breast cancer cells by Steinhilber et al. (1995) and Ram and Hill (1995). Treatment of MCF-7 cells with a melatonin agonist (CGP 52608) specific for these nuclear receptors results in growth inhibition of these cells. Analysis of the 5-flanking region of the ER gene in MCF-7 cells also shows a putative response element for the RORα receptors, an RORE, located at position -868 to -861. Although the functionality of the RORαs as melatonin receptors is questionable, Carlsberg's data may suggest that the RORα receptor pathway may be important for mediating melatonin's effects in breast cancer.

The interaction between melatonin and the immune system could be a third pathway by which melatonin inhibits the development and growth of cancer cells. It appears that melatonin's effects on immune function also may be mediated by both direct and indirect mechanisms. Just as melatonin may affect the development and growth of reproductive tissues via an indirect neuroendocrine pathway by modulating the circulating levels of various hormones, so too could immune function be affected by these same hormones. Membrane receptors for melatonin are reportedly present on T lymphocytes and, with the recent identification of RZR/RORα nuclear receptors, which bind melatonin in B lymphocytes, it is possible that melatonin's oncostatic effects may result from direct interaction with specific immune cells. Whatever the mechanism, it seems clear that stimulation of the pineal gland heightens immune function, whereas inhibition of the pineal or its hormone, melatonin, suppresses immune function, particularly in regard to neoplastic growth.

Based on the evidence presented, it is clear that in a variety of tissues the pineal gland, via its hormone melatonin, is able to suppress and in some cases inhibit the development and growth of specific tumors. Although melatonin is promising as a potential therapeutic tool, a more detailed understanding of its mechanisms of action is needed before this naturally occurring oncostatic hormone can be used in the clinical setting. With the identification and further characterization of melatonin receptors' function and tissue expression, our understanding of how melatonin mediates its effects on normal as well as malignant cells will expand. An increased understanding of the pathways used in a given cell type, the temporal expression pattern of the receptors, and a deeper knowledge of nonreceptor-mediated events will all add to the ability to use melatonin as a potent therapeutic tool. The recent use in clinical studies of melatonin in combination with interleukins in the treatment of patients with gastric cancer and its use as a contraceptive tool are just the beginning of an exciting era of melatonin research that will add melatonin to the ever-expanding list of "biologicals" used in the treatment of cancer.

References

Acuña-Castroviejo D, Pablos MI, Menendez-Pelaez A, et al: Melatonin receptors in purified cell nuclei of liver. Res Commun Chem Pathol Pharmacol 2:253–256, 1993

Acuña-Castroviejo D, Reiter RJ, Menendez-Pelaez A, et al: Characterization of high affinity melatonin binding sites in purified cell nuclei of rat liver. J Pineal Res 16:100–112, 1994

Aldeghi R, Lissoni P, Barni S, et al: Low-dose interleukin-2 subcutaneous immunotherapy in association with the pineal hormone melatonin as a first-line therapy in locally advanced or metastatic hepatocellular carcinoma. Eur J Cancer 30A(2):167–170, 1988

Angeli A, Gatti G, Sartori ML, et al: Effect of exogenous melatonin on human natural killer (NK) cell activity: an approach to the immuno-modulatory role of the pineal gland, in The Pineal Gland and Cancer. Edited by Gupta D, Attanasio A, Reiter RJ. Tübingen, Germany, Muller & Bass, 1992, pp 145–156

Armstrong DK, Issacs JT, Ottavaiano YL, et al: Programmed cell death during regression of the MCF-7 human breast cancer following estro-gen ablation. Cancer Res 51:3418–3424, 1992

Arzt ES, Fernanadez-Castelo S, Finochiaro LME, et al: Immunomodula-tion by indolamines: serotonin and melatonin action on DNA and interferon-γ synthesis by human peripheral blood mononuclear cells. J Clin Immunol 8:513–520, 1988

Banchereau J: Interleukin-4, in The Cytokine Handbook. Edited by Thomason A. London, Academic Press, 1991, pp 119–149

Barlow-Walden LR, Reiter RJ, Abe M, et al: Melatonin stimulates brain glutathione peroxidase activity. Neurochem Int 26:497–502, 1995

Barni S, Lissoni P, Cazzaniga M, et al: Neuroimmunotherapy with subcu-taneous low-dose interleukin-2 and the pineal hormone melatonin as a second-line treatment in metastatic colorectal carcinoma. Tumori 78(6):383–387, 1992

Bartsch C, Bartsch H, Jain A, et al: Urinary melatonin levels in human breast cancer patients. Journal of Neural Transmission 52:281–294, 1981

Bartsch H, Bartsch C, Flehming B: Differential effects of melatonin on slow and fast growing passages of a human melanoma cell line. Neuroendocrinology Letters 8:289–293, 1986

Bartsch H, Bartsch C, Noteborn HPJM, et al: Growth-inhibiting effect of crude pineal extracts on human melanoma cells in vitro is different from that of known synthetic pineal substances. Journal of Neural Transmission 69:299–311, 1987

Bates S, McManaway MR, Lippman ME, et al: Characterization of estro-gen transforming activity in human breast cancer cells. Cancer Res 46:1707–1713, 1986

Bates S, Davidson NE, Valverius EM, et al: Expression of transforming growth factor alpha and its mRNA in human breast cancer: its regula-tion by estrogen and its possible functional significance. Mol Endocri-nol 2:543–555, 1988

Becker J, Veit G, Handgretinger R, et al: Circadian variations in the immunomodulatory role of the pineal gland. Neuroendocrinology Letters 10:65–80, 1988

Becker-André M, Andre E, DeLamarter JF: Identification of nuclear receptor mRNAs by RT-PCR amplification of conserved zinc-finger motif sequences. Biochem Biophys Res Commun 194:1371–1379, 1993

Becker-André M, Wiesenberg I, Schaeren-Wiemers M, et al: Pineal gland hormone melatonin binds and activates an orphan of the nuclear receptor superfamily. J Biol Chem 269:28531–28534, 1994

Beckman JS: Peroxynitrite versus hydroxyl radical: the role of nitric oxide in superoxide-dependent cerebral injury (review). Ann N Y Acad Sci 738:69–75, 1994

Beckman JS, Becman TW, Chen J, et al: Apparent hydroxyl radical production by peroxynitrite: implications for endothelial injury from nitric oxide and superoxide. Proc Natl Acad Sci U S A 87:1620–1625, 1990

Bindoni M, Justisz M, Ribot G: Characterization and partial purification of a substance in the pineal gland which inhibits cell multiplication in vitro. Biochim Biophys Acta 437:577–584, 1976

Birnbaumer LG: G-proteins in signal transduction. Annu Rev Pharmacol Toxicol 30:675–705, 1990

Bittman EL, Weaver DR: The distribution of melatonin binding sites in neuroendocrine tissue of the ewe. Biol Reprod 43:986–993, 1990

Blask DE: The pineal: An oncostatic gland, in The Pineal Gland. Edited by Reiter RJ. New York, Raven, 1984, pp 253–284

Blask DE: Melatonin in oncology, in Melatonin: Biosynthesis, Physiological Effects, and Clinical Applications. Edited by Yu H-S, Reiter RJ. Boca Raton, FL, CRC Press, 1993, pp 447–475

Blask DE, Hill SM: Melatonin and cancer: basic clinical aspects, in Melatonin Clinical Perspectives. Edited by Philbrock MA, Thompson C. Oxford, England, Oxford University Press, 1988, pp 128–173

Blask DE, Nodelman JL: Antigonadotrophic and prolactin-inhibitory effects of melatonin in anosmic male rats. Neuroendocrinology 29:406–414, 1979

Blask DE, Pelletier DB, Hill SM, et al: Pineal melatonin inhibition of tumor promotion in the N-nitroso-N-methylurea model of mammary carcinogenesis: potential involvement of antiestrogenic mechanisms in vivo. J Cancer Res Clin Oncol 117:526–532, 1991

Blask DE, Wilson ST, Lemus-Wilson A: The oncostatic and oncomodulatory role of the pineal gland and melatonin, in Advances in Pineal Research, Vol 7. Edited by Maestroni GJM, Conti A, Reiter RJ. London, John Libbey, 1994, pp 235–241

Brainard GC, Watson-Whitmyer M, Knobler RL, et al: Neuroendocrine regulation of immune parameters: photoperiod control of the spleen in Syrian hamsters. Ann N Y Acad Sci 540:704–706, 1988

Brown AMC, Jeltsch JM, Roberts M, et al: Activation of pS2 gene transcription is a primary response to estrogen in the human breast cancer cell line MCF-7. Proc Natl Acad Sci U S A 81:6344–6348, 1984

Burns DM, Cos C, Blask DE: Demonstration and partial characterization of 2-iodomelatonin binding sites in experimental breast cancer (abstract). Abstracts of the 72nd Annual Meeting of The Endocrine Society 151:62, 1990

Buzzell GR, Amerongen HM, Toma JG: Melatonin and the growth of the Dunning R3327 rat prostatic adenocarcinoma, in The Pineal Gland and Cancer. Edited by Gupta D, Attanasio A, Reiter RJ. Tübingen, Germany, Brain Research Promotion, 1988, pp 295–306

Cardarelli NF: The role of a thymus-pineal axis in an immune mechanism of aging. J Theor Biol 145:397–405, 1990

Carlberg C, Hooft van Huijsduijnen R, Staple JK, et al: RZRs, a new family of retinoid-related orphan receptors that function as both monomers and homodimers. Mol Endocrinol 8:757–770, 1994

Carlson LL, Weaver DR, Reppert SM: Melatonin signal transduction in hamster brain: inhibition of adenylyl cyclase by pertussis toxin-sensitive G protein. Endocrinology 125:2670–2676, 1989

Caroleo MC, Doria G, Nistico G: Melatonin as immunomodulator in immunodeficient mice. Immunopharmacology 23(2):81–89, 1992

Caroleo MC, Frasca D, Nistico G, et al: Melatonin restores immunodepression in aged and cyclophosphamide-treated mice. Ann N Y Acad Sci 719:343–352, 1994

Cavailles V, Augereau P, Garcia M, et al: Estrogens and growth factors induce the mRNA of the 52K-pro-cathepsin-D secreted by breast cancer cells. Nucleic Acids Res 16:1903–1919, 1988

Champney TH, McMurray DN: Spleen morphology and lymphoproliferative activity in short photoperiod exposed hamsters, in Role of Melatonin and Pineal Peptides in Neuroimmunomodulation. Edited by Fraschini F, Reiter RJ. New York, Plenum, 1991, pp 218–223

Chang N, Spaulding TS, Tseng MT: Inhibitory effects of superior cervical ganglionectomy in dimethylbenzanthracene-induced mammary tumors in the rat. J Pineal Res 2:331–340, 1985

Cos S, Blask DE: Melatonin modulates growth factor activity in MCF-7 human breast cancer cells. J Pineal Res 17:25–32, 1994

Cos S, Blask DE, Lemus-Wilson A, et al: Effects of melatonin on the cell cycle kinetics and "estrogen-rescue" of MCF-7 human breast cancer cells in culture. J Pineal Res 10:36–42, 1991

Csaba G, Barath P: Morphological changes of the thymus and the thyroid gland after postnatal extirpation of the pineal body. Endocrinologia Experimentalis 9:59–67, 1975

Danforth DN, Tamarkin L, Lippman ME: Melatonin increases oestrogen receptor binding activity of human breast cancer cells. Science 305:323–325, 1983a

Danforth DN, Tamarkin L, Do R, et al: Melatonin induced increase in cytoplasmic estrogen receptor activity in hamster uteri. Endocrinology 113:81–85, 1983b

Daniel PH, Prichard ML: The response of experimentally induced mammary tumors in rats to ovariectomy. Br J Cancer 17:687–693, 1963

Das Gupta TK, Terz J: Influence of pineal gland on the growth and spread of melanoma in the hamster. Cancer Res 27:1306–1311, 1967

Deguchi T, Axelrod J: Control of circadian change of serotonin N-acetyl-transferase in the pineal organ by β-adrenergic receptor. Proc Natl Acad Sci U S A 70:2411–2414, 1973

del Gobbo V, Libri V, Villani N, et al: Pinealectomy inhibits interleukin-2 production and natural killer activity in mice. Int J Immunopharmacol 11:567–573, 1989

Dickson RB, Lippman ME: Estrogenic regulation of growth and polypeptide growth factor secretion in human breast carcinoma. Endocr Rev 8:29–43, 1987

Dickson RB, McManaway ME, Lippman ME: Estrogen-induced factors of breast cancer cells partially replace estrogen to promote tumor growth. Science 232:1540–1543, 1987

Dubik D, Shiu R: Transcriptional regulation of *c-myc* oncogene expression by estrogen in hormone-responsive human breast cancer cells. J Biol Chem 63:12706–12708, 1988

Dubocovich ML: Pharmacological characterization of melatonin binding sites. Advances in Pineal Research 5:167–173, 1991

Dunn AJ: Psychoneuroimmunology for the psychoneuro-endocrinologist: a review of animal studies of nervous system-immune system interactions. Psychoneuroendocrinology 14:251–274, 1989

Ebisawa T, Karne S, Lerner MR, et al: Expression cloning of a high-affinity melatonin receptor from *Xenopus* dermal melanophores. Proc Natl Acad Sci U S A 91:6133–6137, 1994

Eckert RL, Katzenellenbogen BS: Effects of estrogens and antiestrogens on estrogen receptor dynamics and the induction of progesterone receptor in MCF-7 human breast cancer cells. Cancer Res 42:139–144, 1982

Edwards DP, Chamness GC, McGuire WL: Estrogen and progesterone receptor proteins in breast cancer. Biochim Biophys Acta 5460:457–486, 1979

Forman BM, Chen J, Blumberg B, et al: Cross-talk among RORα1 and the Rev-erb family of orphan receptors. Mol Endocrinol 8:1253–1261, 1994

Fraschini F, Scaglione F, Demartini G, et al: Melatonin action on immune responses, in Advances in Pineal Research, Vol 4. Edited by Reiter RJ, Lukaszyk A. London, John Libbey, 1990, pp 225–233

Giannessi F, Bianchi F, Dolfi A, et al: Changes in the chicken bursa of Fabricius and immune response after treatment with melatonin. In Vivo 6:507–515, 1992

Giguere V, Tini M, Flock G, et al: Isoform-specific amino-terminal domains dictate DNA-binding properties of RORα, a novel family of orphan hormone nuclear receptors. Genes Dev 8:538–553, 1994

Giordano M, Palermo MS: Melatonin-induced enhancement of antibody-dependent cellular cytotoxicity. J Pineal Res 10:117–121, 1991

Gonzalez R, Sanchez A, Ferguson JA, et al: Melatonin therapy of advanced human malignant melanoma. Melanoma Res 1:237–243, 1991

Greene GL, Gilna P, Waterfield M, et al: Sequence and expression of human estrogen receptor complementary DNA. Science 231:1150–1154, 1986

Grossman CJ: Regulation of the immune system by sex steroids. Endocr Rev 5:435–455, 1984

Hanney CS, Kuribayashi K, Kern DE, et al: Interleukin-2 augments natural killer cell activity. Nature 291:335–337, 1981

Heberman RB, Ortaldo JR: Natural killer cells: their role in defense against disease. Science 214:24–25, 1981

Hill SM, Blask DE: Effects of the pineal hormone melatonin on the proliferation and morphological characteristics of human breast cancer cells (MCF-7) in culture. Cancer Res 48:6121–6126, 1988

Hill SM, Spriggs LL, Simon MA, et al: The growth inhibitory action of melatonin on human breast cancer cells is linked to the estrogen response system. Cancer Lett 64:249–256, 1991

Horwitz KB, McGuire WL: Estrogen control of progesterone receptor in human breast cancer: correlations with nuclear processing of estrogen receptors. J Biol Chem 253:2223–2228, 1978

Kothari L: Influence of chronic melatonin on 9,10-dimethyl-1,2-dimethylbenzanthracene-induced mammary tumors in female Holtzman rats exposed to continuous light. Oncology 44:64–69, 1987

Laitinen JT, Saavedra JM: Characterization of melatonin receptors in the rat suprachiasmatic nuclei: modulation of affinity with cations and guanine nucleotides. Endocrinology 126:2210–2215, 1990

Lawson NO, Wee B, Blask DE, et al: Modulation of hypothalamic estrogen receptors by melatonin in female LSH/SsLak golden hamsters. Journal of Biological Reproduction 47:1082–1090, 1992

Lerner AB, Case JD, Heinzelman RV: Structure of melatonin. Journal of the American Chemists Society 81:6084–6085, 1959

Lewinski A, Zelazowski P, Sweerynek E, et al: Melatonin-induced suppression of human lymphocyte natural killer activity in vitro. J Pineal Res 7:153–164, 1989

Lippman ME, Bolan G, Huff K: The effects of estrogen and antiestrogen on hormone-responsive human breast cancer in long-term tissue culture. Cancer Res 36:4595–4601, 1976

Lipton SA, Choi YB, Pan ZH, et al: A redox-based mechanism for the neuro-protective and neurodestructive effects of nitric oxide and related nitroso-compounds. Nature 364:626–632, 1993

Lissoni P, Barni S, Tancini G, et al: Clinical study of melatonin in untreatable advanced cancer patients. Tumori 73:475–480, 1987

Lissoni P, Tisi E, Brivio F, et al: Modulation of interleukin-2-induced macrophage activation in cancer patients by the pineal hormone melatonin. J Biol Regul Homeost Agents 5:154–156, 1991

Lissoni P, Pittalis S, Brivio F, et al: In vitro modulatory effects of interleukin-3 on macrophage activation induced by interleukin-2. Cancer 71:2076–2081, 1993a

Lissoni P, Barni S, Rovelli F, et al: Neuroimmunotherapy of advanced solid neoplasms with single evening subcutaneous injection of low-dose interleukin-2 and melatonin: preliminary results. Eur J Cancer 29A(2):185–189, 1993b

Lissoni P, Barni S, Tancini G, et al: A study of the mechanisms involved in the immunostimulatory action of the pineal hormone in cancer patients. Oncology 50:399–402, 1993c

Lissoni P, Brivio F, Ardizzoia A, et al: Subcutaneous therapy with low-dose interleukin-2 plus the neurohormone melatonin in metastatic gastric cancer patients with low performance status. Tumori 79:401–404, 1993d

Lissoni P, Barni S, Arizzoia A, et al: A randomized study with the pineal hormone melatonin versus supportive care alone in patients with brain metastases due to solid neoplasms. Cancer 73:699–701, 1994

Lissoni P, Barni S, Tancini G, et al: Immunoendocrine therapy with low-dose subcutaneous interleukin-2 plus melatonin on locally advanced or metastatic endocrine tumors. Oncology 52:163–166, 1995

Liu AM, Pang SF: Binding of [^{125}I]-labelled iodomelatonin in the duck thymus. Biol Signals 1:250–256, 1992

Lopez-Gonzalez MA, Calvo JR, Ocuna C, et al: Interaction of melatonin with human lymphocytes: evidence for binding sites coupled to potentiation of cyclic AMP stimulated by vasoactive intestinal peptide and activation of cyclic GMP. J Pineal Res 12:97–104, 1992

Lowenstein CJ, Snyder SH: Nitric oxide: a novel biological messenger. Cell 70:705–707, 1992

Maestroni GJM: The immunoneuroendocrine role of melatonin. J Pineal Res 14:1–10, 1993

Maestroni GJM, Conti A: The pineal neurohormone melatonin stimulates activated CD4+, Thy-1+ cells to release opioid agonist(s) with immunoenhancing and anti-stress properties. J Neuroimmunol 28:167–176, 1990

Maestroni GJM, Conti A: Role of the pineal neurohormone melatonin in the psycho-neuroendocrine immune network, in Psychoneuroimmunology II. Edited by Ader R, Felten DL, Cohen N. San Diego, CA, Academic Press, 1991, pp 495–513

Maestroni GJM, Conti A: Melatonin in relation with the immune system, in Melatonin: Biosynthesis, Physiological Effects, and Clinical Applications. Edited by Yu H-S, Reiter RJ. Boca Raton, FL, CRC Press, 1993, pp 289–311

Maestroni GJM, Pierpaoli W: Pharmacologic control of the hormonally mediated immune response, in Psychoneuroimmunology. Edited by Ader R. New York, Academic Press, 1981, pp 405–428

Maestroni GJM, Conti A, Pierpaoli W: Role of the pineal gland in immunity: circadian synthesis and release of melatonin modulates the antibody response and antagonizes the immunosuppressive effect of corticosterone. J Neuroimmunol 13:19–30, 1986

Maestroni GJM, Conti A, Pierpaoli W: The pineal gland and the circadian, opiatergic, immunoregulatory role of melatonin. Ann N Y Acad Sci 496:76–77, 1987a

Maestroni GJM, Conti A, Pierpaoli W: Role of the pineal gland in immunity, II: melatonin enhances the antibody response via an opiatergic mechanism. Clin Exp Immunol 68:384–391, 1987b

Maestroni GJM, Conti A, Pierpaoli W: The immunoregulatory role of melatonin, in The Pineal Gland and Cancer. Edited by Gupta D, Attanasio A, Reiter RJ. Tübingen, Germany, Muller & Bass, 1988, pp 133–143

Maestroni GJM, Conti A, Lissoni P: Colony-stimulating activity and hematopoietic rescue from cancer chemotherapy compounds are induced by melatonin via endogenous interleukin 4. Cancer Res 54:4740–4743, 1994

Maragos C, Wang JM, Hrabie JA, et al: Nitric oxide/nucleophile complexes inhibit the in vivo proliferation of A375 melanoma cells via nitric oxide release. Cancer Res 53:564–568, 1993

Mayskens FL, Salmon SF: Modulation of clonogenic human melanoma cells by follicle-stimulating hormone, melatonin and nerve growth factor. Br J Cancer 43:111–115, 1981

McGuire WL, Carbone PP, Sears ME, et al: Estrogen receptors in human breast cancer: an overview, in Estrogen Receptors in Breast Cancer. Edited by McGuire WL, Carbone PP, Vollmer EP. New York, Raven, 1975, pp 1–7

Meister A: Glutathione deficiency produced by inhibition of its synthesis and its reversal: applications in research and therapy. Pharmacol Ther 51:155–194, 1991

Menendez-Pelaez A, Reiter RJ: Distribution of melatonin in mammalian tissues: the relative importance of nuclear versus cytoplasmic localization. J Pineal Res 15:59–69, 1993

Misriahi M, Atger M, D'Ariol L, et al: Complete amino acid sequence of the human progesterone receptor deduced from cloned cDNA. Biochem Biophys Res Commun 143:740–748, 1987

Molis TM, Walters MR, Hill SM: Melatonin modulation of estrogen receptor expression in MCF-7 human breast cancer cells. International Journal of Oncology 3:687–694, 1993

Molis TM, Spriggs LL, Hill SM: Modulation of estrogen receptor mRNA expression by melatonin in MCF-7 human breast cancer cells. Mol Endocrinol 8:1681–1690, 1994

Molis TM, Spriggs LL, Jupiter YY, et al: Melatonin modulation of estrogen-regulated proteins, growth factors, and proto-oncogenes in human breast cancer. J Pineal Res 18:93–103, 1995

Morgan DA, Ruscetti FW, Gallo RC: Selective in vitro growth of T lymphocytes from normal human bone marrows. Science 193:1007–1008, 1976

Morgan PJ, Lawson W, Davidson G, et al: Guanine nucleotides regulate the affinity of melatonin receptors in the ovine pars tuberalis. Neuroendocrinology 50:359–362, 1989

Morgan PJ, Williams LN, Davidson G, et al: Melatonin receptors in the pars tuberalis: characterization and autoradiographical localization. J Neuroendocrinol 2:773–776, 1990

Morgan PJ, Perry B, Edward HH, et al: Melatonin receptors: localization, molecular pharmacology and physiological significance. Neurochem Int 24:101–146, 1994

Morrey NM, McLachlan JA, Serkin CD, et al: Activation of human monocytes by the pineal hormone melatonin. J Immunol 153:2671–2680, 1994

Neri B, Fiorelli C, Moroni F, et al: Modulation of human lymphoblastoid interferon activity by melatonin in metastatic renal cell carcinoma. Cancer 73:3015–3019, 1994

Pablos MI, Agapito MT, Gutierrez R, et al: Melatonin stimulates the activity of the detoxifying enzyme glutathione peroxidase in several tissues of chicks. J Pineal Res 19:111–115, 1995

Paciotti GF, Skwerer RG, Tamarkin L: Differential response of rat splenic lymphocytes to short-term and long-term neuroendocrine challenges: possible desensitization of the cellular immune response to corticosteroids. J Neuroimmunol 16:253–259, 1987

Pearson WR: Rapid and sensitive sequence comparison with FASTP and FASTA. Methods Enzymol 183:63–98, 1990

Persengiev SP, Kyurkchiev S: Selective effect of melatonin on the proliferation of lymphoid cells. International Journal of Biochemistry 25:441–444, 1993

Peters BA, Sothmann M, Wehrenberg WB: Blood leukocyte and spleen lymphocyte immune responses in chronically physically active and sedentary hamsters. Life Sci 45:2239–2245, 1989

Philo R, Berkowitz AS: Inhibition of Dunning tumor growth by melatonin. J Urol 139:1099–1102, 1988

Pickering DS, Niles LP: Expression of nanomolar-affinity binding sites for melatonin in Syrian hamster RPMI 1846 melanoma cells. Cell Signal 4:151–168, 1992

Poffenbarger M, Fuller GM: Is melatonin a microtubule inhibitor? Exp Cell Res 103:135–141, 1976

Radi R, Beckman JS, Bush KM, et al: Peroxynitrite oxidation of sulfhydryls. J Biol Chem 266:4244–4250, 1991

Radosevic-Stasic B, Jonjic S, Poliz L, et al: Immune response of rats after pharmacologic pinealectomy. Period Biol 85:119–121, 1983

Ralph CL: Pineal bodies and thermoregulation, in The Pineal Gland. Edited by Reiter RJ. New York, Raven, 1984, pp 193–215

Ram P, Hill SM: Melatonin's inhibition of breast cancer cell proliferation is mediated through the RORα receptor pathway, in Seventh International Congress on Hormones and Cancer, Quebec, Canada, September 1995, p 62

Regelson W, Pierpaoli W: Melatonin: A rediscovered antitumor hormone? its relation to surface receptors, sex, steroid metabolism, immunologic response and chronobiological factors in tumor growth and therapy. Cancer Invest 5:379–385, 1987

Reiter RJ: The pineal and its hormones in the control of reproduction in mammals. Endocr Rev 1:109–131, 1980

Reiter RJ: The melatonin message: duration versus coincidence hypothesis. Life Sci 40:2119–2124, 1987

Reiter RJ: Melatonin: That ubiquitously acting pineal hormone. Psychological Science 6:223–228, 1991a

Reiter RJ: Pineal melatonin: cell biology of its synthesis and of its physiological interactions. Endocr Rev 12:151–180, 1991b

Reiter RJ: Oxidative processes and antioxidant defense mechanisms in the aging brain. FASEB J 9:526–533, 1995

Reiter RJ, Mechiorri D, Sewerynek E, et al: A review of the evidence supporting melatonin's role as an antioxidant. J Pineal Res 18:1–11, 1995

Reppert SM, Weaver DR, Ebisawa T: Cloning and characterization of a melatonin receptor that mediates reproductive and circadian responses. Neuron 13:1177–1185, 1994

Reppert SM, Godson C, Mahle CD, et al: Molecular characterization of a second melatonin receptor expressed in human retina and brain. Proc Natl Acad Sci U S A 92:8734–8739, 1995

Rettori V, Gimeno M, Lyson K, et al: Nitric oxide mediates norpepinephrine-induced prostaglandin E_2 release from the hypothalamus. Proc Natl Acad Sci U S A 89:11543–11546, 1992

Rivkees SA, Carlson LL, Reppert SM: Guanine nucleotide binding protein regulation of melatonin receptors in lizard brain. Proc Natl Acad Sci U S A 86:3882–3886, 1989

Rosenberg SA, Terry WD: Passive immunotherapy of cancer in animals and man. Adv Cancer Res 25:323–334, 1987

Saceda M, Lippman ME, Chambond P, et al: Regulation of estrogen receptor in MCF-7 cells by estradiol. Mol Endocrinol 2:1157–1162, 1986

Sanchez-Barcelo EJ, Corral SC, Mediavilla MD: Influence of pineal gland function on the initiation and growth of hormone-dependent breast tumors. Possible mechanisms, in The Pineal Gland and Cancer. Edited by Gupta D, Attanasio A, Reiter RJ. Tübingen, Germany, Brain Research Promotion, 1988, pp 221–232

Sewerynek E, Melchiorri D, Reiter RJ, et al: A lipopolysaccharide-induced hepatotoxicity is inhibited by the antioxidant melatonin. Eur J Pharmacol 288:327–334, 1995a

Sewerynek E, Melchiorri D, Chen L-D, et al: Melatonin reduces both basal and bacterial lipopolysaccharide-induced lipid peroxidation in vitro. Free Radic Biol Med 19:903–909, 1995b

Stamler JS, Single DJ, Loscalzo J: Biochemistry of nitric oxide and its redox-activated forms. Science 258:1898–1902, 1992

Stanberry LR, Das Gupta TK, Beattie CW: Photoperiodic control of melanoma growth in hamsters: influence of pinealectomy and melatonin. Endocrinology 113:469–475, 1983

Stankov B, Lucini V, Scaglione F, et al: 2-[^{125}]iodomelatonin binding in normal and neoplastic tissues, in Role of Melatonin and Pineal Peptides in Neuroimmunomodulation. Edited by Fraschini F, Reiter RJ. New York, Plenum, 1991, pp 117–125

Stankov B, Biella G, Panara C, et al: Melatonin signal transduction and mechanism of action in the central nervous system: using the rabbit cortex as a model. Endocrinology 130:2152–2154, 1992

Steinhilber D, Brungs M, Werz O, et al: The nuclear receptor for melatonin represses 5-lipoxygenase gene expression in human B lymphocytes. J Biol Chem 270:7037–7040, 1995

Sullivan JS, Cohn CD, Castles CG, et al: Analysis of the 5-flanking region of the estrogen receptor gene in ER-positive and ER-negative breast cancer cell lines (abstract). Abstracts of the 77th Annual Meeting of the Endocrine Society 646:57, 1995

Sutherland RL, Gren MD, Hall RE, et al: Tamoxifen induces accumulation of MCF-7 human mammary carcinoma cells in G_0/G_1 phase of the cell cycle. European Journal of Cancer and Clinical Oncology 19:615–621, 1983

Tamarkin L, Cohen M, Roselle D, et al: Melatonin inhibition and pinealectomy enhancement of 7,12-dimethylbenz[a]nthracene-induced mammary tumors in the rat. Cancer Res 41:4432–4436, 1981

Tamarkin L, Danforth D, Lichter A, et al: Decreased nocturnal plasma melatonin peak in patients with estrogen receptor positive breast cancer. Science 216:1003–1005, 1982

Tan D-X, Poeggeler B, Reiter RJ, et al: The pineal hormone melatonin inhibits DNA-adduct formation induced by the carcinogen safrole in vivo. Cancer Lett 70:65–71, 1993

Tapp E: The pineal gland in malignancy, in Pineal Gland, Vol 3: Extra-Reproductive Effects. Edited by Reiter RJ. Boca Raton, FL, CRC Press, 1982, pp 171–188

Tini M, Fraser A, Giguere V: Functional interactions between retinoic acid receptors, related orphan nuclear receptor (RORα) and the retinoic acid receptors in the regulation of the μF-crystalline promoter. J Biol Chem 270:20156–20162, 1995

Toma JG, Amerongen HM, Hennes SC, et al: Effects of olfactory bulbectomy, melatonin and/or pinealectomy on three sublines of Dunning R3327 rat prostatic adenocarcinomas. J Pineal Res 4:321–326, 1987

Tommasi MS, Brocchi A, Fiorelli C, et al: Effects of melatonin on cytokine production in patients with advanced solid tumors. Euro-Immunoanalyse Lyon, February 4–5, 1993, pp 3–5

Trinchieri G, Perussia B: Human natural killer cells: biologic and pathologic aspects. Lab Invest 50:489–513, 1984

Vakkuri O, Leppaluoto J, Vuolteenaho O: Development and validation of a melatonin radioimmunoassay using radioiodinated melatonin tracer. Acta Endocrinologica (Copenhagen) 106:152–157, 1984

Vanecek J, Pavlik A, Illnerova H: Hypothalamic receptor sites revealed by autoradiography. Brain Res 435:359–363, 1987

Vaughan MK, Hubbard GN, Champney TH, et al: Splenic hypertrophy and extramedullary hematopoiesis induced in male Syrian hamsters by short photoperiod or melatonin injections and reversed by melatonin pellets or pinealectomy. American Journal of Anatomy 179:131–136, 1987

Vermeulen M, Palermo M, Giordano M: Neonatal pinealectomy impairs murine antibody-dependent cellular cytotoxicity. J Neuroimmunol 43:97–101, 1993

Victorin K: Review of the genotoxicity of mitogen oxides. Mutat Res 317:43–55, 1994

Wanebo HJ, Pace R, Hargett S, et al: Production and response to interleukin-2 in peripheral blood lymphocytes of cancer patients. Cancer 57:656–662, 1985

Watson J, Mochizuki D: Interleukin 2: a class of T cell growth factor. Immunol Rev 51:257–260, 1980

Weaver DR, Nanboordiri MAA, Reppert SM: Iodinated melatonin mimics melatonin action and reveals discrete binding sites in fetal brain. FEBS Lett 228:123–127, 1988

Weisz A, Bresciani F: Estrogen induces expression of c-fos and c-myc protooncogenes in rat uterus. Mol Endocrinol 2:816–824, 1988

Welsch CW, Nagasawa H: Prolactin and murine mammary tumorigenesis: a review. Cancer Res 37:951–963, 1977

White BH, Sekura RD, Rollag MD: Pertussis toxin blocks melatonin-induced pigment aggregation in Xenopus dermal melanophores. Journal of Comparative Physiology 157:153–157, 1987

Wiesenberg I, Missbach M, Kahlen J-P, et al: Transcriptional activation of the nuclear receptor RZRα by the pineal gland hormone melatonin and identification of CGP 52608 as a synthetic ligand. Nucleic Acids Res 23:327–333, 1995

Wieser M, Bonifer R, Oster W, et al: Interleukin-4 induces secretion of CSF for granulocytes and CSF for macrophages by peripheral blood monocytes. Blood 73:1105–1108, 1989

Williams LM, Morgan PJ, Hastings MH, et al: Melatonin receptor sites in the Syrian hamster brain and pituitary: localization and characterization using [^{125}]iodomelatonin. J Neuroendocrinol 1:315–329, 1989

Wink DA, Kasprzak KS, Maragos CM, et al: DNA deaminating ability and genotoxicity of nitric oxide and its progenitors. Science 254:1001–1003, 1991

Wurtman RJ, Lieberman HR: Melatonin secretion as a mediator of circadian variations in sleep and sleepiness. J Pineal Res 2:301–303, 1985

Ying S-W, Niles LP, Crocker C: Human malignant melanoma cells express high-affinity receptors for melatonin: antiproliferative effects of melatonin and 6-chloromelatonin. Eur J Pharmacol 246:89–96, 1993

Zhang J, Dawson VL, Dawson TM, et al: Nitric oxide activation of poly (ADP-ribose) synthetase in neurotoxicity. Science 263:687–689, 1994

Chapter 10

The Melatonin Rhythm in Cancer Patients

David E. Blask, M.D., Ph.D.

O ver the past 15 years, melatonin's antineoplastic activity has been explored in both in vivo and in vitro models of carcinogenesis (Blask 1984; Blask and Hill 1988). A variety of neoplasms, particularly those of hormone-sensitive tissues, respond to the oncostatic effects of melatonin. Melatonin has well-known modulatory actions on reproductive function in a variety of species (Reiter 1991); therefore, it is not surprising that this molecule appears to exhibit a strong influence on the growth of hormone-sensitive reproductive neoplasms such as breast cancer (Blask 1993b). Melatonin not only affects the growth and metastatic spread of malignant tumors, but conversely, these tumors also may exert classical neuroendocrine "feedback-like" effects on the pineal production of melatonin (Blask 1993a, 1994b; Blask and Hill 1988). Using breast cancer as a principal focus, I examine in this chapter the anticancer role of physiological levels of melatonin, as well as the nature and potential mechanisms of alterations in the circadian rhythm of physiological melatonin production in cancer patients.

Effects of Physiological Melatonin on Cancer

The circadian rhythm of nocturnal melatonin production may represent a unique regulatory signal for the carcinogenic process. For example, pinealectomy, presumably through the elimination of the circadian melatonin signal, enhances or promotes the development and growth of neoplasms, most notably breast cancer

(Blask 1984; Blask et al. 1991; Shah et al. 1984; Tamarkin et al. 1981). This finding suggests that the nighttime physiological surge of melatonin in the bloodstream or other extracellular fluids may play an important role in carcinogenesis by exerting a "natural restraint" on tumor initiation, promotion, and/or progression. The recent demonstration that melatonin may offer "on-site" protection against free-radical damage by virtue of its antioxidant properties and mitigate against the initiation of cancer adds further credence to this postulate (Reiter et al. 1995). The hypothesis that concentrations of melatonin in the nocturnal physiological range (10 pM–1 nM) have oncostatic effects on tumor growth has been most extensively investigated at the cellular and molecular level in vitro in the human breast cancer cell line MCF-7 (Hill and Blask 1988; Molis et al. 1993, 1994, 1995). It is clear that physiological melatonin suppression of MCF-7 cell growth is highly dependent on the culture conditions (Blask and Hill 1986; Cos and Blask 1990). Moreover, melatonin's antiproliferative effect appears to be limited to estrogen-receptor (ER+) human breast cancer cell lines such as MCF-7 (Hill et al. 1992). Interestingly, a circadian-like presentation of physiological melatonin levels to breast cancer cells in vitro is somewhat more effective than continuous exposure of the cells to this indolamine in suppressing cell growth (Cos and Sanchez-Barcelo 1994).

We are just beginning to acquire some insights into the cellular/molecular mechanisms by which melatonin inhibits breast cancer cell proliferation. For example, flow cytometric studies reveal that physiological melatonin slows the progression of MCF-7 cells, grown in monolayer, from G_0/G_1 to S-phase of the cell cycle, indicating that a cytostatic rather than a cytotoxic effect is being exerted by this molecule (Cos et al. 1991). However, cytotoxic effects of pharmacological concentrations of melatonin have been demonstrated under different culture conditions (Shellard et al. 1989). Moreover, melatonin inhibits estradiol, epidermal growth factor, and prolactin growth-response pathways and also modulates both constitutive and estradiol-induced growth factor activity in these cells (Cos and Blask 1994; Lemus-Wilson et al. 1995). Physiological melatonin levels also suppress ER expression and transcriptional expression of ER messenger RNA (mRNA) in MCF-7 cells, albeit the mechanism by which melatonin down-regulates ER expression is currently unknown (Molis et al. 1993, 1994). Additionally, melatonin alters the steady-state mRNA expression of a variety of other estrogen-regulated proteins, growth factors, and proto-oncogenes in MCF-7 cells (Molis et al. 1995) (see Hill et al., Chapter 9, in this volume).

Although melatonin-binding sites have been identified in a variety of peripheral organs, including neoplastic tissues such as human melanoma cells and carcinogen-induced rat mammary cancers (Burns et al. 1990; Stankov et al. 1991). D. E. Blask and D. M. Burns (unpublished data, June 1990) and others (Stankov et al. 1991) have observed little to no melatonin binding to membrane preparations of MCF-7 cells. Although a high-affinity membrane melatonin receptor was recently isolated, cloned, and sequenced from *Xenopus laevis* dermal melanophores (Reppert et al. 1994), it appears that a membrane-bound melatonin receptor is not involved in conveying physiological melatonin's oncostatic signal to ER+ human breast cancer cells.

In addition to melatonin regulation of growth factor–response pathways, we have recently determined that melatonin blocks calcium-stimulated growth of MCF-7 cells and that melatonin-induced growth inhibition is calcium dependent (D. E. Blask, S. T. Wilson, unpublished data, September 1994). This finding may indicate a fundamental relationship with melatonin's inhibition of growth factor–response pathways because growth factor–stimulated mitogenesis is associated with an increase in cytosolic calcium and growth factors stimulate calcium influx (Moolenaar et al. 1984). Furthermore, in other cell lines and tissues, melatonin alters intracellular calcium/calmodulin homeostasis and prevents calcium-induced microtubule depolymerization and cytoskeletal disruption (Benitez-King and Anton-Tay 1993), which are important elements in calcium/calmodulin-induced cell proliferation (Rasmussen and Means 1987). Additionally, melatonin has been reported to possess calcium-channel-blocking-like effects (Vanecek and Klein 1993) and to influence the activity of the calcium/adenosinetriphosphatase (ATPase) pump (Chen et al. 1992).

Other recent findings (Blask et al. 1997) indicate that the free-radical scavenger and intracellular oxidation-reduction (redox) molecule, glutathione (GSH), is essential for melatonin's inhibitory action on MCF-7 cells. In fact, physiological melatonin itself maintains elevated levels of GSH in these cells during culture. These results may be potentially important in light of strong evidence that melatonin is a highly potent and ubiquitous free-radical-scavenging molecule (Reiter et al. 1995), whereas GSH has a profound impact not only on cancer cell sensitivity to anticancer agents but also on virtually all aspects of cell physiology and metabolism (Meister 1991). Therefore, this simple tripeptide molecule may play a central role in linking melatonin's diverse inhibitory actions on estrogen-, peptide growth factor–, and calcium-induced growth signaling in breast cancer cells.

Circadian Melatonin Rhythm in Cancer Patients

The tumor-promoting effects of pinealectomy, together with the in vitro oncostatic action of physiological melatonin, provide a cogent argument for the role of circadian melatonin production and secretion in the regulation of tumorigenesis. Is there an equally compelling case for a reciprocal regulation of circadian melatonin production in patients with neoplastic disease?

One of the first studies to examine a potential relationship between cancer and circadian melatonin production was by Tamarkin et al. (1982), who assayed plasma immunoreactive melatonin levels every 3 hours over a 24-hour period in pre- and postmenopausal women with clinical stage I and II breast cancer, as well as in age-matched healthy women (Figure 10–1). In aggregate, breast cancer patients exhibited a normal melatonin rhythm, with low levels during the day and high nocturnal levels peaking around 2 A.M. However, when the patients were stratified on the basis of ER status, those with ER– disease had a normal to slightly elevated peak amplitude of melatonin, whereas the amplitude of the nocturnal melatonin peak in ER+ patients was significantly reduced by approximately 40% as compared with that in control subjects. Other parameters of circadian rhythmicity, such as the acrophase or period of the rhythm, were apparently unaltered in both ER+ and ER– breast cancer patients. Interestingly, tumor ER and progesterone receptor (PgR) concentrations were inversely correlated with the peaks of nocturnal melatonin levels in these patients, indicating that women with lower peak melatonin titers have higher ER and PgR levels in their tumors (Danforth et al. 1985). Because elevated tumor ER and PgR concentrations portend a better objective response to endocrine therapy (Wittliff 1988), perhaps decreased nocturnal melatonin levels could be used as yet another marker, in addition to steroid receptor status, to better predict the outcome of hormonal treatment and prognosis of the disease. It is interesting to note that women at high risk for developing breast cancer (either ER+ or ER–) have been reported to exhibit a slightly higher circadian amplitude of melatonin than those at lower risk for developing the disease (Wetterberg et al. 1979). Thus, a slightly higher nocturnal amplitude of melatonin in ER– patients as compared with healthy women (Tamarkin et al. 1982) might also be a marker for a more aggressive and thus less endocrine-sensitive tumor.

Other investigators have found a correlation between tumor size and the nocturnal amplitude of melatonin. For example, Bartsch et al. (1989, 1993), who originally described an alteration in the circadian profile in urinary melatonin levels in breast cancer patients (Bartsch et al. 1981), reported that the peak nocturnal amplitude of melatonin—which was reduced by 50% in patients with primary breast cancer—was inversely correlated with tumor size (Figure 10–2), whereas it was positively correlated with PgR status. However, no correlation was found with ER status. Surprisingly, the melatonin rhythm was completely normal in those patients who developed a secondary recurrence of breast cancer. Because the nocturnal amplitude of the serum 6-sulfatoxymelatonin (major liver melatonin metabolite) rhythm was also depressed in patients with primary breast cancer (Figure 10–3), it appears that decreased pineal melatonin production rather than increased liver metabolism of melatonin was responsible for lower nighttime blood levels of the indolamine (Bartsch et al. 1991).

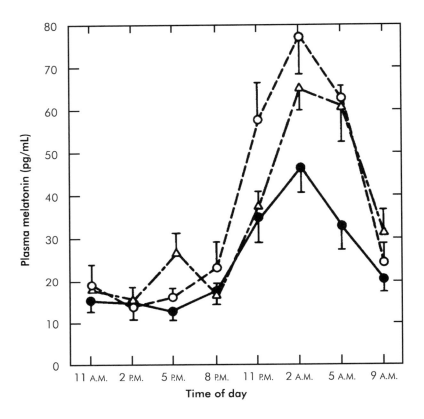

Figure 10–1. Twenty-four-hour circadian profiles of plasma melatonin concentrations in women with either estrogen-receptor-positive (●) or negative (O) breast cancer and in age-matched healthy women (Δ). Data are expressed as the mean ± SEM.

Source. Reprinted from Tamarkin L, Danforth D, Lichter A, et al.: "Decreased Nocturnal Plasma Melatonin Peak in Patients With Estrogen Receptor Positive Breast Cancer." *Science* 216:1003–1005, 1982. Copyright 1982 American Association for the Advancement of Science. Used with permission.

In a similar study of the circadian profile of urinary 6-sulfatoxymelatonin in older postmenopausal women with breast cancer as compared with younger women with benign breast disease, Skene et al. (1990) found a suppression in both the overall 24-hour

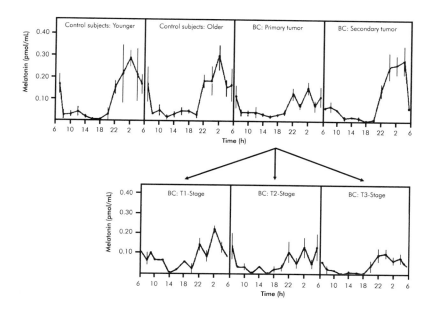

Figure 10–2. Twenty-four-hour circadian profiles of serum melatonin concentrations *(upper panel)* in women with either primary breast cancer (BC: primary tumor) or secondary breast cancer (BC: secondary tumor) as well as in younger and older healthy women (control subjects). Twenty-four-hour circadian profiles of serum melatonin concentrations in women with primary breast cancer divided into subgroups according to increasing size of their tumor *(lower panel)*. Stage T1, small tumors (2 cm or less); stage T2, medium tumors (2–5 cm); stage 3, large tumors (> 5 cm). Data are expressed as the mean ± SEM.

Source. Reprinted from Bartsch C, Bartsch H, Fuchs U, et al.: "Stage-Dependent Depression of Melatonin in Patients With Primary Breast Cancer: Correlation With Prolactin, TSH and Steroid Receptors." *Cancer* 64:426–433, 1989. Copyright 1989 American Cancer Society. Used with permission.

excretion and nocturnal circadian amplitude of 6-sulfatoxymelatonin in the breast cancer patients. However, accurate age matching of the breast cancer patients with healthy women revealed no differences in the circadian profiles in melatonin, indicating that the depressed nocturnal circadian amplitude of 6-sulfatoxymela-

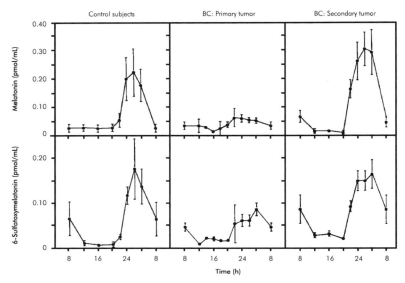

Figure 10–3. Twenty-four-hour circadian profiles of serum melatonin *(upper panel)* and 6-sulfatoxymelatonin *(lower panel)* concentrations in women with either primary breast cancer (BC: primary tumor) or secondary breast cancer (BC: secondary tumor) and in age-matched healthy women (control subjects). Data are expressed as the mean ± SEM.
Source.   Reprinted from Bartsch C, Bartsch H, Bellman O, et al.: "Depression of Serum Melatonin in Patients With Primary Breast Cancer is Not Due to an Increased Peripheral Metabolism." *Cancer* 67:1681–1684, 1991. Copyright 1991 American Cancer Society. Used with permission.

tonin excretion in breast cancer patients was due to the normal, age-associated decline in nocturnal melatonin production (Wald-hauser et al. 1985). Thus, age can be a confounding factor in differentiating between the normal effects of aging and diseases of aging, such as cancer, on melatonin rhythms in an elderly population. Such differences can be addressed only by careful and strict age and gender matching of a healthy control population, with the population harboring the disease under investigation.

Like women with breast cancer, men with clinically detectable adenocarcinoma of the prostate also exhibit a substantially damp-ened nocturnal surge of melatonin in the blood and 6-sulfatoxymelatonin in the urine, as compared with either young men or age-matched patients with benign prostatic hypertrophy (Bartsch et al. 1983, 1985, 1992) (Figure 10–4). Furthermore, the nocturnal, circadian peak of melatonin is inversely correlated with tumor size, as it is in breast cancer patients, suggesting a relationship between the progression of prostate cancer and the development of a defect in the expression of the normal circadian amplitude of melatonin. As in the case of breast cancer patients, no abnormalities in either the phasing or period of the melatonin rhythm were detected (Bartsch et al. 1994).

Alterations in the circadian rhythm of melatonin production are not limited to hormone-responsive cancers of the reproductive tract. For example, Khoory and Stemme (1988) found that in patients with colorectal carcinoma, primarily elderly men, the nocturnal production of melatonin was significantly blunted as compared with age- and gender-matched healthy control subjects. Interestingly, nocturnal melatonin levels appeared to be most markedly reduced in those patients with the highest circulating concentrations of carcinoembryonic antigen (CEA), a tumor marker important in the postoperative follow-up of colorectal cancer.

Potential Mechanism of Circadian Melatonin Suppression in Cancer Patients

What exactly does an altered circadian profile of melatonin production in cancer patients mean in terms of the process of carcinogenesis? If physiological melatonin truly plays an oncostatic role in humans, do some patients develop certain types of cancer because of an underlying defect in the ability of their pineal glands to produce melatonin? Or conversely, does a suppressed nocturnal circadian amplitude of melatonin reflect an influence of tumor growth on the melatonin-generating system of the pineal? Because tumors manufacture a variety of soluble proteins, growth factors, and cytokines, it is conceivable that tumoral secretion of these substances into the circulation could represent a patho-

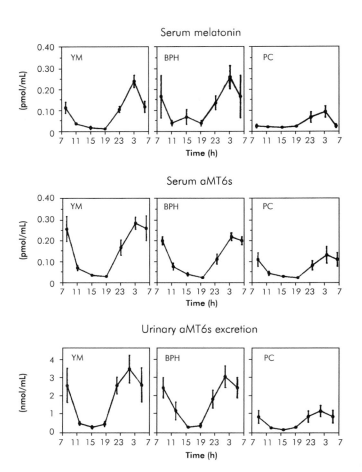

Figure 10–4. Twenty-four-hour circadian profiles of serum melatonin *(upper panel),* serum 6-sulfatoxymelatonin (αMT6s) *(middle panel),* and urinary αMT6s *(lower panel)* concentrations in elderly men with either benign prostatic hyperplasia (BPH) or untreated primary prostate cancer (PC) and in young men (YM). Data are expressed as the mean ± SEM.

Source. Reprinted from Bartsch C, Bartsch H, Fluchter St-H, et al.: "Diminished Pineal Function Coincides With Disturbed Circadian Endocrine Rhythmicity in Untreated Primary Cancer Patients: Consequence of Premature Aging or of Tumor Growth?" in *The Aging Clock: The Pineal and Other Pacemakers in the Progression of Aging and Carcinogenesis (Annals of the New York Academy of Sciences,* Vol 719). Edited by Pierpaoli W, Regelson W, Fabris N. New York, The New York Academy of Sciences, 1994, pp 502–525. Used with permission.

physiological counterpart to a classical neuroendocrine feedback loop regulating the melatonin-generating system anywhere along the neural pathway from the suprachiasmatic nuclei (SCN) to the pineal itself.

In experimental animals, it was initially shown by Lapin and Frowein (1981) that the pineal melatonin content in rats with growing tumors declined as the tumors became larger. Bartsch et al. (1990) described biphasic changes in the nocturnal production of melatonin during the process of carcinogenesis in female rats with chemically induced mammary cancers. They found that both pineal and plasma melatonin levels increased as initially small tumor volumes increased in size to about 10 cm^3, followed by a decline in melatonin levels as the tumors grew to larger volumes. However, like the studies in cancer patients, these experimental investigations did not address the *mechanism* by which melatonin production is altered during the neoplastic process.

Tumors synthesize and secrete a variety of soluble growth factors and cytokines (Osborne and Arteaga 1990; Paciotti and Tamarkin 1995) that may feed back on the neuroendocrine mechanisms controlling melatonin production by the pineal gland. Additionally, tumoricidal or tumoristatic immune cells infiltrating neoplastic tissues produce and release cytokines, which also have been shown to influence pineal melatonin. For example, interferon-γ (IFN-γ) enhances pineal melatonin production in rats, whereas interleukin-2 (IL-2) inhibits melatonin production in humans (Maestroni and Conti 1993). Recently, a tumor-associated melatonin-inhibiting factor (TAMF) was reported to be present in the serum of leukemic mice (Leone and Skene 1994)(see Figure 10–5).

Over a 9-day period, Leone and Skene (1994) sequentially bled mice that had been inoculated with a mouse macrophage/monocyte leukemia cell line. Serum from leukemic mice progressively inhibited isoprenaline-stimulated melatonin production by cultured mouse pineal glands during this 9-day interval. These results indicate that as the leukemia cells proliferated, more TAMF was released into the bloodstream, presumably from the tumor cells, suggesting a direct correlation between tumor stage and the

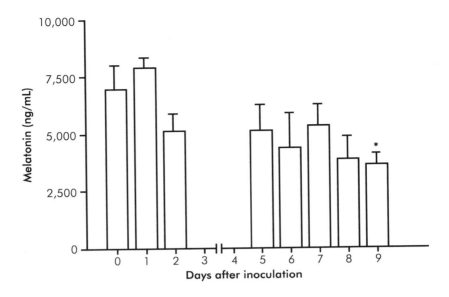

Figure 10–5. Effect of sera, collected from leukemia-bearing mice on different days following inoculation of tumor cells, on isoprenaline (20 μM)-stimulated melatonin concentrations from cultured rat pineal glands 21 hours following exposure to sera. Data are expressed as the mean ± SEM.
Source. Reprinted from Leone AM, Skene D: "Melatonin Concentrations in Pineal Organ Culture Are Suppressed by Sera From Tumor-Bearing Mice." *Journal of Pineal Research* 17:17–19, 1994. Copyright 1994 Munksgaard International Publishers Ltd., Copenhagen, Denmark. Used with permission.

degree of melatonin suppression as originally described in breast cancer patients (Bartsch et al. 1989). Taken together, these results support the postulate that a soluble tumor-derived factor may exert feedback effects directly at the level of the pineal gland to alter circadian melatonin production. It would clearly make sense that such a factor could gain access to the melatonin-generating system at this level because there is no blood-brain barrier within the pineal gland itself (Reiter 1991). Alternatively, such a factor could influence the circadian melatonin-generating system at other sites within the central nervous system devoid of a blood-brain barrier, such as the SCN within the hypothalamus.

Conclusions

Physiological levels of melatonin, resulting from its nighttime surge in the blood and other extracellular fluids, are known to have oncostatic effects on tumorigenesis in both in vivo and in vitro models of experimental carcinogenesis. Reciprocal regulation of pineal melatonin production by tumors during carcinogenesis is suggested by changes that occur in the circadian amplitude of nocturnal melatonin production in patients with cancer of the breast, prostate, and colon/rectum, as well as in those at high risk for developing breast cancer. In cancer patients, the nocturnal surge of melatonin is significantly blunted, with no apparent alteration in either circadian phase or period of the rhythm. Interestingly, in women at particularly high risk for developing breast cancer, the circadian amplitude of melatonin is augmented. Nevertheless, it is quite possible that when the circadian profile of melatonin is examined in a wider array of patients with different tumor types, alterations in the circadian timing might be detected as well. The fact that tumor cells and related cytotoxic and cytostatic immune cells elaborate a variety of soluble factors such as cytokines, which can directly modulate pineal melatonin production, suggests an important "cross talk" between the melatonin-generating system and the tumors themselves. It is tempting to speculate that the ability of tumor-derived substances to compromise nocturnal melatonin production represents yet another cunning means evolved by certain neoplasms to "escape" the natural oncostatic protection seemingly provided by the circadian melatonin signal. If, in fact, dynamic changes occur in the amplitude and timing of the melatonin signal during the course of carcinogenesis, which only prospective longitudinal studies ultimately can address, then the melatonin rhythm may eventually serve as a useful marker for the progression and risk of neoplastic diseases. This marker could potentially have a major impact on the prevention, diagnosis, treatment, and prognosis of cancer. Furthermore, altered circadian melatonin production during carcinogenesis may have important implications for the sleep problems and psychological depression experienced by many cancer patients.

References

Bartsch C, Bartsch H, Jain AK, et al: Urinary melatonin levels in human breast cancer patients. J Neural Transm 52:281–294, 1981

Bartsch C, Bartsch H, Fluchter St-H, et al: Circadian rhythms of serum melatonin, prolactin and growth hormone in patients with benign and malignant tumors of the prostate and in non-tumor controls. Neuroendocrinology Letters 5:377–386, 1983

Bartsch C, Bartsch H, Fluchter St-H, et al: Evidence for modulation of melatonin secretion in men with benign and malignant tumors of the prostate: relationship with the pituitary hormones. J Pineal Res 2:121–132, 1985

Bartsch C, Bartsch H, Fuchs U, et al: Stage-dependent depression of melatonin in patients with primary breast cancer: correlation with prolactin, TSH and steroid receptors. Cancer 64:426–433, 1989

Bartsch C, Bartsch H, Gupta D: Pineal melatonin synthesis and secretion during induction and growth of mammary cancer in female rats, in Neuroendocrinology: New Frontiers. Edited by Gupta D, Wollmann HA, Ranke MB. London, Brain Research Promotion, 1990, pp 326–332

Bartsch C, Bartsch H, Bellman O, et al: Depression of serum melatonin in patients with primary breast cancer is not due to an increased peripheral metabolism. Cancer 67:1681–1684, 1991

Bartsch C, Bartsch H, Schmidt A, et al: Melatonin and 6-sulfatoxymelatonin circadian rhythms in serum and urine of primary prostate cancer patients: evidence for reduced pineal activity and relevance of urinary determinations. Clin Chim Acta 209:153–167, 1992

Bartsch C, Bartsch H, Fluchter St-H, et al: Depleted pineal melatonin production in patients with primary breast and prostate cancer is connected with circadian disturbances of central hormones: possible role of melatonin for maintenance and synchronization of circadian rhythmicity, in Melatonin and the Pineal Gland: From Basic Science to Clinical Application. Edited by Touitou Y, Arendt J, Pevet P. Amstersdam, Elsevier, 1993, pp 311–316

Bartsch C, Bartsch H, Fluchter St-H, et al: Diminished pineal function coincides with disturbed circadian endocrine rhythmicity in untreated primary cancer patients: consequence of premature aging or of tumor growth? in The Aging Clock: The Pineal and Other Pacemakers in the Progression of Aging and Carcinogenesis (Annals of the New York Academy of Sciences, Vol 719). Edited by Pierpaoli W, Regelson W, Fabris N. New York, The New York Academy of Sciences, 1994, pp 502–525

Benitez-King G, Anton-Tay F: Calmodulin mediates melatonin cytoskeletal effects. Experientia 49:635–641, 1993

Blask DE: The pineal: an oncostatic gland? in The Pineal Gland. Edited by Reiter RJ. New York, Raven, 1984, pp 253–284

Blask DE: Integration of neuroendocrine-circadian, pineal, adrenocortical, and immune functions in homeokinesis: implications for host-cancer interactions. Neuroendocrinology Letters 15:117–133, 1993a

Blask DE: Melatonin in oncology, in Melatonin: Biosynthesis, Physiological Effects, and Clinical Applications. Edited by Yu H-S, Reiter RJ. Boca Raton, FL, CRC Press, 1993b, pp 447–475

Blask DE: Neuroendocrine aspects of circadian pharmacodynamics, in Circadian Cancer Therapy. Edited by Hrushesky WJM. Boca Raton, FL, CRC Press, 1994, pp 43–59

Blask DE, Hill SM: Effects of melatonin on cancer: studies on MCF-7 human breast cancer cells in culture. J Neural Transm Suppl 21:433–449, 1986

Blask DE, Hill SM: Melatonin and cancer: basic and clinical aspects, in Melatonin: Clinical Perspectives. Edited by Miles A, Philbrick DRS, Thompson C. Oxford, England, Oxford University Press, 1988, pp 128–173

Blask DE, Pelletier DB, Hill SM, et al: Pineal melatonin inhibition of tumor promotion in the *N*-nitroso-*N*-methylurea (NMU) model of mammary carcinogenesis: potential involvement of antiestrogeneic mechanisms in vivo. J Cancer Res Clin Oncol 117:526–532, 1991

Blask DE, Wilson SM, Zalatan F: Physiological melatonin inhibition of human breast cancer cell growth in vitro: evidence for glutathione-mediated pathway. Cancer Res 57:1909–1914, 1997

Burns DM, Cos-Corral S, Blask DE: Demonstration and partial characterization of 2-iodomelatonin binding sites in experimental mammary cancer (abstract). Abstracts of the 72nd Annual Meeting of the Endocrine Society 151:62, 1990

Chen LD, Tan DX, Reiter RJ, et al: In vivo and in vitro effects of the pineal gland and melatonin on [Ca^{2+} + Mg^{2+}]-dependent ATP-ase in cardiac sarcolemma. J Pineal Res 14:178–183, 1992

Cos S, Blask DE: Effects of melatonin on the anchorage-independent growth of human breast cancer cells (MCF-7) in a clonogenic culture system. Cancer Lett 50:115–119, 1990

Cos S, Blask DE: Melatonin modulates growth factor activity in MCF-7 human breast cancer cells. J Pineal Res 17:25–32, 1994

Cos S, Sanchez-Barcelo EJ: Differences between pulsatile or continuous exposure to melatonin on MCF-7 human breast cancer cell proliferation. Cancer Lett 85:105–109, 1994

Cos S, Blask DE, Lemus-Wilson A, et al: Effects of melatonin on the cell cycle kinetics and estrogen rescue of MCF-7 human breast cancer cells in culture. J Pineal Res 8:21–27, 1991

Danforth DN, Tamarkin L, Mulvihill JJ, et al: Plasma melatonin and the hormone-dependency of human breast cancer. J Clin Oncol 3:941–948, 1985

Hill SM, Blask DE: Effects of the pineal hormone, melatonin, on the proliferation and morphological characteristics of human breast cancer cells (MCF-7) in culture. Cancer Res 48:6121–6126, 1988

Hill SM, Spriggs LL, Simon MA, et al: The growth inhibitory action of melatonin on human breast cancer cells is linked to the estrogen response system. Cancer Lett 64:249–256, 1992

Khoory R, Stemme D: Plasma melatonin levels in patients suffering from colorectal carcinoma. J Pineal Res 5:251–258, 1988

Lapin V, Frowein A: Effects of growing tumors on pineal melatonin levels in male rats. J Neural Transm 50:275–282, 1981

Lemus-Wilson A, Kelly PA, Blask DE: Melatonin blocks the stimulating effects of prolactin on human breast cancer cell growth in culture. Br J Cancer 72:1435–1440, 1995

Leone AM, Skene D: Melatonin concentrations in pineal organ culture are suppressed by sera from tumor-bearing mice. J Pineal Res 17:17–19, 1994

Maestroni GJM, Conti A: Melatonin in relation to the immune system, in Melatonin: Biosynthesis, Physiological Effects, and Clinical Applications. Edited by Yu H-S, Reiter RJ. Boca Raton, FL, CRC Press, 1993, pp 289–309

Meister A: Glutathione deficiency produced by inhibition of its synthesis and its reversal: applications in research and therapy. Pharmacol Ther 51:155–194, 1991

Molis TM, Walters MR, Hill SM: Melatonin modulation of estrogen receptor expression in MCF-7 human breast cancer cells. International Journal of Oncology 3:687–694, 1993

Molis TM, Spriggs LL, Hill SM: Modulation of estrogen receptor mRNA expression by melatonin in MCF-7 human breast cancer cells. Mol Endocrinol 8:1681–1690, 1994

Molis TM, Spriggs LL, Jupiter Y, et al: Melatonin modulation of estrogen-regulated proteins, growth factors, and proto-oncogenes in human breast cancer. J Pineal Res 18:93–103, 1995

Moolenaar WH, Tertoolen LGS, de Laat SW: Growth factors immediately raise cytoplasmic free Ca^{2+} in human fibroblasts. J Biol Chem 259:8066–8069, 1984

Osborne CK, Arteaga CL: Autocrine and paracrine growth regulation of breast cancer: clinical implications. Breast Cancer Res Treat 15:3–11, 1990

Paciotti GF, Tamarkin L: Detection of human breast cancer cell-derived cytokines and their "push-pull" relationship with estrogen in metastatic cancer cell growth (abstract). Abstracts of the 77th Annual Meeting of the Endocrine Society P2-646:452, 1995

Rasmussen CD, Means AR: Calmodulin is involved in regulation of cell proliferation. EMBO J 6:3961–3968, 1987

Reiter RJ: Pineal melatonin: cell biology of its synthesis and of its physiological interactions. Endocr Rev 12:151–180, 1991

Reiter RJ, Melchiorri D, Sewerynek E, et al: A review of the evidence supporting melatonin's role as an antioxidant. J Pineal Res 18:1–11, 1995

Reppert SM, Weaver DR, Ebisawa T: Cloning and characterization of a mammalian melatonin receptor that mediates reproductive and circadian responses. Neuron 13:1177–1185, 1994

Shah PN, Mhatre MC, Kothari LS: Effect of melatonin on mammary carcinogenesis in intact and pinealectomized rats in varying photoperiods. Cancer Res 44:3403–3405, 1984

Shellard SA, Whelan RDH, Hill BT: Growth inhibitory and cytotoxic effects of melatonin and its metabolites on human tumour cell lines in vitro. Br J Cancer 60:288–290, 1989

Skene DJ, Bojkowski CJ, Currie JE, et al: 6-Sulphatoxymelatonin production in breast cancer patients. J Pineal Res 8:269–276, 1990

Stankov B, Lucini V, Scaglione F, et al: 2-[^{125}I]iodomelatonin binding in normal and neoplastic tissues, in Role of Melatonin and Pineal Peptides in Neuroimmunomodulation. Edited by Fraschini F, Reiter RJ. New York, Plenum, 1991, pp 117–125

Tamarkin L, Cohen M, Roselle D, et al: Melatonin inhibition and pinealectomy enhancement of 7,12-dimethylbenz[a]anthracene-induced mammary tumors in the rat. Cancer Res 41:4432–4436, 1981

Tamarkin L, Danforth DN, Lichter A, et al: Decreased nocturnal plasma melatonin peak in patients with estrogen receptor positive breast cancer. Science 216:1003–1005, 1982

Vanecek J, Klein DC: Melatonin inhibits gonadotropin-releasing hormone-induced elevation of intracellular Ca^{2+} in neonatal rat pituitary cells. Endocrinology 130:701–707, 1993

Waldhauser F, Weiszenbacher G, Tatzer E, et al: Alterations in nocturnal serum melatonin levels in humans with growth and aging. J Clin Endocrinol Metab 66:648–652, 1985

Wetterberg L, Halberg F, Tarquini B, et al: Circadian variation in urinary melatonin in clinically healthy women in Japan and the United States of America. Experientia 35:416–418, 1979

Wittliff JL: Steroid receptor analyses, quality control, and clinical significance, in Cancer of the Breast. Edited by Donegan WL, Spratt JS. Philadelphia, WB Saunders, 1988, pp 303–335

Chapter 11

Meditation, Melatonin, and Cancer

Ann O. Massion, M.D., Jane Teas, Ph.D., and
James R. Hebert, Sc.D.

M editation generally can be described as the process of intentionally focusing attention on the present moment with nonjudgmental awareness (Kabat-Zinn 1982, 1990, 1994). In this chapter, we will expand on the definition of meditation, using additional details on the types of meditation used in our studies, with emphasis on mindfulness meditation.

Components of Meditation Practice

Most meditative traditions include two, not necessarily exclusive, categories or components of practice: concentration and mindfulness (Kabat-Zinn et al., in press). Concentrative practices are used to develop one-pointed attention. Mindfulness practices begin

The authors gratefully acknowledge permission to report their studies and technical assistance from Kenneth G. Walton, Ph.D., Maharishi University of Management, Department of Chemistry, Neurochemistry Laboratory, Fairfield, IA; and Gregory A. Tooley, M. Clin. Psych., Deakin University, Department of Psychology, Burwood, Australia; technical assistance from Melissa Blacker, M.A., University of Massachusetts Medical Center, Department of Medicine, Division of Preventive and Behavioral Medicine, Worcester, MA; data analytic assistance from Yunsheng Ma, M.D., M.P.H., University of Massachusetts Medical Center, Department of Medicine, Division of Preventive and Behavioral Medicine, Worcester, MA; project coordination from Susan K. Druker, M.A., project director, BRIDGES study, University of Massachusetts Medical Center, Department of Medicine, Division of Preventive and Behavioral Medicine, Worcester, MA; and expertise from Jon Kabat-Zinn, Ph.D., director, Stress Reduction Clinic, University of Massachusetts Medical Center, Department of Medicine, Division of Preventive and Behavioral Medicine and Director, Center for Mindfulness in Medicine, Health Care, and Society, Worcester, MA. The BRIDGES study was supported by the U.S. Army Medical Research and Material Command under Grants DAMD 17-94-J-4261 and DAMD 17-94-J-4475.

with one-pointedness and then expand the field of awareness to include a range of inner and outer experience of the present moment that shifts from moment to moment (Kabat-Zinn et al., in press).

Concentrative and Mindful Meditation

The following is an excerpt on the differences between concentrative and mindfulness practices from work we and other colleagues published elsewhere:

> Examples of concentrative practices include: the use of mantras (sounds or phrases used repetitively to concentrate attention); koans (phrases or questions in the Zen tradition that are aimed at cutting through discursive thinking); and the breath, when . . . [these] serve as the singular, invariant focus of attention. Concentration practices can bring about profound states of calmness, inner stillness and nonreactivity of mind.
>
> Mindfulness practices, exemplified in the vipassana (Goldstein 1976; Goldstein and Kornfield 1987; Kornfield 1993; Levine 1979; Thera 1962) and Soto Zen (C. Beck 1989, 1993; Suzuki 1970) traditions, cultivate an intentionally nonreactive, nonjudgmental moment-to-moment awareness of a changing field of objects [of attention]. Rather than becoming absorbed, as in concentrative practices which to a degree shut out the world, the practitioner attends to the full range of whatever is present in the field of his or her unfolding experience, no matter what it is. This makes mindfulness a highly practical inner orientation for people with busy, engaged lives, especially if they are faced with a life-threatening illness and all its accompanying emotional turbulence in addition to other life stressors. Mindful attention helps in facing and embracing all aspects of life, however painful or frightening, with increasing degrees of equanimity and wisdom. These qualities develop as the practitioner spends time each day in periods of silence and nondoing (formal meditation practice), with the focus on present-moment experience as it unfolds and then as the practitioner carries that moment-to-moment awareness into various aspects of daily living (informal practice). (Kabat-Zinn et al., in press, italics in original)

At some point, concentration and mindfulness may merge and become indistinguishable, as does the distinction between the meditator and the object of attention. As a result, meditation becomes a direct experience in the moment and *of* the moment, a way of being fully present, which can expand beyond the period of formal meditation to simply a way of being. In fact, one insight that can arise from the practice is the experience of connectedness, the sense of separation dissolving, whether it be between the "I" who is meditating and the object of attention (Kabat-Zinn et al., in press) or between the individual and the entire universe of beings, both animate and inanimate. Some teachers talk about reaching the space between thoughts. This dissipation of emotional reactivity, self-absorption, and self-preoccupation can give rise to profound feelings of well-being and unity (Epstein 1995; Kabat-Zinn et al., in press).

Transcendental Meditation

Although the transcendental meditation (TM) technique may or may not be the same as mindfulness, some aspects of both concentrative meditation and mindfulness appear to be present in this technique. In TM, derived by Maharishi Mahesh Yogi from the Vedic tradition (Roth 1994; Maharishi 1990), the mantra is used in a way that frees the mind from a specific focus, which Maharishi (1990) described as allowing the attention to turn "inwards towards the subtler levels of a thought until the mind transcends the experience of the thought and arrives at the source of the thought" (p. 470). He noted that his systematic technique is "neither a matter of contemplation nor of concentration," asserting that both these activities "hold the mind on the conscious thinking level, whereas Transcendental Meditation systematically takes the mind to the source of thought, the pure field of creative intelligence" (Maharishi 1990, p. 471). Another description given by an experienced teacher trained by Maharishi is that the TM technique "allows mental activity to settle down to a silent state of awareness where the mind is calm, collected, yet fully expanded, fully awake, . . . the simplest form of human awareness" (Roth 1994, p. 11).

In other schools of meditation, the practitioner may be trained first to stabilize attention through concentrative practice and then expand awareness through mindfulness practice.

Goal- and Non–Goal-Directed Meditation

Confusion often arises around the question of whether meditation has a goal, largely because the answer is a paradox. In forms of meditation such as mindfulness and Zen, there is no particular state or goal to be achieved in meditation. The overall orientation is one of nonstriving and nondoing (Kabat-Zinn 1994; Kabat-Zinn et al., in press) in the context of being fully present and nonjudgmentally aware from moment to moment. This means observing and experiencing the full range of *all* sensations, emotions, thoughts, and states as they arise. The process is one of embracing experience rather than detaching from it, creating distance by judging it, or diminishing it by harnessing the present to the goals of the future.

The paradox lies in the fact that people *do* have various goals and motivations for learning meditation and for life in general. They may want to reduce their pain or anxiety, achieve a relaxed state, or develop an improved ability to cope with stress. They may even achieve some of these goals as part of their practice. However, part of meditation practice involves the insight that goals can come and go like "thought formations, something like clouds in the sky, beyond their personal meaning and content, just like all other thoughts in the field of awareness" (Kabat-Zinn et al., in press). As described by one meditation teacher (M. Blacker, personal communication, March 1996), goals can be "lightly held," in the sense that they are held for a time and then released when their time is over, in a tapestry of permutation and change. Just noticing that one has goals and at times is attached to them can be part of the practice. A revered Thai meditation teacher, Achaan Chah, was quoted as saying "Your only job is to stay in your seat (meditation seat). You will see it all arise and pass, and out of this, wisdom and understanding will come" (Kornfield 1993, p. 31).

Certainly, there are specific meditation practices that involve embodying or developing specific states or qualities, such as loving-kindness or compassion. But none of these are presented as the overall goal of practice. The TM technique involves the experience of transcendent or higher states of consciousness, but these are said to develop spontaneously and naturally as a result of the practice, not from individual effort to bring them about (Alexander et al. 1990).

Nondoing can be best explained as intention without effort. An example is the drowning person and the rescuer. The more the drowning person flails about in the water, trying harder and harder to stay afloat, the more he or she is in danger of drowning both himself or herself and the rescuer. However, in actuality, all the person needs to do is float, which requires no rescue at all but simply the intention to float and the disbanding of effort. Some action still is required in order to float, but it is different from trying harder.

Meditation is often taught through the use of paradox embedded in stories, particularly stories that end with a riddle or seemingly impossible question. One such story comes from the Zen tradition:

> A young man went to the sensei (Zen master) at a monastery and said, "I wish to study to become like you, master. How long must I study?"
>
> "Ten years," replied the sensei.
>
> "Ten years! But what if I study twice as hard as the other students, master?"
>
> "Well, then it will take you 20 years," replied the master.
>
> "Twenty years! But what if I study night and day, master?"
>
> "Then it will take you 30 years," replied the master.
>
> "I don't understand," said the young man. "Why does it take longer if I work harder?"
>
> "Because the task is not to work harder but to work *softer*. If you keep one eye fixed on your destination, it will take you twice as long, because then you will have only one eye left with which to find your way."

Orientations of Meditation Practice

Along with the two components of practice, most meditative traditions have two possible orientations: meditation for the benefit, awakening, or enlightenment of oneself and meditation with the intention to transmit the benefit from oneself to all beings. There may be an emphasis of one over the other or a progression from one *to* the other. These two orientations, relationship to oneself and to others, are linked through the practice itself or the teaching. They are closely related to the "three jewels" of the Buddhist tradition (Gyatso 1985, p. 56): 1) the sense of being fully awakened (*buddha*), 2) the teaching (*dharma*), and 3) the community of beings (*sangha*) (Yeshe 1979). These three jewels can be seen as woven into the universal aspects of all human experience.

First is the direct experience of one's inherent wisdom and through that the realization of the vast potential inherent in all human beings. The word *buddha* actually refers to a "totally opened mind" (Yeshe 1979, p. 11), with the understanding that that capacity already exists in everyone and simply needs to be realized or revealed.

Second are the teachings that underlie the practice. The word *dharma* refers simply to understanding reality (Yeshe 1979), including understanding the nature of impermanence, of suffering, and of the ways to stop suffering. The literal meaning of dharma, a Sanskrit term, is "that which holds" (Gyatso 1984, p. 1). In this sense, dharma can be viewed as outer teachings that become inner realizations that hold, protect, and sustain the individual in daily life. For a person with cancer, it might mean the realization that he or she is more than someone with a disease, that the illness really is more background than foreground. Or it might mean the understanding that pain is not the same as suffering (i.e., that pain is the physical sensation and suffering is the perception of it), that the pain may be chronic but not necessarily the suffering. In understanding the nature of change and impermanence, a person with panic attacks may be able to let go of the need for controlling the attacks and instead learn to cope by "floating" through them (Weekes 1969, p. 35).

Third is a sense of connection with a larger community beyond oneself and of being supported by this community. "Sangha consists of those who are endowed with wisdom and can help us along the way" (Yeshe 1979, p. 11). This term might mean people who support one another in their practice and are committed to fostering each other's personal growth, or it might mean a group of friends, doctors, nurses, or other health care professionals who help an individual cope with or recover from his or her illness (Yeshe 1979).

Meditation is sometimes mistaken for a solitary experience, as in the ascetic hermit meditating for years in a cave to the point of being unaware that bugs are eating his skin. Solitary experiences can be true in some cases or some traditions, but most traditions contain various aspects of the three elements described above. In this context, meditation is very much a practice done *in* the world, and the experience of practice can have therapeutic benefits similar to psychotherapy. In the following discussion, meditation is compared with relaxation strategies, such as biofeedback, progressive muscle relaxation, and visual imagery, and to two specific psychotherapies, cognitive-behavior and supportive-expressive therapy.

The major differences between schools of meditation practice often are more stylistic differences in the *emphasis* placed on one of the two components or orientations, or differences in the *order* of their presentation during meditation training. Other differences often can be explained by cultural and historical factors.

Finally, most meditative traditions have some schema or description of different stages or levels of consciousness that may be experienced at various stages of practice. These include the more commonly known levels of consciousness, such as waking, sleeping, and half-awake or hypnagogic states, but with additional levels beyond these, which are seen as evolving states according to the length or depth of practice.

In terms of meditation research, different effects may be seen depending on the particular stage of training of the subjects, the particular orientation at the time the measurements are taken, and the particular level or state of consciousness.

Meditation Compared With Self-Regulatory/Relaxation Strategies and With Other Psychotherapies

Meditation, as used in clinical settings, can be distinguished from self-regulatory or relaxation strategies, such as biofeedback, progressive muscle relaxation, or visual imagery, primarily by the fact that in meditation there is no explicit goal, for relaxation or anything else. The actual practice may look similar; the focus on the breath, for example, might be done both as part of a meditation practice and as part of relaxation training.

Breathing retraining also is taught as part of cognitive-behavior therapy used to treat anxiety disorders (Moras et al. 1990). The difference is that, as with relaxation training, there is an explicit goal, namely to reduce anxiety or bring about a change in avoidance or phobic behavior. Also, breathing retraining, as taught in either relaxation strategies or cognitive-behavior therapy, usually is not presented as a way of being or general lifestyle, nor is it presented in the larger context of meditative practice as described previously.

Supportive-expressive group therapy (Classen et al. 1994; Spiegel and Spira 1991) originally was developed as a way to cope with recurrent cancer, again an explicit goal. However, part of the approach is to encourage patients to live as fully as possible, which has some similarity to the approach taught in mindfulness meditation. In addition, a breathing technique based on self-hypnosis is taught. This technique shares some features with meditation practice in the focus on the breath, but in supportive-expressive group therapy it is taught mostly for pain control. There is a large component of group support in supportive-expressive therapy, although in this case the community is defined by the illness. In meditation practice, group support is inherent in the concept of community but with a different focus than that of coping with cancer. In mindfulness-based stress reduction programs, often taught in clinical settings in a group format, group support may occur but is not the predominant focus or stated goal.

Other differences between meditation and self-regulatory/relaxation strategies are presented in Table 11–1. Differences among meditation, cognitive-behavior therapy, and supportive-expressive group therapy are presented in Table 11–2. Both tables were adapted from work published by us and other colleagues (Kabat-Zinn et al., in press).

Meditation, Melatonin, and Cancer

Because the many functions of melatonin have been well covered in the other chapters of this book, we will confine this discussion to our proposed relationship between melatonin and meditation, with the exception of a brief section on melatonin and cancer. Previously, we published our hypothesis and preliminary data suggesting that the pineal gland not only is photosensitive but also psychosensitive (Massion et al. 1995). The correlate would be that a psychosocial intervention such as meditation could influence melatonin levels. It should be noted that increased melatonin production might not necessarily reflect pineal activity alone, as there is some indication in the literature that some melatonin may be produced in extrapineal sites such as the gastrointestinal tract (Huether 1993, 1994).

Melatonin and Meditation Studies

Various studies from the literature on either meditation or melatonin indicate that the two share several physiological effects, which are summarized in Table 11–3. For at least three of these effects, pain reduction, insomnia reduction, and anxiety reduction, a common underlying mechanism is suggested by the literature. Some of melatonin's effects have been shown to be mediated through the opioid system (Guerrero and Reiter 1992; Maestroni and Conti 1993). The mindfulness-based Stress Reduction and Relaxation Program (SR and RP) (Kabat-Zinn 1990, 1994; Kabat-

Table 11–1.   Meditation versus self-regulatory/relaxation strategies: major differences

Meditation	Other self-regulatory/relaxation strategies
Orientation of nondoing, nonstriving, nonattachment to specific goals	Relaxation or coping with some specific condition is targeted as the goal (e.g., reducing anxiety, coping with cancer, visualizing overcoming cancer cells)
Experiencing whatever is present in the moment, allowing present sensations, thoughts, and feelings to be as they are, without having to hold on to them or push them away	Attempting to create a change in the present and future (e.g., by creating relaxation or reducing anxiety or pain)
Practiced as a way of being rather than a technique; a way to live fully and include all experience, pleasant or unpleasant	Usually presented as a technique for solving or coping with a condition
Practiced daily, for its own sake, as part of learning to be awake and nonjudgmentally aware; not based on an attempt to induce a change in state	Often practiced as needed, to relieve or cope with a particular condition or mood state (e.g., tension, anxiety, or pain)

Zinn et al., in press), first developed by Jon Kabat-Zinn, Ph.D., at the Stress Reduction Clinic of the University of Massachusetts Medical Center (UMMC), has been shown to be effective for chronic pain (Kabat-Zinn 1982; Kabat-Zinn et al. 1985, 1986). Amelioration of pain is known to involve the opioid system. Therefore, the opioid system may be the common mechanism for both meditation and melatonin.

The SR and RP also was found to be effective for patients with panic disorder and generalized anxiety disorder (Kabat-Zinn et al. 1992; Miller et al. 1995). The etiology of generalized anxiety disorder has been shown to be related to the γ-aminobutyric acid (GABA) receptor (Dubovsky 1990). One of the main pharmacological treatments for both generalized anxiety disorder and insomnia

Table 11–2. Comparison of meditation with other psychosocial interventions[a]

Meditation	Cognitive-behavior therapy[b]	Supportive-expressive therapy[c]
Goal		
Presented as a way of being or general lifestyle approach. Group support is present but is not a stated goal or predominant focus. Emphasis is on living life fully and being in touch with the full range of emotions. Nonattachment to goals is taught (e.g., lightly held goals).	Generally presented as a way to cope with a particular mood, feeling state, or illness (e.g., depression, anxiety, or cancer). Group support usually occurs spontaneously and may or may not be a stated goal.	Goals are to 1) facilitate full expression of emotions and thoughts about the illness, based on the assumption that this will be therapeutic; 2) provide a support system to alleviate social isolation; and 3) live life as fully as possible.
Individual/group format		
Can be taught in large or small groups of people with either homogeneous or diverse problems and concerns.	Usually presented to individuals or groups with one overall concern (e.g., depression or anxiety).	Usually provided in small intimate groups that are homogeneous for a particular illness or common concern.
Taught as a class to large or small groups (up to 40 people).	Provided as individual or small-group therapy (6–10 people).	Provided as group therapy, usually with smaller groups (8–10 people).

(continued)

Table 11–2.   Comparison of meditation with other psychosocial interventions (*continued*)

Meditation	Cognitive-behavior therapy	Supportive-expressive therapy
Skills/practices presented		
Coping skills are presented in the larger framework of everyday life, as a practice for living, using formal and informal practices and demonstrating how these are mirrored in everyday life. The practices are used for the purpose of cultivating greater present-moment awareness and self-acceptance rather than as technique-based coping strategies.	Coping skills are presented largely in relation to the mood or feeling state to be dealt with and may be secondarily related to a more general lifestyle change.	Coping strategies specific to the common illness or concern are learned by hearing what other group members have found helpful, by suggestions from the group leaders, or both. Uses a breathing technique based on self-hypnosis that shares some features with sitting meditation practice, including a primary focus on the breath.
No attempt is made either to monitor or reframe particular thoughts or feeling states. Whatever appears in awareness is simply held as the salient aspect of the present-moment experience. If there is a change in perception, it emerges spontaneously.	Thoughts and reactions to physical sensations are monitored, reframed, and sometimes induced (e.g., symptoms of panic attacks). Through systematically looking at thought patterns or attributions to sensations, a change in perception is facilitated that may be associated with improvement (e.g., less anxiety or depression,	A forum for expressing feelings and concerns is presented, usually oriented around a specific illness; thoughts and feelings are not specifically induced or systematically monitored and reframed. Changes in lifestyle or perception usually are related to coping with the illness.

greater ability to cope with the illness) and may secondarily include greater self-acceptance.

[a] Adapted from Kabal-Zinn et al., in press.
[b] A. Beck et al. 1979; Greer et al. 1992; Moorey and Greer 1989; Moorey et al. 1994; Moras et al. 1990.
[c] Classen et al. 1994; Spiegel and Spira 1991.

is the benzodiazepines, which interact at this receptor (Dubovsky 1990). The pineal gland has $GABA_A$ receptors and actively synthesizes and metabolizes GABA (Demisch 1993). Also, melatonin has been shown to significantly increase the inhibitory effect of GABA and to have a benzodiazepine-like activity (Stankov et al. 1993). This finding suggests that the GABA system might be one common mechanism by which meditation and melatonin exert their anti-anxiety and anti-insomnia effects.

To the best of our knowledge, melatonin has not been used as an outcome measure for any psychosocial intervention in a published peer-reviewed study before the 1995 preliminary study described in the discussion in the following section "Research on Meditation, Melatonin, and Cancer." The most closely related study was one using regular practitioners of the TM technique, showing higher daytime levels of the serotonin metabolite 5-hydroxyindoleacetic acid (5-HIAA) compared with that in control subjects and showing that the levels increased following meditation (Bujatti and Riederer 1976). However, the report was based on 5-HIAA urine concentration for a 2-hour period rather than total excretion. In a separate review that commented on this study, the author hypothesized that the reported rise in serotonin was due to enhanced pineal activity (Romijn 1978).

Melatonin and Cancer

Melatonin has been shown to have oncostatic properties and to inhibit the growth of a wide range of neoplasms in animal and human in vivo and in vitro models, with the most compelling evidence being in the area of breast cancer (see Hill et al., Chapter 9, and Blask, Chapter 10, in this volume).

Based on the theory of pineal/melatonin involvement in the etiology of certain cancers, a group of Italian investigators has conducted several preliminary and two randomized trials of groups of patients with a variety of cancers, administering either oral melatonin alone or melatonin with a series of interleukin-2 (IL-2) injections (Lissoni et al. 1989, 1991, 1992a, 1992b, 1992c, 1993, 1994a, 1994b). Most of the patients were unresponsive to standard

Table 11–3. Similarities in effects of meditation and melatonin based on literature review

Effect	Meditation	Melatonin
Analgesia	Kabat-Zinn et al. 1985, 1986	Maestroni and Conti 1993
Antistress	*Pain:* Kabat-Zinn et al. 1985, 1986	*Psychological:* Katz et al. 1995
	General: Kabat-Zinn et al. 1989	*Physical:* Khan et al. 1990, Maestroni and Conti 1993, Monteleone et al. 1992, 1993
Anti-insomnia/ hypnotic	Woolfolk et al. 1976	Dollins et al. 1994
Decreased anxiety	Kabat-Zinn et al. 1992	*Based on GABA receptor:* Stankov et al.
Decreased heart rate	Delmonte 1984	Chuang et al. 1993
Decreased blood pressure	Alexander et al. 1996, Delmonte 1984, Schneider et al. 1995	Chuang et al. (1993)

Note. GABA = γ-aminobutyric acid.

chemotherapy or other anticancer therapies. In one of the randomized studies on patients with brain metastases due to solid neoplasms, those treated with melatonin, compared with supportive care alone, had a significantly greater survival at 1 year, longer free-from-brain-progression period, and longer mean survival time, along with significant improvement in their Karnofsky Performance Status Score (Lissoni et al. 1994b). In the second randomized study, melatonin combined with IL-2 was associated with a significant improvement in immune parameters and a higher rate of survival at 1 year, compared with IL-2 given alone (Lissoni et al. 1994a). In a separate study, increasing melatonin levels were predictive of a favorable response to chemotherapy in a group of cancer patients, some of whom had breast cancer (Lissoni et al. 1988).

Psychosocial Interventions and Cancer

We were unable to find a published study using meditation as the primary component in a psychosocial intervention for cancer patients. However, at least two randomized studies have used psychosocial interventions in which relaxation/self-regulatory strategies were one component: one study in women with metastatic breast cancer followed for 10 years (Spiegel et al. 1989) and the other study in postsurgical patients with malignant melanoma followed for 6 years (Fawzy et al. 1990a, 1990b, 1993). Both showed improved survival associated with the psychosocial interventions.

In the following discussion, we present preliminary data from an ongoing randomized study of women with stages I and II breast cancer, using a modified form of the SR and RP as one of two interventions and melatonin as one of the biological outcome parameters.

Research on Meditation, Melatonin, and Cancer

In 1995, we published preliminary studies showing that regular practice of meditation may be associated with increased levels of melatonin as measured in the urine. In this preliminary cross-sectional study we compared 12-hour overnight (8 P.M.–8 A.M.) levels of the urinary metabolite of melatonin, 6-sulfatoxymelatonin (αMT6s), in healthy women, eight of whom regularly meditated and eight who did not (Massion et al. 1995). After controlling for age and the nonsignificant effect of menstrual period interval, the meditators were found to have significantly higher αMT6s levels ($t = 2.60$, $P = .02$). We suggested that melatonin would be a relevant outcome variable in assessing psychosocial interventions, particularly for subjects with breast or prostate cancer.

Since that time, we conducted another preliminary study of healthy men and women before and after an intensive meditation retreat (A. O. Massion et al., unpublished observations, 1995). We also began a larger randomized study of women with stage I or II breast cancer, using a modified form of the SR and RP as one of the intervention arms and melatonin as one of the biological outcome variables.

In the meditation retreat study, 12-hour overnight (8 P.M.–8 A.M.) urinary αMT6s levels were measured on the first and last days of either an 11-day or 21-day mindfulness meditation retreat in late May to June 1994, in Barre, Massachusetts. Samples were collected from 11 retreat participants (six from the 11-day retreat and five from the 21-day retreat) and from 9 staff members. The staff were practicing the same form of meditation on a less intensive schedule and living at the same location, with a similar lifestyle and food intake (mainly vegetarian), but were not participating in the retreat schedule. Subjects were healthy men and women, all of whom agreed to go to bed by midnight.

The retreats were overlapping so that the two retreat groups were together for the last 11 days. The majority of the retreat was conducted in silence, with walking and sitting meditations beginning at approximately 5:45 A.M. and ending at approximately 9 P.M. In contrast, the staff were meditating on their own for an average of 50 minutes per day.

A general linear model (linear regression), with the general linear models procedure (PROC GLM) in the *Statistical Analysis System (SAS) Users Guide* (1993), was used for this study. The change in αMT6s total excretion amount was the dependent variable (the change score was calculated by subtracting the baseline value from the value on the last day of the retreat). The covariates or independent variables were groups (fitting indicator variables for retreat groups together and separately in two separate models), sex, age, daily rate (in minutes per day) of average meditation practice prior to the retreat, and baseline level of αMT6s excretion. Also modeled as independent variables were the interactions between retreat group and both gender and rate of meditation practice prior to the retreat.

Exploratory analyses showed that there were no significant differences between αMT6s levels or other differences between the two retreat groups, so they were combined in subsequent analyses. After we controlled for covariates, the results showed a significant increase in αMT6s excretion between pre- and post-measurements for the retreat group but not the staff. However, the difference between the retreat group and the staff group was not significant. The results are summarized in Table 11–4.

Of the covariates fitted, only the daily rate of average meditation practice before the retreat was predictive of the change in αMT6s excretion. The association was inverse, with greater practice before the retreat being predictive of a smaller change during the retreat (i.e., −0.015 μg of αMT6s/minute of meditation/week, $t = 2.15, P = .05$).

The significant difference between pre- and post-αMT6s levels in the retreat group seems especially notable given the small sample size. For the staff group, there was a suggestion but no significant difference between pre- and postrates of excretion. Because both groups were eating essentially the same food and going to bed by midnight, the differences between groups are unlikely to be explained by sleep or dietary factors. The results are consistent with a dose-dependent effect of meditation because 1) the staff were involved in some aspects of the retreat and doing some meditating on their own for much shorter periods than the retreat participants, and 2) the difference in αMT6s levels was approximately twofold higher for the retreat participants, although this difference was not significant. The lack of statistical significance between the retreat group and staff group appears to be a consequence of the small sample size in relation to the magnitude of the difference in αMT6s, which may in turn reflect the difference in meditation time.

The fact that the maximal change apparently was reached by the end of the 11-day retreat suggests a plateau effect for at least the period of meditation represented in the study. Regular meditation over a period of years also may show such an effect.

Increase of Serum Melatonin After Meditation

A study in Australia by G. A. Tooley et al. (unpublished observations) measured serum melatonin levels taken serially at six time points before and after a period of meditation beginning at midnight and lasting up to 60 minutes. They hypothesized that medi-

Table 11–4. Differences in pre- and postretreat total 12-hour (8 P.M.–8 A.M.) 6-sulfatoxymelatonin (αMT6s) excretion in retreat group versus staff in the Meditation Retreat Study, Barre-Worcester, Massachusetts, 1994

	Retreat group ($n = 11$)			Staff ($n = 9$)			Intergroup comparison
	Mean	(SE)	P^a	Mean	(SE)	P^a	P^b
Baseline αMT6s (μg/12 hours)	9.96	(5.03)		10.36	(6.79)		.88
Follow-up αMT6s (μg/12 hours)	15.49	(8.45)		12.86	(10.65)		.57
Crude difference[c] (μg/12 hours)	5.73	(1.67)	.008	2.70	(1.76)	.17	.22
Adjusted difference[d] (μg/12 hours)	5.78	(1.56)	.004	2.90	(1.73)	.12	.24

[a]P value for the test of the hypothesis that the difference between baseline and follow-up = 0.
[b]P value for the test of the hypothesis that the group mean values are the same, based on two-sample t test for continuous variables.
[c]Based on the simple intergroup difference (i.e., subtracting the baseline from the value obtained at the end of the intervention). This value represents all those subjects for whom we had complete data to compute an adjusted score.
[d]The adjusted difference is obtained as the least means square (LSMEANS) using the general linear model in the *Statistical Analysis System* (PROC GLM). This difference is based on the same simple intergroup difference as above in c. The value is adjusted for previous rate of meditation (minutes/week), gender, baseline production of melatonin (to control for regression to the mean), and interactions between retreat group and both sex and previous rate of meditation. None of these covariates was independently predictive of changes in melatonin amount.

tation would be associated with an acute rise in serum melatonin. There were three groups of healthy subjects: 1) 11 long-term TM practitioners, 2) 7 practitioners of an internationally well-known form of meditative-based yoga who participated on the condition that their organization was not identified, and 3) 10 volunteers with no prior meditation or yoga experience (nonmeditator group). Both the TM and yoga groups were long-term practitioners (mean of 12.3 ± 6.43 years for the TM group; 5.77 ± 4.45 years for the yoga group). During the study, the TM group meditated for an hour and the yoga group for approximately 45 minutes. A repeated-measures crossover design was used, with random allocation to control or intervention conditions on two separate nights 2 weeks apart. The TM and yoga groups were randomly assigned to meditate beginning at midnight on one night and to the control condition (no meditation) on the alternate night. Instead of meditating, the nonmeditator group was instructed to sit with their eyes closed for 1 hour beginning at midnight on the intervention night. On the control night, all groups were asked to sit quietly but otherwise could engage in any activities they chose, such as talking or watching television.

Lighting levels were monitored throughout the experiment and did not exceed 15 lux, which was below the level known to influence melatonin secretion (Lewy et al. 1980; McIntyre et al. 1988). Blood was sampled via a butterfly needle inserted in a vein in the cubital fossa region of the forearm at the following times: 1) four samples before meditation at 10 P.M., 11 P.M., 11:30 P.M., and midnight and 2) six samples taken 20 minutes apart postmeditation (10 samples total).

The mean paired differences between meditation and control night melatonin levels were significant for both the TM and yoga groups for both major outcome measures, the maximum melatonin peak after baseline ($P < .05$) and total cumulative melatonin production ($P < .05$). The results indicated that the average postbaseline melatonin levels peaked higher on the meditation compared with the control night and that more melatonin was secreted overall during the postbaseline sampling period on the meditation night. For the nonmeditator group, no differences were noted between intervention and control nights. Although both the TM and yoga groups appeared to show a decline from the peak after approximately 1 A.M., in the nonmeditator group the peak appeared to be higher than the TM and yoga groups and not completely defined in that it occurred toward the end of the interval. Of note, the nonmeditator group was, on average, more than 12 years younger than the other two groups, which may account for the apparent higher average peak production in the nonmeditator group. Also, the last sample was taken at 2:40 A.M., which is earlier than the end of the normal range for the circadian melatonin peak, namely, between midnight and 3 A.M., with considerable interindividual variability (McIntyre et al. 1987; Reiter 1991). Taking the last sample before 3 A.M. may explain why the peak was not completely captured. Finally, midnight is an unusual time for people to meditate and was chosen mainly to maximize the influence on peak melatonin production. However, the main finding was that both the TM and yoga groups had a significant acute increase in melatonin levels on the meditation nights compared with the control nights and the nonmeditator group did not, which would seem to rule out an effect due to simple rest or relaxation.

Acute and Chronic Stress and Melatonin

A second study, by K. G. Walton et al. (1990; unpublished observations) compared long-term TM-practicing college students (mean years of practice 8.5 ± 5.1 years) from Maharishi University of Management with a group of nonmeditating college students from a different university, both universities being in Iowa. Apparently unlike the previous studies, K. G. Walton et al. (1990; unpublished observations) assessed the students during a relatively stressful time, approximately 2 weeks before final examinations. The investigators proposed that because meditation has been reported to reduce psychological and biochemical indicators of acute and chronic stress and because it has been postulated that melatonin increases with acute stress, that the long-term TM group would have lower indicators of chronic stress and correspondingly reduced indicators of melatonin level or turnover. Melatonin levels were measured using 24-hour urinary αMT6s excretion. Indicators of chronic stress were excretion rates of cortisol, vanillylmandelic acid, and sodium, along with scores on the Profile of Mood States (POMS; McNair et al. 1971) and State-Trait Anxiety Inventory (STAI; Spielberger and Sydeman 1994). On the basis of these indicators, the 22 college students in the TM group were found to have lower stress (designated as the LS group) than the 31 nonmeditating college students who were felt to have average stress levels (designated as the AS group). Ages were similar in both groups. αMT6s excretion rates were significantly higher for the AS group (nonmeditators) compared with the LS group (TM practitioners), as reflected by the 24-hour urine samples (AS = 508 ± 49 ng/h and LS = 318 ± 58 ng/h; $F = 6.11$, $P = .017$). These results were independent of the use of alcohol, nicotine, and caffeine. Higher αMT6s excretion correlated directly with higher stress indicators, both within each group and across all subjects.

The results of this latter study appear to be inconsistent with the first three studies in that the meditating groups had higher rather than lower melatonin levels in the two studies by Massion et al. (1995, in submission) and the study by G. A. Tooley et al. (unpublished observations). The difference in types of meditation (TM and mindfulness) does not account for the results because G. A. Tooley et al. and K. G. Walton et al. (1990; unpublished observations) both used subjects practicing the TM technique, as well as the more advanced TM-Sidhi program. Because the study by Walton et al. was cross-sectional, it is possible that variables other than TM practice, such as lifestyle or dietary factors, were responsible for the difference in melatonin levels. Also, Walton et al. used college students in a situation that would be experienced as stressful by most people, a condition apparently absent from the other studies. Furthermore, the college students may have been experiencing both acute and chronic stress simultaneously, which makes the issue more complicated, especially considering the reported variability of the effects of stress on human melatonin levels according to the nature and timing of the stress. As a case in point, a study of 23 pregnant women showed higher αMT6s levels on work versus nonwork days based on within-subjects comparisons (Katz et al. 1995), which would seem to be an indicator of acute psychological stress.

Other reports have suggested that the human pineal is unresponsive to acute physical stress induced either during the day or 3 hours after the beginning of darkness but does respond to acute physical stress induced in the second half of the dark phase (Monteleone et al. 1992, 1993). Reports on circulating melatonin levels in various groups of cancer patients, presumably under chronic stress levels ranging from mild to severe, have shown both increased and decreased levels (Blask 1993).

Obviously, all of the previously mentioned meditation studies need to be replicated, preferably with larger samples. The only conclusion that can be made at this point is that meditation does seem to influence melatonin levels; the majority of the studies suggest enhanced or increased melatonin levels, but certainly the direction of the effect is not well established at this point.

None of these were randomized studies. Although randomized studies are testing hypotheses and estimating effects, this approach seems unusually difficult for examining the relationship between melatonin and meditation because self-selection factors play such an important role in the motivation to practice intensive meditation, particularly of the kind used in these studies. The disadvantages of a randomized clinical trial are that subjects are asked to sustain effort, attention, and practice for concentrated or prolonged periods and that they are likely to have strong treatment preferences (Brewin and Bradley 1989). Motivation plays a crucial role in compliance with the intervention.

Breast Cancer, Meditation, and Melatonin

Despite this difficulty with randomized studies, we and other colleagues in a multidisciplinary research group at the University of Massachusetts Medical Center (UMMC) did design and initiate a larger multisite study—the BRIDGES (*B*reast *R*esearch *I*nitiative for *D*evelopin*G* *E*ffective *S*kills) study—of women, ages 20–65 years, with stages I or II breast cancer and within 2 years of diagnosis. The aims of the study are to identify effective skills for coping with breast cancer and measure psychosocial and biological outcome parameters over 2 years of follow-up. Outcome measures include psychosocial variables (quality of life, coping methods, anxiety, depression), immunological parameters (interferon-γ [IFN-γ], soluble IL-2 receptor, and interleukin-4 [IL-4]), and melatonin.

Study participants are randomized to one of three arms: 1) a modified form of the SR and RP, expanded to address issues specific to breast cancer; 2) a nutrition education intervention originally intended to act as an attention control but also with the hypothesis that it might have therapeutic effects; and 3) a usual-treatment control group. Subjects have had no prior experience in either intervention. They are randomized according to strata of age (< 55 years or $\geq$ 55 years), disease status (stage I or II), and institution. Each subject is followed for 2 years. A description of the SR and RP has been provided elsewhere (Kabat-Zinn 1990, 1994; Kabat-Zinn et al., in press), but briefly, this is a well-developed psychosocial intervention that has been in operation for the past 17 years as an outpatient service of the UMMC Stress Reduction Clinic in the Department of Medicine, Division of Preventive and Behavioral Medicine. More than 8,000 patients with a wide range of chronic medical conditions, many life threatening, have been physician-referred to the program. Research on the SR and RP has shown clinically significant short- and long-term improvement in physical and psychological symptoms, as well as enhanced psychological well-being, in patients with chronic conditions, including chronic pain (Kabat-Zinn 1982; Kabat-Zinn et al. 1985, 1986), anxiety disorders (Kabat-Zinn et al. 1992; Miller et al. 1995), and psoriasis (Bernhard et al. 1988).

The program is structured as an 8-week course given to heterogeneous groups of 25–40 people referred for problems, including cancer, hypertension, gastrointestinal problems, chronic pain, and anxiety. Classes meet for 2 ½ hours once a week and one intensive daylong silent meditation retreat on the weekend during the sixth week. The core curriculum is intensive training in mindfulness meditation (formal practice) and its applications to daily living (informal practice). Classes include training in sitting and walking meditation, hatha-yoga, experiential exercises, and discussion.

The SR and RP was modified for use in the BRIDGES study by adding six sessions, one before and five after the standard 8-week SR and RP. Only women with breast cancer who are in the study attend these six sessions. The sessions are used to reinforce the meditation training and practice, and to address issues specific to breast cancer.

The nutrition education program (NEP) was designed to reduce dietary fat to 20% or less. The NEP is presented as 14 weekly class sessions and one all-day session in order to be attentionally equivalent to the SR and RP. The NEP is used to introduce participants to nutritional concepts, techniques, and group cooking/eating experiences that broaden rather than restrict dietary options. Although the NEP is equivalent in time commitment to the SR and RP and includes an important aspect of group support, it includes no element of mindfulness meditation. The usual care group may include attendance in community support groups but otherwise has none of the elements of either the SR and RP or the NEP.

Currently, we have 160 women enrolled in the study. Preliminary data on 24-hour αMT6s levels have been collected on 84 subjects for the baseline and 4-month (2–3 weeks postintervention) assessment points. These data do not include the immunological parameters because those assays will not be done until the final year of the study for quality control reasons.

A total of 84 women had complete data at both the baseline and 4-month assessment points. Of these, two had taken melatonin supplementation at some time during this study interval. Although we chose to analyze the data according to the intention-to-treat paradigm of randomized clinical trials, we decided to exclude the two users of melatonin from these analyses because of the direct relationship between the intake of melatonin supplements and increased excretion of αMT6s. Because of the stratified method of randomization by age and severity of disease, these factors were controlled by design. Of the 82 subjects on whom we had complete data for this analysis, 23 had completed the NEP, 30 were in the SR and RP arm, and 29 were assigned to usual care.

We found that there was a suggestion that both the NEP and SR and RP were associated with increases in αMT6s excretion in the study period. In the usual-care group, we observed a mean *decrease* of 1.06 μg/24 hours, whereas in the SR and RP and the NEP groups, we observed mean *increases* of 1.58 μg/24 hours and 3.26 μg/24 hours, respectively. Mean baseline and 4-month values are shown in Table 11–5.

Because of the relatively large variability in the data, the overall effect was not statistically significant ($P = .33$), nor was the effect due to either of the interventions relative to usual care (NEP [$P = .15$] and SR and RP [$P = .34$]). We believe these results warrant as much attention as the statistically significant results of the previous studies because they were obtained in a randomized trial in which background factors are controlled by design and in which we would expect less of an effect than in a highly self-motivated group of experienced meditators; hence, there is more relevance to the experience of average people. In addition, an effect of this magnitude would be statistically significant in even a slightly larger sample and probably is of clinical significance. Finally, these results cover only the first 4 months of follow-up and may reflect more immediate postintervention changes. These results may

Table 11–5.   BRIDGES study: baseline and 4-month (postintervention) 24-hour 6-sulfatoxymelatonin (αMT6s) values (μg/24 hours)

Group	N	Mean baseline (SD)	Mean 4-month (SD)	Mean difference (SD)[a]	Effect relative to usual care (P value)
SR and RP	30	9.83 (9.23)	11.41 (10.99)	+ 1.58 (11.87)	.34
NEP	23	9.63 (6.08)	12.89 (12.50)	+ 3.26 (9.03)	.15
Usual care	29	11.20 (10.15)	10.16 (5.68)	− 1.06 (10.30)	

Note.   SR and RP = Stress Reduction and Relaxation Program; NEP = Nutrition Education Program.
[a]Crude mean difference for each group with the standard deviation of the difference (not the overall standard deviation) shown in parentheses.

change over the course of the 2-year follow-up period.

Table 11–6 summarizes the results of the meditation/melatonin studies discussed in this chapter. All but one study showed increased melatonin levels associated with meditation practice. In terms of pineal function, an elevation in endogenous melatonin could reflect a change in circadian amplitude, circadian phase, or liver metabolism. However, all the studies had healthy subjects without liver disease; the only exception was the BRIDGES study in which the subjects had early stage breast cancer. Therefore, an effect on liver metabolism seems unlikely. All but one of the studies used total excretion of urinary αMT6s and therefore were not able to address directly the question of amplitude versus phase. G. A. Tooley et al. (unpublished observations) did use serum melatonin levels and characterized the circadian phase, but not definitively because the sample collection ended shortly before 3 A.M. Overall, the results appear to favor a change in circadian amplitude as the most likely explanation.

Conclusions

In general, the results of the preliminary studies reported in this chapter suggest that meditation practice is associated with enhanced endogenous melatonin levels. The results need to be replicated with larger samples and/or a randomized trial. A number of related questions are still to be answered, such as whether this effect 1) holds true for both long-term and short-term meditation practitioners, 2) persists over long-term follow-up, and 3) can be explained by a change in circadian amplitude or phase. If meditation can influence pineal activity, this in turn could influence the course of certain diseases for which melatonin plays a role, such as breast or prostate cancer. The potential value of meditation for people with such conditions remains to be investigated.

Recently, there has been a great deal of interest in the use of oral melatonin supplements for disorders such as insomnia and jet lag (see Lewy et al., Chapter 4, in this volume). Often, these supplements are taken in doses resulting in blood levels that are higher

Table 11–6. Summary of preliminary meditation/melatonin studies

Author/study	Type of meditation	Short- or long-term practice	Population	Melatonin measurement	N	Melatonin levels[a]
Massion et al. (1995), cross-sectional, nonrandomized	Mindfulness	Long-term	Healthy women	12-hour[b] αMT6s, urine	16	Increased
Massion et al. (in submission), retreat study, nonrandomized	Mindfulness	Variable	Healthy men/women	12-hour[b] αMT6s, urine	20	Increased
Tooley et al. (in submission), pre-post on two nights, nonrandomized	Transcendental meditation	Long-term	Healthy men/women	Serum	25	Increased
K. G. Walton et al. (1990; unplublished observations) cross-sectional, nonrandomized, college students	Transcendental meditation	Long-term	Healthy men/women	24-hour αMT6s, urine	53	Decreased
Preliminary analysis 1996, BRIDGES study, pre-post over 4 months, randomized	Mindfulness	Short-term	Women with breast cancer	24-hour αMT6s, urine	82	Increased

Note. αMT6s = 6-sulfatoxymelatonin; BRIDGES = Breast Research Initiative for Developing Effective Skills.
[a]Melatonin levels in meditators relative to comparison or control groups; all results were statistically significant except for BRIDGES study.
[b]Overnight collection from 8 P.M. to 8 A.M.

than the physiological range. Our hope is that this chapter has at least raised the thought-provoking possibility of influencing melatonin production by using capacities that are inherent in all people and that act within our own physiological and psychological homeostatic resources for being in the world. Certainly, melatonin is not the only biological outcome measure that could be used in meditation research, but it is one porthole into the fascinating interface between psyche and soma.

References

Alexander CN, Davies JL, Dixon CA, et al: Growth of higher states of consciousness: the Vedic psychology of human development, in Higher States of Human Development: Perspectives on Adult Growth. Edited by Alexander C, Langer E. New York, Oxford University Press, 1990, pp 286–340

Alexander CN, Schneider RH, Staggers F, et al: Trial of stress reduction for hypertension in older African Americans. Hypertension 28:228–237, 1996

Beck A, Rush A, Shaw B, et al: Cognitive Therapy of Depression. New York, Guilford, 1979

Beck C: Everyday Zen. San Francisco, CA, HarperCollins, 1989

Beck C: Nothing Special. San Francisco, CA, HarperCollins, 1993

Bernhard JD, Kristeller J, Kabat-Zinn J: Effectiveness of relaxation and visualization techniques as an adjunct to phototherapy and photochemotherapy of psoriasis. J Am Acad Dermatol 19:572–573, 1988

Blask DE: Melatonin in oncology, in Melatonin: Biosynthesis, Physiological Effects, and Clinical Applications. Edited by Yu H-S, Reiter R. Boca Raton, FL, CRC Press, 1993, pp 447–475

Brewin CR, Bradley C: Patient preferences and randomised trials. BMJ 299:313–315, 1989

Bujatti M, Riederer P: Serotonin, noradrenaline, dopamine metabolites in transcendental meditation-technique. J Neural Transm 39:257–267, 1976

Chuang JI, Chen SS, Lin MT: Melatonin decreases brain serotonin release, arterial pressure and heart rate in rats. Pharmacology 47:91–97, 1993

Classen C, Hermanson KS, Spiegel D: Psychotherapy, stress, and survival in breast cancer, in The Psychoimmunology of Cancer. Edited by Lewis C, O'Sullivan C, Barraclough J. Oxford, England, Oxford University Press, 1994, pp 123–162

Delmonte MM: Physiological concomitants of meditation practice. Int J Psychosom 31:23–36, 1984

Demisch L: Clinical pharmacology of melatonin regulation, in Melatonin: Biosynthesis, Physiological Effects, and Clinical Applications. Edited by Yu H-S, Reiter R. Boca Raton, FL, CRC Press, 1993, pp 513–540

Dollins AB, Zhdanova IV, Wurtman RJ, et al: Effect of inducing nocturnal serum melatonin concentrations in daytime on sleep, mood, body temperature and performance. Proc Natl Acad Sci U S A 91:1824–1828, 1994

Dubovsky SL: Generalized anxiety disorder: new concepts and psychopharmacologic therapies. J Clin Psychiatry 51 (suppl 1):3–10, 1990

Epstein M: Thoughts Without a Thinker. New York, Basic Books, 1995

Fawzy FI, Cousins N, Fawzy NW, et al: A structured psychiatric intervention for cancer patients, I: changes over time in methods of coping and affective disturbance. Arch Gen Psychiatry 47:720–725, 1990a

Fawzy FI, Kemeny ME, Fawzy NW, et al: A structured psychiatric intervention for cancer patients, II: changes over time in immunological measures. Arch Gen Psychiatry 47:729–735, 1990b

Fawzy FI, Fawzy NW, Hyun CS, et al: Malignant melanoma: effects of an early structured psychiatric intervention, coping and affective state on recurrence and survival 6 years later. Arch Gen Psychiatry 50:681–689, 1993

Goldstein J: The Experience of Insight. Boston, Shambhala, 1976

Goldstein J, Kornfield J: Seeking the Heart of Wisdom. Boston, MA, Shambhala, 1987

Greer S, Moorey S, Baruch et al: Adjuvant psychological therapy for patients with cancer: a prospective randomized trial. BMJ 304:675–680, 1992

Guerrero J, Reiter R: A brief survey of pineal gland-immune system interrelationships. Endocr Res 18:91–113, 1992

Gyatso GK: Buddhism in the Tibetan Tradition: A Guide. Boston, Routledge & Kegan Paul, 1984

Gyatso GK: Meaningful to Behold: A Commentary to Shantideva's Guide to the Bodhisattva's Way of Life. London, Tharpa Publications, 1985

Huether G: The contribution of extrapineal sites of melatonin synthesis to circulating melatonin levels in higher vertebrates. Experientia 49:665–670, 1993

Huether G: Melatonin synthesis in the gastrointestinal tract and the impact of nutritional factors on circulating melatonin, in The Aging Clock: The Pineal and Other Pacemakers in the Progression of Aging and Carcinogenesis (Annals of the New York Academy of Sciences, Vol 719). Edited by Pierpaoli W, Regelson W, Fabris N. New York, The New York Academy of Sciences, 1994, pp 146–158

Kabat-Zinn J: An out-patient program in behavioral medicine for chronic pain patients based on the practice of mindfulness meditation: theoretical considerations and preliminary results. Gen Hosp Psychiatry 4:33–47, 1982

Kabat-Zinn J: Full Catastrophe Living. New York, Delacorte, 1990

Kabat-Zinn J: Wherever You Go, There You Are. New York, Hyperion, 1994

Kabat-Zinn J, Lipworth L, Burney R: The clinical use of mindfulness meditation for the self-regulation of chronic pain. J Behav Med 8:163–190, 1985

Kabat-Zinn J, Lipworth L, Burney R, et al: Four-year follow-up of a meditation-based program for the self-regulation of chronic pain: treatment outcomes and compliance. Clin J Pain 2:159–173, 1986

Kabat-Zinn J, Skillings A, Santorelli SF: Sense of coherence and stress hardiness as predictors and measures of outcome of a stress reduction program. Poster presented at the annual meeting of the Society of Behavioral Medicine, San Francisco, CA, March 31, 1989

Kabat-Zinn J, Massion AO, Kristeller J, et al: Effectiveness of a meditation-based stress reduction program in the treatment of anxiety disorders. Am J Psychiatry 149:936–943, 1992

Kabat-Zinn J, Massion AO, Hebert JR, et al: Meditation, in Textbook of Psycho-oncology. Edited by Holland J. London, Oxford University Press, in press

Katz VL, Ekstrom RD, Mason GA, et al: 6-sulphatoxymelatonin levels in pregnant women during workplace and nonworkplace stresses: a potential biologic marker of sympathetic activity. Am J Perinatol 12:299–302, 1995

Khan R, Daya S, Potgieter B: Evidence for a modulation of the stress response by the pineal gland. Experientia 46:860–862, 1990

Kornfield J: A Path With Heart. New York, Bantam, 1993

Levine S: A Gradual Awakening. New York, Doubleday, 1979

Lewy AJ, Wehr TA, Goodwin FK, et al: Light suppresses melatonin secretion in humans. Science 210:1267–1269, 1980

Lissoni P, Tancini G, Barni S: Melatonin increase as predictor for tumor objective response to chemotherapy in advanced cancer patients. Tumori 74:339–345, 1988

Lissoni P, Barni S, Crispino S, et al: Endocrine and immune effects of melatonin therapy in metastatic cancer patients. European Journal of Cancer and Clinical Oncology 25:789–795, 1989

Lissoni P, Barni S, Cattaneo G, et al: Clinical results with the pineal hormone melatonin in advanced cancer resistant to standard antitumor therapies. Oncology 48:448–450, 1991

Lissoni P, Tisi E, Barni S, et al: Biological and clinical results of a neuroimmunotherapy with interleukin-2 and the pineal hormone melatonin as a first line treatment in advanced nonsmall cell lung cancer. Br J Cancer 66:155–158, 1992a

Lissoni P, Barni S, Ardizzoia A, et al: Immunological effects of a single evening subcutaneous injection of low-dose interleukin-2 in association with the pineal hormone melatonin in advanced cancer patients. J Biol Regul Homeost Agents 6(4):132–136, 1992b

Lissoni P, Barni S, Ardizzoia A, et al: Randomized study with the pineal hormone melatonin versus supportive care alone in advanced nonsmall cell lung cancer resistant to a first-line chemotherapy containing cisplatin. Oncology 49:336–339, 1992c

Lissoni P, Barni S, Tancini G, et al: Immunotherapy with subcutaneous low-dose interleukin-2 and the pineal indole melatonin as a new effective therapy in advanced cancers of the digestive tract. Br J Cancer 67:1404–1407, 1993

Lissoni P, Barni S, Tancini G, et al: A randomised study with subcutaneous low-dose interleukin-2 alone versus interleukin-2 plus the pineal neurohormone melatonin in advanced solid neoplasms other than renal cancer and melanoma. Br J Cancer 69:196–199, 1994a

Lissoni P, Barni S, Ardizzoia A, et al: A randomized study with the pineal hormone melatonin versus supportive care alone in patients with brain metastases due to solid neoplasms. Cancer 73:699–701, 1994b

Maestroni GJM, Conti A: Melatonin in relation to the immune system, in Melatonin: Biosynthesis, Physiological Effects, and Clinical Applications. Edited by Yu H-S, Reiter R. Boca Raton, FL, CRC Press, 1993, pp 289–309

Maharishi: Maharishi Mahesh Yogi on the Bhagavad-Bita. London, Arkana, 1990

Massion AO, Teas J, Hebert JR, et al: Meditation, melatonin and breast/prostate cancer: hypothesis and preliminary data. Med Hypotheses 44:39–46, 1995

McIntyre IM, Norman TR, Burrows GD, et al: Melatonin rhythm in human plasma and saliva. J Pineal Res 4:177–183, 1987

McIntyre IM, Norman TR, Burrows GD, et al: Human melatonin suppression by light is intensity dependent. J Pineal Res 6:149–156, 1988

McNair D, Lorr M, Droppleman L: Manual for the Profile of Mood States. San Diego, CA, Educational and Industrial Testing Service, 1971

Miller JJ, Fletcher K, Kabat-Zinn J: Three-year follow-up and clinical implications of a mindfulness meditation-based stress reduction intervention in the treatment of anxiety disorders. Gen Hosp Psychiatry 17:192–200, 1995

Monteleone P, Maj M, Fuschino A, et al: Physical stress in the middle of the dark phase does not affect light-depressed plasma melatonin levels in humans. Neuroendocrinology 55:367–371, 1992

Monteleone P, Maj M, Franza F, et al: The human pineal gland responds to stress-induced sympathetic activation in the second half of the dark phase: preliminary evidence. J Neural Transm 92:25–32, 1993

Moorey S, Greer S: Psychological Therapy for Patients With Cancer: A New Approach. Washington, DC, American Psychiatric Press, 1989

Moorey S, Greer S, Watson M, et al: Adjuvant psychological therapy for patients with cancer: outcome at one year. Psycho-oncology 3:39–46, 1994

Moras K, Craske MG, Barlow DH: Behavioral and cognitive therapies for panic disorder, in Handbook of Anxiety, Vol 4: The Treatment of Anxiety. Edited by Noyes RJ, Roth M, Burrows G. Amsterdam, Elsevier Science, 1990, pp 311–325

Reiter RJ: Pineal melatonin: cell biology of its synthesis and of its physiological interactions. Endocr Rev 12:151–180, 1991

Romijn HJ: Minireview: the pineal, a tranquilizing organ? Life Sci 23:2257–2274, 1978

Roth R: Maharishi Mahesh Yogi's Transcendental Meditation. New York, Primus, Donald I Fine, 1994

Schneider RH, Staggers F, Alexander CN, et al: A randomized controlled trial of stress reduction for hypertension in older African Americans. Hypertension 26:820–827, 1995

Spiegel D, Spira J: Supportive-Expressive Group Therapy: A Treatment Manual of Psychosocial Intervention for Women With Recurrent Breast Cancer. Stanford, CA, Psychosocial Treatment Laboratory, Stanford University School of Medicine, 1991

Spiegel D, Bloom J, Kraemer H, et al: Effect of psychosocial treatment on survival of patients with metastatic breast cancer. Lancet 2:888–891, 1989

Spielberger CD, Sydeman ST: State-Trait Anxiety Inventory and State-Trait Anger Expression Inventory, in The Use of Psychological Testing for Treatment Planning and Outcome Assessment. Edited by Marvish ME. Hillsdale, NJ, Lawrence Earlbaum Associates, 1994, pp 292–321

Stankov B, Fraschini F, Reiter RJ: The melatonin receptor: distribution, biochemistry, and pharmacology, in Melatonin: Biosynthesis, Physiological Effects, and Clinical Applications. Edited by Yu H-S, Reiter R. Boca Raton, FL, CRC Press, 1993, pp 156–186

Statistical Analysis System (SAS) Users Guide. Cary, NC, SAS Institute, 1993

Suzuki S: Zen Mind, Beginner's Mind. New York, Weatherall, 1970

Thera N: The Heart of Buddhist Meditation. New York, Weiser, 1962

Walton KG, Brown GM, Pugh N, et al: Indole-mediated adaptation: does melatonin mediate resistance to stress in humans? (abstract). Society of Neuroscience Abstracts 16:273, 1990

Weekes C: Hope and Help for Your Nerves. New York, Signet, 1969

Woolfolk RL, Carr-Kaffashan L, McNulty TF, et al: Meditation training as a treatment for insomnia. Behavior Therapy 7:359–365, 1976

Yeshe LT: Wisdom Energy 2. Ulverston, Cumbria, England, Wisdom Culture, 1979

Index

Page numbers printed in **boldface** *type refer to tables or figures.*

Achaan Chah, 264
Acquired immunity, and melatonin, 217–219
ACTH. *See* Adrenocorticotropic hormone
Activity-rest cycle, and bipolar disorder, 113
ADCC. *See* Antibody-dependent cellular cytotoxicity
Adenosinetriphosphatase (ATPase), 245
Adenosine triphosphate (ATP), 44
Administration, of supplemental melatonin to children, 178
Adolescence. *See also* Age; Puberty
    changes in melatonin production during, 151–155
    depression and melatonin levels in, 157–162
    prevalence of eating disorders and anxiety disorders in, 126
Adrenal lung tumors, 222
Adrenocorticotropic hormone (ACTH), 133
Advanced sleep phase syndrome (ASPS), 88–91

Affective disorders, phase-advance theory of, 45. *See also* Depression
Age. *See also* Adolescence; Aging; Children; Elderly
    abnormalities of bone, 179
    cancer and melatonin rhythms, 250, **252**
    depression and decrease in melatonin production by, 55–56
    influence of on melatonin production, 47–48
Age-related sleep inefficiency, 12
Aging, changes in circadian melatonin cycle related to, 10, **11**. *See also* Age; Elderly
Agoraphobia, panic disorder and cortisol levels, 134
Algae, and melatonin, 28
Alkoxyl radical, **13**
Aluminum-induced neuropathy, **15**
Alzheimer's disease, 3, **15**, 17
Amenorrhea, and eating disorders, 131, 132
Amphibians, and pineal gland, 27

Amplitude hypothesis, and light
   therapy for depression, 58,
   65–66
Amytrophic lateral sclerosis
   (ALS), **15**, 17
Analgesia, effects of meditation
   and melatonin, **275**
Androgen-sensitive tumors, 194
Anorexia nervosa. *See also* Eating
   disorders
   comorbidity with panic
      disorder, 127, 128
   depression and melatonin
      levels in, 156
   pineal gland function and,
      129–131, 132
Anoura caudifer, 36
Antibody-dependent cellular
   cytotoxicity (ADCC), 215
Anticonvulsants, 178
Antidepressants
   influence of on production
      and secretion of
      melatonin, 47, 111
   light therapy for seasonal
      affective disorder as, 93,
      96
   sleep deprivation as treatment
      for depression, 46, 108
   sleep deprivation as treatment
      for rapid-cycling bipolar
      patients, 110–111, 117
Antioxidant, melatonin as
   cancer and effects of, 211–214,
      244
   free radicals and, 8, 13, 16
Antisocial behavior, and
   depression in children and
   adolescents, 157

Antitumorigenic activity, of
   melatonin, 192
Anxiety, effects of meditation
   and melatonin on, **275**. *See
   also* Anxiety disorders
Anxiety disorders
   comorbidity with bulimia
      nervosa, 127
   prevalence of, 126
   sleep disorders in children
      and, 175
Apomorphine, 136
Arteries, and blood supply to
   pineal gland, 33
Attention-deficit/hyperactivity
   disorder, 175
Atypical depression, in children
   and adolescents, 158–160
Autism, 175, 176
Auto-oxidation, process of, 16

β-adrenergic receptors, 8, 44, 58
Bats, pineal concretions in, 36
Batten's disease, **15**
Behavior, and sleep disorders in
   multidisabled children, 180.
   See also Antisocial behavior
Benign prostatic hypertrophy,
   251
Benzodiazepines, 8, 274
Biological clock, melatonin and
   regulation of, 44–45
Biological marker, melatonin as,
   53
Bipolar disorder
   circadian rhythm disturbances
      in, 105–111
   melatonin secretion and,
      111–116
Birds, and pineal gland, 28, 192

Bladder carcinoma, 194, **195**
Blastogenesis, 216, 217, 219
Blindness
    altered sleep-wake cycles and,
        12
    sleep disorders in children
        and, 169, 170, 175
Blood pressure, effects of
    meditation and melatonin
    on, **275**
B lymphocytes, 226
Body-rhythm regulator,
    melatonin as, 70
Bone age, abnormalities of, 179
Brain
    damage to by free radicals,
        12–13
    damage to and sleep disorders
        in children, 169
    tumors of and sleep disorders
        in children, 175
Breast cancer. *See also* Cancer;
    MCF-7 breast cancer cell line
    antitumorigenic action of
        melatonin and, 193
    circadian melatonin rhythm
        in, 246–250, 255
    effects of melatonin on, **195**,
        196–198, 223, 225
    estrogen-response pathway of
        breast tumor cells and,
        205–210
    meditation and, 276, 283–287,
        289
Breathing retraining, 268
BRIDGES (**B**reast **R**esearch
    Initiative for **D**evelopin**G**
    Effective **S**kills) study,
    283–287, 289

British Columbia Children's
    Hospital Visually Impaired
    Program, 170
BSO. *See* Buthionine sulfoximine
Buddhist tradition, of meditation
    practice, 266
Bulimia nervosa. *See also* Eating
    disorders
    comorbidity with anxiety
        disorders, 127
    comorbidity with panic
        disorder, 127, 128
    neurotransmitters and pineal
        gland function in, 132
    prevalence of, 126
Buthionine sulfoximine (BSO),
    212

Calcareous concretions, in pineal
    gland, 35–36
Calcium, and growth of MCF-7
    cells, 245
Calcium channel blockers, 15
Calcium channels, and free
    radicals, **14**
Calmodulin, and cell
    proliferation, 245
CAMP. *See* Cyclic adenosine
    monophosphate
Cancer, and melatonin. *See also*
    Breast cancer; Tumors
    antioxidant effects of, 211–214
    effects of on neoplastic cells,
        193–198, **224**
    effects of physiological on
        circadian rhythm,
        243–256
    estrogen-response pathway of
        breast tumor cells and,
        205–210

Cancer, and melatonin *(continued)*
  as immunotherapeutic agent,
    220–223
  meditation and levels of,
    269–270, 274–289
  rhythm of as marker for,
    255–256
  tissue and subcellular
    localization and binding
    sites for, 198–205
Carbohydrates, and light therapy
  for depression, 64
Carcinoembryonic antigen
  (CEA), 251
Carcinoid tumor, 222
Caregivers, of
  neurodevelopmentally
  disabled children with sleep
  disorders, 171, 173, 176–177,
  181
Cathepsin D, 208
CEA. *See* Carcinoembryonic
  antigen
Cerebral blood flow, and light
  therapy for depression, 67
Cerebral ischemia, 15–16
Cerebral palsy, 175
Cerebrospinal fluid, and
  measurement of melatonin
  levels, 158
C-*fos* gene, 206, 209
CGMP. *See* Cyclic guanosine
  monophosphate
Children. *See also* Age
  changes in melatonin levels
    during development of,
    9, 151–155
  depression and melatonin
    levels in, 157–162

  psychic trauma and melatonin
    levels, 54–55
  sleep disorders in
    neurodevelopmentally
    disabled and melatonin,
    169–185
Chlorpromazine, 47
Chromogranin A, 36
Chronobiological mood
  disorders, melatonin and
  light therapy for, 92–97
Chronobiological sleep disorders,
  melatonin and light therapy
  for, 84–85, 88–91
Circadian rhythm. *See also*
  Diurnal rhythm; Internal
  body rhythms
  bipolar disorder and
    disturbances of, 105–111
  blood levels of melatonin and,
    7
  cancer and effects of
    physiological melatonin
    on, 243–256
  light therapy for depression
    and, 58–60
  melatonin as marker of phase
    position in relation to
    light, 61–62, 67
  neurobiology of melatonin
    production and, 4–6
  phase-advance theory of
    manic-depressive illness
    and, 45
  sleep disorders associated
    with dyssynchronized
    and supplemental
    melatonin, 12
Clonidine-growth hormone
  challenge test, 134, 135, 137

C-*myc* gene, 206, 209, 210

Cognitive-behavior therapy, 268, **271**

Cognitive skills, and sleep disorders in multidisabled children, 180

Colchicine, 193

Colon carcinoma, 194, 223

Colony-stimulating factors, 219

Colorectal carcinoma, 221, 251

Comprehensive Psychopathological Rating Scale (CPRS), 49, 51

Concentration, and meditation, 261–263

Concretionary deposits, and pineal gland, 35–36

Consciousness, meditation and levels of, 267

Contraceptives, and melatonin, 227

Coping skills, and meditation, **272**

Corticotropin-releasing hormone (CRH), 133

Cortisol
  chronic stress and, 282
  depression and secretion of, 44, 50, 51
  hypothalamic-pituitary-adrenal axis and, 133–134
  melatonin and monoamine oxidase in platelets as markers for depression, 56–57

CRH. *See* Corticotropin-releasing hormone

Cyclic adenosine monophosphate (cAMP), 44, 216

Cyclic guanosine monophosphate (cGMP), 216

Cystic fibrosis, 181

Cysts, of pineal gland, 33–35

Cytokines, 255

Darkness. *See also* Light
  melatonin synthesis as chemical expression of, 4–5
  regulation of melatonin production by, 43–44, 191–192

Dawn simulation, for seasonal affective disorder, 93, 96

Day length, melatonin and timing of reproduction, 192

DBD. *See* DNA-binding domain

Death, melatonin levels in victims of sudden, 156–157

Decarboxylase, 4, **5**

Delayed sleep-onset disorder, 175–176

Delayed sleep phase syndrome, 12, 88–91

Depression, and melatonin. *See also* Affective disorders; Mood disorders
  adults and levels of, 155–157
  age and decrease in production of, 55–56
  amplitude of secretion in, 112
  anorexia nervosa and, 129–130
  bulimia nervosa and, 127
  children and adolescents and levels of, 157–162
  and cortisol or monoamine oxidase in platelets as markers for, 56–57
  diagnosis and, 48–49

Depression, and melatonin
    (continued)
    diurnal rhythm disturbances
        and, 45–46
    factors influencing production
        of and, 47–48
    internal body rhythms and,
        44–45, 107
    light therapy and, 57–69
    low-melatonin syndrome and,
        49–55
    phase shift in unipolar and
        bipolar patients and, 108
    seasonal variations in, 46–47
    sleep deprivation and, 46, 108
    as therapeutic agent for, 69–70
Desferrioxamine, 17–18
Desipramine, 8
Dexamethasone suppression test
    (DST), 49–52, 56–57, 133, 155
Dharma, meditation and concept
    of, 266–267
Diabetes mellitus, 161
Diagnosis, melatonin levels and
    psychiatric
    depressive disorders and, 69
    mood disorders and, 48–49
Diarrhea, nonspecific chronic, 181
7,12-Dimethylbenzanthracene
    (DMBA), 194, 197, 207
Dimethyl phthalate, 47
Dim light melatonin onset
    (DLMO)
    phase shifts of as function of
        circadian time, 89
    seasonal affective disorder
        and, 93
Diurnal rhythm, depression and
    disturbances of, 45–46. See
    also Circadian rhythm;

Internal rhythms
Divorce, and shift work, 91. See
    also Family
DLMO. See Dim light melatonin
    onset
DMBA. See 7,12-Dimethylbenz-
    anthracen
DNA-binding domain (DBD), 203
DNA
    damage to by oxidative stress
        and free radicals, 211–212
    markers for bipolar disorder
        and, 109
Dopamine system, and anorexia
    nervosa, 137
Dosage, of supplemental
    melatonin. See also
    Pharmacotherapy;
    Supplemental melatonin
    for insomnia and jet lag, 287,
        289
    for neurodevelopmentally
        disabled children with
        sleep disorders, 177–178,
        183–184
    for seasonal affective disorder,
        98
    soporific side effects and, 88, 92
Down's syndrome, 15, 169
Drosophila melanogaster, 28, 109
Drowsiness, as side effect of
    supplemental melatonin, 88,
        92, 179
Drug interactions, with
    supplemental melatonin,
    180. See also
    Pharmacotherapy;
Supplemental melatonin
DSM-III-R, and melancholia,
    52–53

DSM-IV, diagnostic categories of and melatonin as biological marker, 53

Duration, of melatonin therapy for children with neurodevelopmental disabilities, 181–182. *See also* Pharmacotherapy; Supplemental melatonin

Dysthymic disorder, in children and adolescents, 158–160

Eating disorders. *See also* Anorexia nervosa; Bulimia nervosa
  comorbidity with panic disorders and
    epidemiological aspects of, 125–129
    neuroendocrine abnormalities in, 132–137
    pineal gland function, 129–131
    neurotransmitters and pineal gland function, 132

ECP. *See* Endogenous circadian pacemaker

EGF. *See* Epidermal growth factor

Ehrlich's tumor, 194

Elderly. *See also* Age; Aging
  age-related decline in melatonin production in, 10–11
  cancer and melatonin rhythms in, 250

Endogenous circadian pacemaker (ECP), **90**

Environmental factors
  for comorbidity in eating disorders and panic disorders, 126
  in melatonin production and depression, 54

Epidemiology, of panic and eating disorders, 125–129

Epidermal growth factor (EGF), 209, 210, 244

Epidermoid carcinoma, 194

Epilepsy
  free radicals and, 14–15
  melatonin for neurodevelopmentally disabled children and, 181, 183

Epithalamus, and pineal gland, 29

ER. *See* Estrogen-receptor breast cancer

Esophageal reflex, 180, 183

Estradiol, 197, 244

Estrogen, melatonin and circulating levels of, 225

Estrogen-receptor breast cancer (ER), 197–198, 205–210, 244, 247, **248**

Estrogen-regulated genes, modulation of by melatonin, 208–210

Evening light, and seasonal affective disorder, 96, 97

Evolution, of pineal gland, 27–29

Eyes, neural connections to pineal gland, 6

Family, and neurodevelopmentally disabled children with sleep disorders, 176–177, 181, 184. *See also* Divorce; Parents

Fast-release oral melatonin, 184
Feeding formulas, and
    administration of
    supplemental melatonin to
    children, 178
Fenfluramine, 134, 136, 137
Fetus, melatonin levels in, 8
Fibrosarcomas, 194, **195**
Fluoxetine, 66, 67
Fluvoxamine, 66
Follow-up studies, of eating and
    panic disorders, 128–129
Free radicals
    DNA damage induced by,
        211–212, 213
    melatonin and neutralization
        of toxic, 3, 12–13, 244, 246
    neuronal disorders and, 14–18
    types damaging neuronal
        tissue, **13**
Free-running rhythm, hypothesis
    of failure in subtypes of
    depression, 44–45

GABA system, 271, 274
Gas chromatography mass
    spectrometry, 150
Gastric carcinoma, 221, 227
Gastrointestinal tract
    melatonin and function of, 181
    synthesis of melatonin in, 150
Gender, and melatonin levels
    during puberty, 151–152
Generalized anxiety disorder,
    and Stress Reduction and
    Relaxation Program, 269
Genetics
    bipolar disorder and
        disruptions of circadian
        rhythms, 109–111, 117

comorbidity of eating and
    panic disorders and,
    126–127
influence of on melatonin
    production, 47, 110
nocturnal melatonin levels in
    depressed patients and, 54
responsiveness to light and
    seasonal depression, 68
GFAP. *See* Glial fibrillary acidic
    protein
GHRH. *See* Growth
    hormone-releasing hormone
Glial cells, 33
Glial fibrillary acidic protein
    (GFAP), 36
Glutamate, 6, **14**
Glutamyl cycle, 212
Glutathione (GSH), 211–212, 246
Goal-directed meditation,
    264–265
Golgi complex, 31
Gonyaulax polyedra, 28
G-protein-linked membrane
    receptors, 200–202, 225–226
Group therapy, 268, **271**
Growth hormone
    eating disorders and, 135–136,
        137
    immune system and, 220
Growth hormone-releasing
    hormone (GHRH), 135
GSH. *See* Glutathione
GTP. *See* Guanosine
    5'-triphosphate
Guanosine 5'-triphosphate
    (GTP), 199

Hamilton Depression Rating
    Scale (HDRS), 48, 60, 63, **95**

HBD. *See* Hormone-binding domain

Head injury, and sleep disorders in children, 175

Health benefits, of melatonin therapy for sleep disorders in multidisabled children, 180–181

Heart rate, effects of meditation and melatonin on, **275**

Hemoglobin, 214

Hepatocellular carcinoma, 221

5-HIAA. *See* 5-Hydroxyindoleacetic acid

Hibernation, and melatonin production, 151

High melatonin major depression (HMMD), 161–162

HIOMT. *See* Hydroxyindole-*O*-methyltransferase

History, of research
  on neurobiology of pineal gland and melatonin production, 149–151
  on role of melatonin in circadian phase sleep and mood disorders, 82–85

HMMD. *See* High melatonin major depression

Hormone-binding domain (HBD), 203

Hormone response elements (HREs), 203–204

HREs. *See* Hormone response elements

Huntington's disease, 17

5-Hydroxyindoleacetic acid (5-HIAA), 274

Hydroxyindole-*O*-methyltransferase (HIOMT), 4, 44, 149

Hydroxyl radical, **13**

6-Hydroxymelatonin sulfate, 10–11

5-Hydroxytryptophan, 4, **5**

Hyperbaric hyperoxic injury, 14, **15**

Hypermelatoninemia, 161–162

Hypoglycemia, and anorexia nervosa, 130

Hypomania, and sleep deprivation, 107

Hypomelatoninemia, 162

Hypothalamic-pituitary-adrenal (HPA) axis, 44, 52, 133–134

Hypothalamic-pituitary-ovarian axis, 132–133

Hypothalamic-pituitary-thyroid axis, 134–135

Hypothalamus. *See* Suprachiasmatic nucleus

IFNs. *See* Interferons

ILs. *See* Interleukins

I-MEL, radioligand, 198–199, 201, 202–203

Immune system, and role of pineal gland in immunity, 214–223

Immunotherapeutic agent, cancer and melatonin as, 220–223

Infantile lipofuscinosis, 9

Infants. *See also* Newborns
  circadian melatonin cycle in, 8–9
  melatonin levels in, 152, **153**

Insect repellents, 47

Insomnia. *See also* Sleep disorders
  melatonin supplements for,
    287
  Stress Reduction and
    Relaxation Program for,
    270, 274
Insulin
  expression of estrogen and, 206
  synthesis of melatonin and, 160
Insulin-like growth factors
  (IGFs), 206
Interferons (IFNs), 219, 222, 253
Interleukins (ILs), 215, 218,
  219–220, 221–222, 227, 253,
  274, 275
Internal body rhythms,
  melatonin and monitoring
  of, 44–45. *See also* Circadian
  rhythm;
Diurnal rhythm
Internal desynchronization, in
  bipolar illness, 106–107
*International Classification of
  Diseases* (ICD-9-CM; World
  Health Organization 1980), 56
Ipsapirone, 134
Ischemia-reperfusion injury, **15**
Isoproterenol, 8

Jet lag
  internal desynchronization
    and, 106
  light therapy for, 85–88
  melatonin levels and, 11–12, 45
  melatonin supplements for, 287

Karnofsky Performance Status
  Score, 275

Learning disabilities, 175

Leukemia, 194, **195**, 219, **254**
LH. *See* Luteinizing hormone
LHRH. *See* Luteininzing
  hormone-releasing hormone
Life cycle, changes in melatonin
  levels throughout, 8–11,
  151–155
Life events, and circadian
  rhythm disruption, 109
Light. *See also* Darkness; Light
  therapy
  exposure to at night and
    decline in melatonin
    production, 6, 46
  history of research on
    melatonin and, 82–85
  melatonin as marker of phase
    position in relation to,
    61–62
  regulation of melatonin
    production by, 43–44,
    191–192
  suppression of melatonin by
    bright, 63–64
Light therapy. *See also* Light
  bipolar disorder and nocturnal
    light-suppression
    studies, 114–116
  for chronobiological mood
    disorders, 92–97
  for chronobiological sleep
    disorders, 88–91
  for depression, 57–68
  history of research on, 84–85
  for jet lag, 85–88
  need for future research on
    depression and, 68–69
  for rapid-cycling bipolar
    disorder, 113

for seasonal affective disorder, 92–97

for shift-work maladaptation, 91–92

Light visor, 96

Lipid peroxide, **13**

Lipofuscinosis, 9, **15**

Lipopolysaccharide (LPS)-induced lipid peroxidation, 214

5-Lipoxygenase, 216

Lithium, 107, 111, 116

Liver, metabolism of melatonin in, 158, 160

LMMD. *See* Low melatonin major depression

Locusta migratoria, 28

Low melatonin major depression (LMMD), 161–162

Low-melatonin syndrome, and depression, 49–55

Lung carcinoma, 194, 222

Luteinizing hormone (LH), 132–133, 152

Luteinizing hormone-releasing hormone (LHRH), 133

Lymphocytes. *See* B lymphocytes; T lymphocytes

Lymphokines, 218, 219

Macrophages, 220

Maharishi Mahesh Yogi, 263

Mammals, melatonin production in hibernating, 151. *See also* Vertebrates

Mania, and internal desynchronization, 106, 107

Manic-depressive disorder circadian rhythm and, 105

desynchronization of sleep-wake cycle in, 106

phase-advance theory of, 45

Marriage. *See* Divorce; Family

MCF-7 breast cancer cell line, 205, 207, 208–209, 210, 213–214, 225, 244–246

M-CPP. *See* Metachloro-phenylpiperazine

Meditation

cancer and melatonin levels, 269–270, 274–289

compared with self-regulatory/relaxation strategies and psychotherapy, 268–269

components of practice of, 261–263

goal- and non-goal-directed, 264–265

orientations of practice of, 266–268

psychosocial interventions compared to, **271–273**

transcendental, 263–264, 274, 280–283, **288**

Melancholia, and low-melatonin syndrome, 52–53

Melanoma, 192, 195–196, 221, 223, 276

Melatonin. *See also* Pineal gland

acquired immunity and, 217–219

bipolar disorder and circadian rhythm disturbances, 105–111

bipolar disorder and secretion of, 111–116

Melatonin (continued)
  cancer and
    antioxidant effects of,
      211–214
    effects of on neoplastic cells,
      193–198, **224**
    effects of physiological on
      circadian rhythm,
      243–256
    estrogen-response pathway
      of breast tumor cells
      and, 205–210
    meditation and levels of,
      269–270, 274–289
    melatonin rhythm as
      marker for, 255–256
    tissue and subcellular
      localization and
      binding sites for,
      198–205
  changes in levels of
    throughout life cycle,
    8–11, 151–155
  circadian phase sleep and
    light therapy for mood
    disorders
    chronobiological mood
      disorders and, 92–97
    chronobiological sleep
      disorders and, 88–91
    history of research on, 82–85
    jet lag and, 85–88
    shift-work maladaptation
      and, 91–92
  depression and
    adults and levels of, 155–157
    age and decrease in
      production of, 55–56
    children and adolescents
      and levels of, 157–162

and cortisol or monoamine
      oxidase in platelets as
      markers for, 56–57
    diurnal rhythm
      disturbances and, 45–46
    factors influencing
      production of, 47–48
    internal body rhythms and,
      44–45
    light therapy for, 57–69
    low-melatonin syndrome
      and, 49–55
    seasonal variations and,
      46–47
    as therapeutic agent for,
      69–70
  eating and panic disorders and
    epidemiological aspects of,
      125–129
    neuroendocrine
      abnormalities in,
      132–137
    pineal gland function and,
      129–131
  evolution and secretion of,
    28–29
  genetic influence on secretion
    of, 47, 110
  jet lag and, 11–12, 45, 85–88,
    106, 287
  light/darkness and regulation
    of production, 4–5, 43–44,
    191–192
  natural immunity and, 219–220
  neurobiology of production
    and secretion of, 3–8,
    149–151, 191–192
  neurochemical mechanisms of
    increased pineal
    function, 131–132

neurodegenerative diseases and, 12–18

panic disorder and increased levels of, 131

sleep disorders in children with neurodevelopmental disabilities and, 169–185

Mental retardation, 169, 175, 176

Metachlorophenylpiperazine (m-CPP), 134, 136

Metaclopramide, 136

Metanephrine, 132

3-Methoxy-4-hydroxyphenylglycol (MHPG), 108

Methoxypsoralen, 8

1-Methyl-4-phenyl-1,2,3,6-tetra-hydropyridine (MPTP), 16–17

MHPG. *See* 3-Methoxy-4-hydroxyphenylglycol

Mindfulness, and meditation, 261–263, **288**

Mitral valve prolapse, and comorbidity of eating and panic disorders, 128

MK-801, 8

Monoamine oxidase (MAO) , 16, 56–57

Monocytes, and melatonin, 218

Mood disorders, and melatonin. *See also* Depression

amplitude of in patients with, 112–113

chronobiological aspects of, 69

depression in children and adolescents and, 157

diagnosis and, 48–49

jet lag and, 45, 85–88

light therapy for chronobiological, 92–97

risk of suppression in, 115

seasonal variations in, 46

as therapeutic agent for subgroups of, 70

Mood state, and sleep disorders in multidisabled children, 180

Morning light, and seasonal affective disorder, 93, 96–97

Motivations, for learning meditation, 264

MPTP. *See* 1-Methyl-4-phenyl-1,2,3,6-tetrahydropyridine

Multiple sclerosis, 17–18

Multipolar pinealocytes, 31

Muscular dystrophy, **15**

Mutation studies, and genetic factors in circadian rhythms, 109–110

Myasthenia gravis, **15**

N-acetylserotonin, 149, 150

N-acetyltransferase (NAT), 4, **5**, 44

Naloxone, 134, 136

NAT. *See N*-acetyltransferase

National Cancer Institute Cooperative Human Tissue Network, 29

Natural immunity, and melatonin, 219–220

Natural killer (NK) cells, 216, 217, 218, 219–220

Neoplastic cells, effects of melantonin on, 193–198, 211–214, **224**

Neopterin, 220, 222

Nerves, and structure of pineal gland, 33

Neurobiology, and melatonin
neurodegenerative diseases
and, 12–18
production and secretion of,
4–8, 149–151, 191–192
roles of melatonin and, 3–4
Neuroblastoma, 194
Neurochemistry, and
mechanisms of increased
pineal function, 131–132
Neurodegenerative diseases, and
melatonin, 12–18
Neurodevelopmental disabilities,
and sleep disorders in
children, 169–185
Neuroendocrine lung tumors, 222
Neuroendocrinology,
abnormalities of in eating
and panic disorders, 132–137
Neurofilaments, in
pineocytomas, 36
Neuromelanin, 16
Neuropsychoendocrine
dysfunctions, and seasonal
variations in melatonin
levels, 47
Neurospora, 109
Neurotoxic damage, **15**
Neurotransmitters, and pineal
function in eating disorders,
132
Newborns. See also Infants
melatonin levels in, 8, 152, 153
pineal gland in, 29
Nitric oxide, 15–16, 212–214
NK cells. See Natural killer cells
NMDA receptors, **14**
NMMA. See N-mono-
methyl-L-arginine

NMMD. See Normal melatonin
major depression
N-monomethyl-L-arginine
(NMMA), 213–214
NMU. See N-nitrosomethylurea
(NMU)-induced mammary
tumors
N-nitrosomethylurea
(NMU)-induced mammary
tumors, 194
Nocturnal light-suppression
studies, and bipolar disorder,
114–116
Noise, and treatment of sleep
disorders in multidisabled
children, 183
Non-goal-directed meditation,
264–265
Noradrenaline, 43–44
Normal melatonin major
depression (NMMD), 161–162
Norpinephrine, 6, 191
Nuclear melatonin receptors,
202–205
Nuclear orphan receptors, 199–200
Nutrition education program
(NEP), 284–287, 289

Oligomenorrhea, and bulimia
nervosa, 132
ONOO–. See Peroxynitrite anion
Opioids, and eating disorders,
134, 136
Optic nerve gliomas, 183
Optic nerve hypoplasia, 175
Ovarian carcinoma, **195,** 223

Pain, and sleep disorders in
neurodevelopmentally
disabled children, 175, 183

Pancreatic islet cell carcinoma, 222
Pancreatic spasmolytic polypeptide (pS2) mRNA, 206, 209, 210
Panic disorders
    epidemiological aspects of comorbidity with eating disorders, 125–129
    melatonin levels and, 131
    neuroendocrine abnormalities and comorbidity with eating disorders, 132–137
    neurotransmitters and pineal gland function in, 132
    Stress Reduction and Relaxation Program and, 269
Parenchyma, pineal, 30–31, **34–35**
Parents. *See also* Caregivers; Family
    loss of as childhood trauma and melatonin levels, 54–55
    sleep charting for children and, 171, 173
Parkinson's disease, 3, **15,** 16–17
Peroxyl radical, **13**
Peroxynitrite anion (ONOO–), 213
PgR. *See* Progesterone receptor
Pharmacotherapy. *See also* Dosage; Drug interactions; Duration; Side effects; Supplemental melatonin; Toxicity
    low-melatonin syndrome and, 69

melatonin as immunotherapeutic agent in cancer, 220–223
melatonin as therapeutic agent for depression, 69–70
Phase advances. *See also* Phase-shift hypothesis
    bipolar disorder and, 108–109
    theory of affective illness and, 45
Phase delay, and bipolar disorder, 109
Phase-response curves (PRCs), and light therapy, 85, **86, 87,** 88
Phase-shift hypothesis. *See also* Phase advances
    of bipolar disorder, 108–109, 113–114
    of depression, 58–59, 67, 93
Phobia, and bulimia nervosa, 127
Photoreceptor cells, in retina, 6
Phototherapy. *See* Light therapy
Pinealectomy, immunodepression following, 218
Pineal gland. *See also* Melatonin
    aging and decline in melatonin production, 10
    Alzheimer's disease and, 17
    anorexia nervosa and function of, 129–131
    concretionary deposits in, 35–36
    evolution of, 27–29
    immunity and role of, 214–223
    neurobiology of melatonin and, 4–8, 149–151, 191–192

Pineal gland *(continued)*
   neurochemistry of increased
      function of, 131–132
   as oncostatic endocrine organ,
      192
   pineal cysts and, 33–35
   puberty and tumors of, 149
   structure of, 29–33
   sudden infant death
      syndrome (SIDS) and
      development of, 9
   tumors of, 36, 149
Pinealocytes, 6, 7, 30–31, 191
Pineocytomas, 36
Pituitary gland
   abnormalities of in children
      with neurodevelop-
      mental disabilities, 179
   actions of melatonin at cellular
      level and, 192
   tumors of, 194, **195**
Plasticizers, and melatonin
   production, 47
Platelets, and melatonin, cortisol,
   and monoamine oxidase as
   markers for depression, 56–57
Polysomnographic studies, in
   children with multiple
   disabilities, 171
Polyunsaturated fatty acids, 13
Population-based surveys, of
   eating disorders and panic
   disorders, 126–127
PRCs. *See* Phase-response curves
Prepubescence, and melatonin
   levels, 152, 154
PRL. *See* Prolactin
Profile of Mood States (POMS),
   282

Progesterone, and expression of
   estrogen, 206
Progesterone receptor (PgR), 206,
   208, 209, 247
Prolactin (PRL)
   eating disorders and, 136–137
   immune system and, 220
   melatonin and circulating
      levels of, 225
   tumor growth and, 197, 244
Propranolol, 215
Prostate cancer, 194–195, 223,
   250–251, **252**
pS2. *See* Pancreatic spasmolytic
   polypeptide mRNA
Psychoactive drugs, and
   melatonin secretion, 111
Psychotherapy, and meditation,
   268–269, **271–273**, 276
Pterygophora, 28
Puberty. *See also* Adolescence
   bone age abnormalities and
      precocious, 179
   melatonin levels during, 9, **11**,
      151–155, 159
   pineal gland tumors and, 149

Quantitative trait loci (QTL), and
   circadian rhythms, 110

Radioimmunoassay (RIA), 150
Rapid-cycling bipolar disorder
   antidepressant effects of sleep
      deprivation for, 110–111,
      117
   internal desynchronization
      and, 107
   light therapy for, 113
   melatonin secretion amplitude
      in, 112

oral melatonin for, 113–114
Rapid eye movement (REM)
  sleep, 46, 108
RAR. *See* Retinoic acid receptors
Reactive oxygen species, and
  damage to neuronal tissue, **13**
Receptors, binding sites for
  melatonin and tissue or
  subcellular localization,
  198–205
Relaxation strategies, and
  meditation, 267, 268–269, **270,**
  276
Reproduction, melatonin and
  photoperiodicity of, 192
Reptiles, and pineal gland, 27–28,
  192
Research
  history of on neurobiology of
    pineal gland and
    melatonin, 149–151
  history of on role of melatonin
    in circadian phase sleep
    and mood disorders,
    82–85
  light therapy for depression
    and need for future,
    68–69
  on meditation, melatonin, and
    cancer, 276–289
Research Diagnostic Criteria
  (RDC), 48, 49, 56, 156
Retina
  neural connections between
    eye and pineal gland, 6
  synthesis of melatonin in, 150
Retinoic acid receptors (RARs),
  193, 199–200, 203

Retinoid orphan response
  elements (ROREs), 205, 208,
  226
Retinoid X receptors (RZRs),
  202–205, 216, 226
Rett's syndrome, 169
Rhythm-regulatory hormone,
  melatonin as, 70
RORα receptors, 203–205, 208,
  216, 226
RORE. *See* Retinoid orphan
  response elements
RZR. *See* Retinoid X receptors

SAD. *See* Seasonal affective
  disorder
Safety, of melatonin as drug, 12.
  See also Pharmacotherapy;
  Supplemental melatonin
Saliva, and measurement of
  melatonin, 158
Sangha, meditation and concept
  of, 267
Schizophrenia, free radicals and
  neuronal dysfunction in, 18
SCN. *See* Suprachiasmatic nucleus
Seasonal affective disorder
  (SAD). *See also* Seasonal
  variations
  history of research on light
    therapy for, 84–85
  low-melatonin syndrome and,
    69
  phase-delay of internal
    rhythms and, 45
  recommendations on light
    therapy for, 92–97

Seasonal variations, in melatonin
    levels and depression, 46–47,
    58–60, 64, 65, 68. *See also*
    Seasonal affective disorder
Seizure disorders, 14, 183
Self-regulatory strategies, and
    meditation, 268–269, **270**, 276
Serotonin and serotonin system
    dysregulation of
        neurotransmission in
        seasonal depression and,
        66–67
    metabolic pathway of
        conversion to melatonin,
        4, **5**
    panic disorder and pineal
        function, 136–137
Serotonin-specific reuptake
    inhibitors, 67
Severe sleep myoclonus, 175
Shift work
    circadian rhythm disturbances
        and, 110
    disturbances in melatonin
        levels and, 12
    internal desynchronization
        and, 106–107
    light therapy for, 88, 91–92
Side effects, of supplemental
    melatonin, 88, 92, 179, 184,
    185. *See also*
    Pharmacotherapy;
Supplemental melatonin
Signal transduction pathways,
    192–193
Singlet oxygen, **13**
Skeleton, development of in
    children and melatonin
    levels, 154
Sleep charting, 171, 173

Sleep deprivation
    internal desynchronization
        and mood states, 107
    as treatment for depression,
        46, 108
    as treatment for rapid-cycling
        bipolar disorder,
        110–111, 117
Sleep disorders, and melatonin.
    See also Insomnia;
    Sleep-wake cycles
    children with
        neurodevelopmental
        disabilities and, 169–185
    light therapy for
        chronobiological, 84–85,
        88–91
Sleep-wake cycles. *See also* Sleep
    disorders
    altered in blind individuals, 12
    disturbances of in children
        with
        neurodevelopmental
        disabilities, **172–173**, 179
    internal desynchronization in
        bipolar illness and,
        106–107
    phase-advanced and
        depression, 59
Slow-release oral melatonin,
    183–184
Sodium, stress and excretion
    rates of, 282
Sodium nitroprusside, 214
Somatostatin, 136
SR and RP. *See* Stress Reduction
    and Relaxation Program
Starvation, and melatonin release
    in anorexia nervosa, 130
State marker, melatonin as, 55

State-Trait Anxiety Inventory (STAI), 282

Steroid/thyroid hormone receptor superfamily, 200, 203–204, 210

Stress
effects of meditation and melatonin on, **275,** 281–283
shift work and, 91

Stress Reduction and Relaxation Program (SR and RP), 269–270, 274, 276–277, 284–287, 289

Subcellular localization, and melatonin receptors, 198–205

Substance abuse
depression in children and adolescents and, 157
shift work and, 91

Substantia nigra, 16

Sudden infant death syndrome (SIDS), 9

Suicide
melatonin levels in victims of, 156–157
seasonal variations in depression and, 46–47

6-Sulfatoxymelatonin, 247, 248–250, **252,** 276, **279, 286**

Superoxide anion radicals, **13,** 213

Supplemental melatonin. *See also* Dosage; Drug interactions; Duration; Pharmacotherapy; Side effects; Toxicity
for jet lag, 12
for rapid-cycling bipolar disorder, 113–114
for shift work maladaptations, 12

for sleep disorders in children with neurodevelopmental disabilities, 177–182

Supportive-expressive therapy, 268, **271**

Suprachiasmatic nucleus (SCN), of hypothalamus, 6, **90,** 116, 150, 158, 183

Suprapineal recess, 29

Synaptic ribbons, and pineal tumors, 36

Synaptophysin, 36

Tamoxifen, 198, 212, 225

Tardive dyskinesia, **15,** 18

Temperature
bipolar disorder and rhythms in, 107
phase advance and temperature-REM cycle, 108
sleep deprivation and body rhythms in, 46

Testosterone, 194–195

TGFs. *See* Transforming growth factors

Therapeutic agent, melatonin as, 69–70. *See also* Pharmacotherapy; Supplemental melatonin

Thrombocytopenia, 220

Thymus gland, 217

Thyroid carcinomas, 222

Thyroid-stimulating hormone (TSH), 134–135

Thyrotropin-releasing hormone (TRH), 135

Thyroxine, 134

Tissue localization, and
melatonin receptors, 198–205
T lymphocytes, 218, 219, 226
TM. *See* Transcendental
meditation
Tourette's syndrome, 169
Toxicity, lack of in melatonin as
drug or supplement, 12. *See
also* Pharmacotherapy;
Supplemental melatonin
Trait marker, melatonin as, 55
Transcendental meditation (TM),
263–264, 274, 280–283, **288**
Transforming growth factors
(TGFs), 206, 208, 209, 210
Trauma, psychic in childhood
and melatonin levels, 54–55
TRH. *See* Thyrotropin-releasing
hormone
Tricyclic antidepressants, 66
Tryptophan, 4, **5**, 134, 136
TSH. *See* Thyroid-stimulating
hormone
Tuberous sclerosis, 169
Tumors. *See also* Breast cancer;
Cancer
antitumorigenic actions of
melatonin and, 192
of brain and sleep disorders in
children, 175
of pineal gland, 36, 149
Two oscillators hypothesis, for
melatonin regulation and
depression, 67

UFC. *See* Urinary-free cortisol
Ulcerative colitis, 175, 180–181
Unipolar depression, melatonin
secretion amplitude in, 112
University of Massachusetts
Medical Center (UMMC),
270, 283
Urinary-free cortisol (UFC), 133
Uterine tumors, 194, 223

Vanillylmandelic acid, 282
Vertebrates, evolution of pineal
gland in, 27–28. *See also*
Mammals
Vigabatrin, 180
Vitamin E deficiency, **15**, 18

Walter 256 transplantable
tumors, 194
WD. *See* Seasonal affective
disorder
Weight, and melatonin release in
anorexia nervosa, 130
Werdnig-Hoffman disease, **15**
Winter depression (WD). *See*
Seasonal affective disorder

Xenobiotic nerve damage, **15**
Xenopus laevis, 200–201, **202**, 245

Yoga, 280–281. *See also* Meditation

Zen tradition, of meditation, 265
Zonulae adherentes, 31